THE PRACTICE OF CLINICAL ENGINEERING

CLINICAL ENGINEERING SERIES

CESAR A. CACERES, M.D., *Series Editor*

Clinical Systems Associates, Inc.

Washington, D. C.

Walmor C. De Mello. Electrical Phenomena in the Heart. 1972

Anthony Sances, Jr., and Sanford J. Larson. Electroanesthesia: Biomedical and Biophysical Studies. 1975

Herbert H. Roth, Erwin S. Teltscher, and Irwin M. Kane. Electrical Safety in Health Care Facilities. 1975

Cesar A. Caceres (Ed.). The Practice of Clinical Engineering, 1977

THE PRACTICE OF CLINICAL ENGINEERING

Edited by

CESAR A. CACERES, M.D.

Clinical Systems Associates
Washington, D.C.

With the assistance of

ALBERT ZARA

Clinical Engineering News
Washington, D.C.

ACADEMIC PRESS New York San Francisco London 1977

A Subsidiary of Harcourt Brace Jovanovich, Publishers

ACADEMIC PRESS, INC.
111 Fifth Avenue, New York, New York 10003

United Kingdom Edition published by
ACADEMIC PRESS, INC. (LONDON) LTD.
24/28 Oval Road, London NW1

Library of Congress Cataloging in Publication Data

Main entry under title:

The Practice of clinical engineering.

(Clinical engineering series)
Bibliography: p.
1. Biomedical engineering. I. Caceres, Cesar A.
II. Zara, Albert N.
R856.P7 616'.0028 76-42966
ISBN 0-12-153860-5

PRINTED IN THE UNITED STATES OF AMERICA

This volume is dedicated to Julius A. Rippel. Through his wisdom, foresight and efforts, the practice of clinical engineering has received the stimulus needed to become an effective tool in the fields of medicine and health.

CONTENTS

PART VII / MAINTENANCE

LIST OF CONTRIBUTORS

J. C. ALLER—National Science Foundation, Washington, D.C.
G. ARBONA—University of Puerto Rico, Rio Piedras, Puerto Rico
M. ARNOLD—Pennsylvania State University, University Park, Pennsylvania
N. ANDERSON—Oak Ridge National Laboratory, Oak Ridge, Tennessee
S. ARONOW—Massachusetts General Hospital, Boston, Massachusetts
J. H. U. BROWN—Southwest Research Consortium, San Antonio, Texas
H. S. BENNET—Electrical Engineering Dept., Army Electronics Command, Dept. of the Army, Fort Monmouth, New Jersey
J. H. BUSSER—Formerly, Alliance for Engineering in Medicine and Biology, Chevy Chase, Maryland
R. F. BRIDGMAN—Inspecteur general des Affaires Sociales France, Paris, France
A. BRODZIAK—Wewnetrzynch Slaskiej Akademic Medyczej, Katowice, Poland
J. BRAY—Doctors Hospital, San Diego, California
D. BUCHMUELLER—St. Luke's Hospital, Chicago, Illinois
A. BENNETT—United Hospital Fund of New York, New York
R. J. BOSTON—University of Maryland, College Park, Maryland
C. BERKLEY—Ramapo College of New Jersey, Mahwah, New Jersey
C. A. CACERES—Clinical Systems Associates, Washington, D.C.
J. K. CYWINSKI—Massachusetts General Hospital, Boston, Massachusetts
J. CAVALLARI—Memorial Sloan—Kettering Cancer Center, New York, New York
G. R. COOPER—Communicable Disease Center, U.S. Department of Health, Education and Welfare, Atlanta, Georgia
A. COLOMBO—Dosapro—Milton Roy S.A., Switzerland
G. D. DEVEY—National Science Foundation, Washington, D.C.
P. DeSALVO—Massachusetts General Hospital, Boston, Massachusetts
D. DJORDJEVIC—Federal Institute of Public Health, Belgrade, Yugoslavia
B. S. DUNBAR—George Washington University Medical Center, Washington, D.C.
J. DONAHUE—Medtronic, Inc., Minneapolis, Minnesota
R. DAVIS—Hospital Association of New York State, Inc., Albany, New York
M. EDEN—Massachusetts Institute of Technology, Cambridge, Massachusetts
L. A. GEDDES—Purdue University, West Lafayette, Indiana
J. T. GRISNER—Minneapolis Veterans Hospital; Minneapolis, Minnesota
L. GOODMAN—Medtronic Inc., Minneapolis, Minnesota
G. R. GOODMAN—Texas Heart Institute, Houston, Texas
F. I. GILBERT—The Pacific Health Research Institute, Honolulu, Hawaii

W. HOBSON—World Health Organization, Alexandria, United Arab Republic
J. HOPPS—International Federation for Medical and Biological Engineering, Ottawa, Canada
T. S. HARGEST—Medical University of South Carolina, Charleston, South Carolina
G. S. HAMMER—Association for the Advancement of Medical Instrumentation, Arlington, Virginia
D. JURELA—City Public Health Institute, Zagreb, Yugoslavia
S. JACOBS—American Hospital Association, Chicago, Illinois
J. E. JACOBS—Northwestern University, Chicago, Illinois
P. KLATELL—City University of New York, New York, New York
K. L. KAYSER—Milwaukee Heart Surgery Associates, Milwaukee, Wisconsin
A. E. HERTZLER KNOX—The Hartford Insurance Group, Hartford, Connecticut
J. K. KEREKES—Association of Biomedical Technologists, Monterey Park, California
I. M. KANE—Nyack Hospital, Nyack, New York
K. S. KAGEY—Peter Bent Brigham Hospital, Boston, Massachusetts
D. LEE—U.S. Department of Labor, Washington, D.C.
H. LAUFMAN—Albert Einstein College of Medicine, New York, New York
C. LASZLO—McGill University, Montreal, Canada
J. LENIHAN—Western Regional Hospital Board, Glasgow, Scotland
A. D. LEWIS—Department of Defense, Washington, D.C.
D. LUBIN—Sinai Hospital, Baltimore, Maryland
I. M. METH—City University of New York, New York, New York
J. VAN DER MASS—Philips—Liechti A.G., Ostermundigen, Switzerland
I. MARGAN—Setaliste Karla Masksa, Zagreb, Yugoslavia
J. MATAUSCHEK—VEB Kombinat Medizinund Labortechnik, Dresden, German Democratic Republic
J. McCORMICK—Pelam, Inc., Hinsdale, Illinois
M. MYERS—National Institutes of Health, Bethesda, Maryland
M. J. MILLER—Association for the Advancement of Medical Instrumentation, Arlington, Virginia
M. MILOSEVIC—Institute for Nuclear Science, Belgrade, Yugoslavia
J. A. McLAREN—Evanston Hospital, Evanston, Illinois
V. L. NEWHOUSE—Purdue University, Lafayette, Indiana
F. NORMAN—United Nations Industrial Development Organization, Vienna, Austria
J. W. OWEN—St. Thomas Hospital, London, England
B. PARKER—Montefiore Hospital and Medical Center, Bronx, New York
L. PETROVIC—University of Belgrade, Yugoslavia
M. PRYWES—University of the Negev, Beer-Sheva, Israel
P. PARASKEVOPOULOS—Greek Atomic Energy Commission, Athens, Greece
B. PENDIC—Klinicka Bolnica Grada, Belgrade, Yugoslavia
S. POCOCK—Medical Research Council, Middlesex, England
S. PADWO—Department of Commerce, Washington, D.C.
M. RIDGWAY—Hospital Council of Southern California, Los Angeles, California
J. A. RIPPEL—Fannie E. Rippel Foundation, Morristown, New Jersey
R. REDER—Massachusetts General Hospital, Boston, Massachusetts
A. REMOND—International Institute for Medical Electronics and Biological Engineering, Paris, France
J. J. RIORDAN—Private Consultant, Washington, D.C.

I. P. STAPP—University of Kentucky Medical Center, Lexington, Kentucky
A. SCHWAN—Northwest Ohio Clinical Engineering Center, Toledo, Ohio
H. H. SUN—Drexel University, Philadelphia, Pennsylvania
P. E. STANLEY—Purdue University, Lafayette, Indiana
D. SALINAS—Hotel Dieu, Paris, France
W. SELIGMAN—Princeton Hospital, Princeton, New Jersey
M. J. SHAFFER—George Washington University Medical Center, Washington, D.C.
R. SWANSON—Veterans Administration, Washington, D.C.
W. STAEWEN—Sinai Hospital, Baltimore, Maryland
L. C. SHEPPARD—University of Alabama, Birmingham, Alabama
G. THOMAS—World Health Organization, Copenhagen, Denmark
R. TOMOVIC—Yugoslav Committee for Electronics and Automation, Belgrade, Yugoslavia
M. J. VAN TROMMELL—Erasmus University, Rotterdam, Holland
R. THORNER—Department of Health, Education and Welfare, Rockville, Maryland
J. H. TOLBERT—Hospital Research and Educational Trust of New Jersey, New Jersey
B. VAN EIJNSBERGEN—Institute of Medical Physics, Utrecht, The Netherlands
G. WEBB—Johns Hopkins Hospital, Baltimore, Maryland
H. R. WEED—Ohio State University, Columbus, Ohio
J. WEINMAN—Hadassah Medical School, Jerusalem, Israel
M. WHITE—Hewlett Packard Co., Waltham, Massachusetts
T. WILLIAMS—U.S. Army Medical Optical and Maintenance Agency, Denver, Colorado
J. O. WEAR—Veterans Administration Hospital, Little Rock, Arkansas
W. E. WILLIAMS—Director of Hospital Services, Baltimore, Maryland
A. ZARA—Clinical Engineering News, Washington, D.C.
G. ZARKNOIC—University of Sarajevo Medical School, Sarajevo, Yugoslavia
T. ZEREN—Murmara Scientific and Industrial Research Institute Cebze, Istanbul Turkey

PREFACE

This book is intended for the individual concerned with the utilization of diagnostic and therapeutic medical instrumentation or systems, and engineers concerned with clinical medicine. The orientation is interdisciplinary to meet both engineering and medical requirements. The book aims to supply an overview as well as details required for each discipline.

Clinical engineering is a new field. The concepts of technology as an integral part of medicine and engineers as part of the health care team was until recent years literally unknown. The term ''clinical engineering'' is itself new and was coined a decade ago to aid in identification of the people involved with and in recognition of the field itself. The term is now used internationally to focus on the needs that can be fulfilled through the application of technology to patient care.

The book first defines the field, its educational requirements, the requirements for accreditation, and practice, including legislation and liability. The book then proceeds to identify the areas wherein clinical engineering interacts with the administrative operational problems of a hospital and the various specialized care facilities. The modes by which one can apply technology to patient care are detailed so that not just concepts but methodologies are outlined. This is done to make the book useful to the student as well as to the practitioner. The book should be of value in engineering schools and in medical schools that have courses involving medical instrumentation. The areas of maintenance, hospital safety, and clinical fields are dealt with, keeping in mind that the engineer, the physician, the nurse and the paramedical person along with those in industry responsible for the instrumentation and systems must all be able to speak a common language to understand such areas.

Government agencies now are concerned with instrumentation in the medical field. Personnel involved in the practice of clinical engineering and utilization of instrumentation need guides to meet regulatory requirements, particularly, for hospital safety. Increasingly, in the future, requirements for patient education in these areas will have to be met as well. The book is intended to provide a foundation in such fields.

This book is intended for use in areas in which the application of technology to patient care now exists or potentially exists. This potential must be recognized in considering medical instrumentation and systems in diagnostic as well as in therapeutic areas, such as intensive care, operating room emergencies, etc. The book contains chapters by authorities on the various topics and covers and codifies the field of clinical engineering. It brings together information previously scattered and not found in a single publication. The materials are, to some extent, abstracted and re-edited from *Clinical Engineering News,* but have been recompiled according to functional topics and edited in a uniform style. Additional contributions have been obtained from materials presented at recent conferences, some of which were sponsored by the AAMI.

ACKNOWLEDGMENTS

I wish to acknowledge the stimulus and assistance of many individuals in the development of this book. Its beginning dates back to the mid-1960s, when I directed of the Medical Systems Development Laboratory of the Public Health Service. It then became apparent that technologically oriented physicians and nurses, could work better together with engineers, statisticians, mathematicians and a variety of persons in ancillary fields in medicine if all recognized that technological efforts in medicine, by definition, have to be goal-oriented to clinical care.

The formalization of the concept was possible through the recognition of the need for the concept by Julius A. Rippel, who with Herbert C. Englert conveyed the potential merit that they saw to the trustees of the Fannie E. Rippel Foundation. It authorized a grant allowing formation of the first department of clinical engineering in a university.

Throughout that early period, Gilbert Devey and James Aller participated in formulation of plans and brought together a number of individuals including George Webb, Carl Berkely, David Lubin, Anthony Sances, and Saul Aronow in a group sponsored by the Engineering Foundation. The deliberations of that group were carried on with stimuli from many others, including David Simmons, then of the Veterans Administration, to the point that it was possible to seek the support of a broad technology–technologist–clinician oriented association, the Association for the Advancement of Medical Instrumentation (AAMI).

Without the guidance and attention given the concept by Michael Miller, Executive Director of the Association, and his constant and nonwavering support, along with backing from Harold Laufman, past AAMI president, among others, it would not have been possible to bring the concept of clinical engineering to national scrutiny and acceptance.

With the support of the AAMI, backed by the Rippel Foundation's contributions, it was possible to distribute *Clinical Engineering News* to all hospitals in the United States and more recently to medical students as well as to faithful and welcome subscribers.

Acknowledgment is hereby made to AAMI for use of material from its journals as well as to the American Institute of Biological Sciences for use of material from its International Bio-Medical Engineering Workshop Series whose proceedings were sponsored by the Fannie E. Ripple Foundation, and to the National Academy of Engineering for use of material from its Committee on the Interplay of Engineering with Biology and Medicine.

This book would not have been possible without the cooperation of a great number of clinical engineers, physicians, and others as well as a number of organizations including Academic Press, which ventured into this field early on with this series on clinical engineering.

Throughout this effort, there has been meticulous care given each of these publications and proceedings by Albert Zara, Assistant Editor of *Clinical Engineering News*. Without his assistance, much of the work entailed in the completion of this book could not have reached conclusion.

Appreciation must also be expressed to all of the authors, whose work is reprinted here, for their cooperation and their efforts in this field. The editor assumes the blame for any errors that may be present from putting a variety of authors and topics together.

Thanks are also due to the staff of the first department of Clinical Engineering. These include Anna Lea Weihrer, James Landoll, David Weiner, David Lee, and William Ayers. They aided in the development of the concept and must be acknowledged for their pioneering efforts. Unfortunately, the pioneering efforts were unsuccessful in the initial setting due to some conventional pressures, on which were superimposed outside pressures from government agency personnel that opposed the concept. Nevertheless, that opposition allowed the framework of the concept to be tested so that success, if not in the initial hoped for nidus, has been possible in a number of other locations in this country and now, beginning in other areas of the world.

Throughout this effort and in the hectic period of transition of the concept from its onset within a government agency, to a university and the private sector much personal support and backing has been indispensible. My deepest appreciation is expressed to William Raymond Mize, Jr.

C. A. Caceres

THE PRACTICE OF CLINICAL ENGINEERING

INTRODUCTION

C. A. Caceres

Why Technology and Medical Service Delivery?

"The lack of technology transferral to the providers of health care is the most crucial element facing medicine today." That is a strong statement. Indeed, health providers in the United States and other nations are for the most part not yet aware of the technological opportunities available to augment directly their capability in health-care delivery.

Health-care delivery ultimately means that a decision has to be made by a responsible physician in charge of a patient who has sought assistance. That fact is basic. It is also basic that delivery is intimately involved with payment for the services, which means costs passed on to the recipient in some form. Today's political question is: "Can those costs be reduced?"

One cannot answer the question regarding reduction of costs until it is determined why technology, an almost universal solution to many human problems in the 1970s, is not in widespread use in health and medicine today.

Some who try to solve the cost-reduction problem alone attempt to differentiate a one-to-one patient/physician method of health-service delivery from various types of medical-group practices. However, in each of these, a patient-care decision is still ultimately dependent on a one-to-one relationship. Can it be otherwise? The key fact that there must be a one-to-one patient/physician relationship in medicine is responsible for (*a*) the benefits; and (*b*) the problems in health-care delivery.

To solve the cost problems, one cannot ignore that in the final analysis a one-to-one medical-care relationship must exist. The real problem is that to attain the benefits the recipient wants, that is, personalization as required in any quality service involving human life, one must investigate and cure, as necessary, the factors that are the problems. With a nontechnological-assisted approach, one-to-one medical care means difficulty with availability, costs, and quality as the population increases.

Providers and Technology

The health-care delivery system is composed both of providers of health care and those that supply the providers with instrumentation and systems. Some providers have realized that technology can help them solve the problems in health-care delivery by assisting them in improving their one-to-one medical decisions by adding personalization. Some health-care providers, assisted by suppliers that realize the importance of the providers, are developing the techniques by which technology may be used wisely. Many groups are trying to foster that development and communicate the results of the provider's achievement to those providers of health care not currently taking advantage of technology. It is felt that there is a need to make known achieved technological results and organize educational means to stimulate other providers to use technology. It is indeed a lack of education that has caused the present lack of technology use. In addition, the strength of the health-care system of the future will depend to a great extent on whether its users will be able to properly communicate to those not yet taking advantage of technology.

Freedom from Hospitalization?

Those of us who live in a complex era of developed and underdeveloped communities must show that the problem implicit in one-to-one medical care can be solved. It is felt that with a technological approach the quality of health care that can be delivered can be maintained or increased while its availability to expanding populations is increased. It must be shown that by technology and productivity human comfort can increase. If this can be achieved, the costs to the ultimate recipient can be sustained within the levels of standards of living required by the recipients. These standards may involve the recipients' freedom from hospitalization, freedom from disease throughout his or her working life, etc. Such concepts cannot be considered for future reality by providers who today do not use technology.

At times, it becomes apparent that the health planner and some technologists are impatient and want to bypass the knowledge available from the background and intuition of the accepted provider of health-care delivery. Attempts were made not too many years ago when screened health testing was being stimulated in the United States, for example, to suggest that if payment could be made directly to nonmedical operators of centers providing health tests, those owners could order more technology to be used by hired physicians. That would, of course, be the use of technology for the sake of using technology and not for the sake of providing what the provider knows the recipient needs—one-to-one care.

In the same vein, there have also been attempts in the United States to suggest that payments be made for preventive medical techniques without consideration that the real problem is not the payment but the lack of education on the part of the providers and recipients to use preventive medicine properly. Payment is only an incentive and, if not coupled to educational efforts, a waste. Preventive medicine should be used because the provider can best accomplish the one-to-one needs of the recipient through it.

Many advanced technological projects have begun that have forgotten the basic need for education and a one-to-one patient/physician relationship. The instigators of such projects are more involved with their own status needs and not community fulfillment and environmental requirements. But concerned as we now are with many multiple communities and their total environment, it can be clearly seen that education of the provider and through the provider and education of the recipient must be a preeminent goal.

The Physician and Technology

About 10 years ago it was suggested that one suitable goal for technology in public health was to have 250,000 physicians in the United States (about the number in practice), each with a technological center at his command, that is, in each of their offices. There is, by such means, an alternative to grouping physicians into types of practices they do not wish. Practices they intuitively know result in impersonal approaches that are not satisfying to the recipients of care. The proposed solution was to have each physician develop a center in the way he saw fit but with technological assistance to increase productivity, availability, and quality. He would use technology if he understood the opportunities. In addition, he would use technology if sufficient education about the possibilities were available to him. The physician in history has never rejected advances he comprehends to aid him in patient care.

It is crucial not to ignore the central issue that what the public wants first is quality care, and this directly implies personalization and one-to-one care. What the physician wants to provide, *in part because of his own human need,* is also personalization! The solution to attain these goals is obviously education of all concerned. If the health planner wants to decrease cost, he cannot ignore the human element.

The Stimulus to Technology Use

We often see proposals for computer usage in the health field rejected if they are of a practical nature, for example, to link community facilities, to study and document the methods being used, or to develop communication and other techniques to improve health delivery. It is common to see proposals accepted that are oriented to technology for technology's sake. The overwhelming acceptance of such projects from the research community over practical efforts by the providers themselves makes it difficult to show the opportunities to the one who ultimately is responsible—the physician. The physician in practice, where technology should be, cannot become aware of what a small number of his peers have achieved unless demonstrations, within his understanding, can be implemented.

In the past 10 to 15 years, technology utilization has not succeeded in health and medicine. It is appropriate to face the reality and look at the central issues and not skirt about them. There are good reasons for the failures. The providers know one reason: many health planners do not know certain answers and do not ask the providers the questions. It is basically that technological health planners have tried to solve their own problems and not the critical issue in health care.

The issue is really how to increase the desired one-to-one relationship in health-care delivery. Only that result can maintain or increase the quality of health-care delivery. If those who have used technology believe they have found the solution, it is now necessary to define and educate others as regards the methods. The solution is not simply to create more physicians but to augment their end product—health- and medical-service delivery. This is being shown possible through clinical engineering.

The term *clinical engineering* was coined in 1967. It was first used in discussions that eventually led to the establishment of a department of clinical engineering at the George Washington University Medical School. The department was set up in the clinical-science area, establishing that it would not be oriented toward basic research or basic science. The term *medical engineering* was not used to reemphasize that the department was not to be preoccupied with those areas encompassed by the broad connotation of the term "medicine" as used in medical schools (which includes such basic sciences as physiology and microbiology) or restricted to the narrower meaning as delimited by a department of medicine. The department was established through the assistance of the Fannie A. Rippel Foundation (a medical foundation), whose leaders stressed their concern for both health- and medical-care delivery. They recognized, as did the initial planners of the department, that it was appropriate to orient engineers and other disciplines into the practical areas of health- and medical-care delivery.

The Engineering Foundation also recognized that fact and funded a study within the department to assist in the development of concepts on what could be done for patient care through technology. That study focused on what could be used to solve the problem of interfacing engineering to health and medical care.

The study recognized the need for a transferral agency for implementation of the concepts. The clinical concept involves not a single-discipline-oriented group but a broad range of disciplines to encompass the total complexity of health and medical delivery as well as consumer areas. The concept of clinical engineering is not limited to a specific engineering discipline. It is broader in its implication and reaches the community at large.

The Meaning of Words

The definition of engineering in its simplest form suggests a discipline that is oriented to problem solving through the use of technology. The word *technology* verbalizes the concept of the art and science of industry. The word *industry* conveys a field concerned with mass production. The word *clinical* is precise in its meaning. It is used to denote direct patient care.

Some question whether an engineer can supply direct patient care. It is easy to define that the internist or surgeon is involved in direct patient care. It is also easy to reason that a nurse on the wards, although administering or supervising groups of nurses, practical nurses, or orderlies, is also taking care of patients. We also recognize that the clinical pathologist, who might spend the majority of his time in the laboratory, rarely sees a patient, and perhaps has contact with only a portion of the patient under a microscope, is involved in clinical care.

Criteria for Evaluation of a Clinical Engineer

With that background, it is possible to look at clinical engineers and realize that a current need is to define the criteria required to evaluate attributes that peers believe prove an engineer to be a good clinical engineer. The word *attribute* is a good one to use because it does not strictly denote a qualification, rather a qualification plus human factors.

It is usual to judge qualifications in engineering to establish suitability to practice engineering. A variety of tests or examinations are commonly used. A degree from an engineering school, a license granted by a state, or a test that demonstrates that the individual could pass courses in an engineering school or could pass the qualification requirements of a licensing examination are steps that allow one to judge that an individual can be considered for recognition by his peers regarding his engineering qualifications.

A more complex question is what criteria to use to consider attributes that allow one to judge whether a person with established engineering qualifications can serve in a field that involves direct patient care.

From the viewpoint of peers in the field, three criteria stand out. The first criterion involves ethics. This qualitative field can be judged by (*a*) demonstrated ability to accept responsibility; and (*b*) demonstrated knowledge of limitations.

The second criterion is that the subject be able to show effective results of past performance in the field(s) in which (s)he has been engaged. This can be accomplished best through references by those who have actually seen evidence of his professional status. The third criterion is that the individual be able to demonstrate comprehension of the total field of clinical engineering and to differentiate as well, for practical utilization and evaluation, his or her specific expertise and in-depth knowledge in a portion thereof.

The Means by Which Instrumentation and Technology Can Be Used for Health-Service Delivery

We must call on several disciplines to define the technology we can use in health care. The basic question to be asked of each is: ''What can be done *now* to brighten the future of health services?''

We have begun to use technology in medical signal analysis, hospital information systems, medical records, patient monitoring systems, and multiphasic screening. From what has been achieved, we believe short- and long-term projections can be made.

Planning Viewpoints

To begin, one must consider two *practitioner* viewpoints. The first is that technology groups should accept the prime responsibility for demonstrating that systems developed function in service. The second is that technological groups must actively participate in the implementation of the systems they have developed. The practitioner expects the involvement required so that he will be able to practice at a defined and consistent standard level of performance with this assistance. Insufficient numbers of qualified members of other disciplines now play an active role in the areas.

The simultaneous performance of both service and development is always difficult. One must build up actual working experience to develop a usable system. Furthermore, the basic step to technology transfer from the laboratory to the service operations is generation of acceptance, which requires constant communication and coordination of feedback information in educational systems.

Clinical engineering implies generating the means for an interface between the old and the new. Clinical engineering implies the necessity for reference to alternative methods. It acknowledges that one's work cannot be for a single group but for differing groups, each with viewpoints unlike the other. There are several major types. (*a*) One group is primarily interested in a *service;* (*b*) there are other groups concerned with the improvement in *quality* or (*c*) extending the *availability* of services; (*d*) there are groups primarily concerned with *cost;* (*e*) another is simply interested in *research*.

Basic Interfaces

It is vital that there be a gradual transition between new and the established systems. While we introduce new ideas, we must understand what existed before. The established system provides the first basis for feedback. Communication between old and new must be a part of system design.

We need first to survey user needs and define the objectives of the system to be built, based on the system in use. Once we have those objectives, then we can define requirements. The clinical engineer must engage in research, market analysis, and user consultation before attempting to make old systems efficient or to interface new ideas with the user. In other words, the first need is a system analysis of the old system before trying to make a new one.

In studying the user, we cannot neglect the nonuser and the reason he's a nonuser. Priorities and funding, for example, must take the fact of their existence into consideration. In other words, our work is not for 100% of people but for a percentage that must be well defined.

The Engineering Viewpoint

Medical engineering is emerging from an initial preoccupation with machines treated as gadgets to a broader concern with the needs of society. This is an important step and the focus of clinical engineering. The clinical engineer has established himself as a creative applications-oriented person to differentiate him from one who wants to solve an interesting problem only for its academic interest. He can apply himself to almost any problem by using the interdisciplinary approach that he has learned to follow.

Engineering is beginning to be called on to do more in health because we have a significant problem. Just as exploitation of the sea for minerals is too important to leave only in the hands of chemists, or oil exploration to leave in the hands of geologists, the needs of medicine are really too important to leave only in the hands of physicians.

The engineer trained in a systems approach is concerned with the interrelationship of such things as quality, quantity, economics, and manpower. He is trained to improve existing methods, design useful new machines or standards, and reduce costs.

Thus, faced with the necessity of planning a health-care system for a whole city, where should we turn for help to provide the system? Certainly the answer is to a multidisciplined team.

No single group is entirely familiar with all the concepts of new technology. There are many components of systems that we have to pull together. If we are asked to define health from an engineering viewpoint, one would include elements of mathematics, statistics, and physics, as well as applied science, to form the composite of *clinical engineering*.

The Community Viewpoint

Our socioeconomic environment is ready to accept words such as "technological," "interdisciplinary," and "industrial" as adjectives to "health." It began to realize the vastness of health through crude tools like X-ray and screening tests. We once felt that simply adding tests gave us a system. We later added concepts like "mass screening." Doing things on a mass basis helped in getting results without long time gaps. The entrance of mass screening focused on case finding and preventive techniques. Epidemiologists began to identify risk factors. The statistician's role has devised methods or tools by which physiological parameters can be better understood.

In the 1970s, these techniques can finally be used "on line" and in "real time" with the availability of the computer. Now we are beginning to build up massive amounts of data. We had to be satisfied before with a minimum amount. Long-term longitudinal studies will be a thing of the past with cross-sectional probability estimates. Our initial hypothesis used to require much time to prove or disprove. With massive and easily obtained amounts of data, we start on a higher level and can work faster.

The dictionary tells us technology refers to a systematic approach as well as to the art and science of industry. Clinical engineering uses technology in the development of systems in health care, which means organizations of men, machines, and procedures, as well as interplays of personality designed to perform a specific task.

The impact of technology will be most felt by the system concept. The system will consider all information available when needed with the intercorrelations physicians require to make decisions with greater accuracy.

How Will Clinical Engineering Work?

What can be done by clinical engineers? They will first develop an overview of the situation, then decide where and at what level to enter the picture. The mark of success will depend on visible impact on the problems that face the nation—the health problems of the whole community.

It is not obvious how one decides where to intervene and what kinds of intervention are going to have what kind of predictable effects? The logical choice is to develop groups of multidisciplinary clinical enginnering groups that would pick the levels, priorities, and magnitude of effort. One of the errors of the past has been that our decisions have been glamorous and not political, in the best sense of the word. Political decisions are those that effect the greatest public good. Since this requires that we consider the simple idea of interfacing with the existing system, clinical engineers must, at the same time they bring in new ideas, become a reference of methods and detect wherein the old is as good as the new.

The public is waiting for whole systems and coordinated programs. The health profession has not yet developed them.

We need, for example, to manage efficiently all the information involved in caring for a patient in the hospital and showing results quickly, but that demands an early data base.

The clinical engineer is aware that a medical system already exists and that we are changing it, not developing a new one. Our problem is that we do not have enough clinical engineers but do have an excess of well-trained manpower.

PART I

A DEFINITION FOR CLINICAL ENGINEERING

1

AN INTRODUCTION TO CLINICAL ENGINEERING

A. Zara, B. Parker, D. Lee, D. Lubin, and I. P. Stapp

The patient is the focus and his well-being the purpose of all clinical engineering. It is the direct and immediate application of technology to health care that distinguishes clinical engineering from bioengineering. The clinical engineer works primarily in close association with physicians, nurses, and allied specialists having direct patient contact. Social purpose and responsibility have long been the foundation of engineering ethics, a commitment that is especially demanding when engineering theory and practice are applied to patient care.

It has been said that all professions are a conspiracy against the laity. All concerned must ensure that this charge can never be levied against clinical engineering. In particular, there is the requirement not to profess expertise in areas outside one's training or experience, a sobering thought for anyone with the temerity to offer to judge their peers.

Within the past half century, scientific disciplines such as physics, chemistry, genetics, and biology have collaborated with medicine to produce a continuing succession of spectacular advances in research and clinical practice.

In the last decade, as a result of the marriage of particular engineering fields with the medical field, such innovations as the intensive-care unit (ICU), the open-heart operation, the artificial organ, computerized electrocardiography, and a host of other new diagnostic and therapeutic techniques have evolved. The fundamental changes, new concepts, and approaches created by the overlap of many of these disciplines are generally taken for granted.

It has become particularly apparent, however, that the collaborative effort that has evolved between engineers and medical practitioners offers revolutionary potentialities for extending our capabilities in medicine. New frontiers have opened in precise analysis and the interrelation of intricate functional relationships that possess the potential to accelerate and improve the techniques by which disease is diagnosed and cared for.

Many new titles and corresponding definitions of those who are actively engaged in these new fields have evolved. For example, titles such as *bioengineer, biomedical engineer, medical engineer, clinical engineer,* and *hospital engineer* are encountered. There is also an array of titles at the technician level.

If we recognize that the older, more established professions have necessarily gone through a lengthy period of time before clear definition was possible, then the same must invaribly hold true for those new professionals who have evolved as a result of the marriage between the engineering and medical sciences. It is difficult to be logical and to define these professionals in any exact, specific manner. Their educational or job requirements and certification or accreditation will remain in a state of flux for some time. However, some of the more common professional titles that are most frequently encountered may be defined in terms of what is required of them.

Initial attention should be focused on the definition of two professionals: the biomedical engineer and the clinical engineer. An attempt to differentiate between them aids in clarifying basic goals.

Biomedical Engineering. This field is concerned with the application of engineering and medicine to biological and medical problems. The field often must deal with many problems of a theoretical nature, often requiring the individual to have a doctoral degree or equivalent. In most instances, the biomedical engineer conducts research and development in areas of applied physiology. This professional may work in such complex areas as muscle dynamics, hormonal control, neurophysiology of vision, audition of somatesthesia, cardiovascular physiology, or the development of heart-assist devices. He may be part of a team whose members include competent researchers in the life sciences and medicine, or he may be a fully independent researcher capable of relying on his own ability in a complex multidisciplinary field.

Clinical Engineering. In general, the professional in this field applies a broad spectrum of knowledge toward services in health-service delivery, and may also function as a researcher. But there the clinical engineer is application oriented rather than theoretically oriented. Thus, the clinical engineer may be more likely to be working toward becoming a registered professional or licensed engineer as opposed to receiving a doctoral degree.

The clinical engineer must be capable of solving problems in his field using a systems approach. This approach requires that the individual not only exhibit competence in established engineering fields but also have capabilities in other areas, for example, mathematics, statistics, or business administration as they apply to a clinical area. Thus, the clinical engineer must evolve into a ''hybrid'' individual. However, at the outset, the clinical engineer must be a firmly based professional who must want to utilize the essential areas of several fields to solve effectively problems in the clinical area. Nevertheless, a clinical engineer must be an individual who has demonstrated evidence of having met the requirements of an engineer.

Several basic educational requirements can be considered sufficient to prepare one for an apprenticeship or supervisory period. One requirement might be the successful completion of a full 4-year professional engineering curriculum leading to a bachelor's degree in engineering from an accredited college or university. The curriculum would have to include courses such as differential and integral calculus, statistics, dynamics, strength of materials (stress–strain relationships), fluid mechanics, hydraulics, thermodynamics, electrical fields and circuits, nature and properties of materials (relating particle and aggregate structure to properties), and other comparable areas of fundamental engineering science or physics, such as optics, heat transfer, mechanics, or electronics. Four years of college-level education, training and/or technical experience, which provides a thorough knowledge of the physical and mathematical sciences underlying professional engineering and a good understanding, both theoretical and practical, of the engineering sciences and techniques and their applications to one of the branches of engineering, could be substituted. The knowledge and understanding gained, however, must be equivalent to that provided by a full 4-year professional engineering curriculum. Successful completion in an accredited college of a full 4-year or longer related curriculum leading to a bachelor's degree in an appropriate professional field such as physics or architecture might be acceptable in lieu of a degree in engineering, provided the individual has had professional engineering experience acquired under professional engineering supervision and guidance. The adequacy of such a background, however, must be demonstrated.

Subsequent to this background, one must add the knowledge of particular engineering fields, which must be available to understand properly and work in the professions of health and medicine.

For a medical setting, clinical engineering assumes a broad definition. In this setting, the clinical engineer is one who may

1. Specifically assist medical-center personnel in defining their problems and needs in connection with biomedical instrumentation
2. Design and supervise the construction and testing of special-purpose electronic equipment when requirements cannot be met by commercially available apparatus
3. Conduct continuing study and research in contemporary developments, designs, and construction methods as applied to medical and health care
4. Develop methods for calibrating and performance-checking biomedical instrumentation, maintaining a set of fundamental electrical standards and instruments adequate for this work
5. Supply background in physics, chemistry, mechanical engineering, control theory, and mathematics provide informal instruction in electronic theory and practice to instrumentation section specialists and other medical-center electronics technicians for improved understanding of current developments (i.e., integrated circuits, digital techniques, computer interfaces)

6. Provide technical supervision for those aspects of a medical-center electrical safety program that involve the instrumentation section
7. Provide direction to service personnel in the diagnosis and solution of maintenance problems
8. Develop and conduct instructional courses in instrument electronics
9. Represent the medical center in dealings with outside organizations involving professional engineering responsibilities
10. Act as a consultant and adviser to research and clinical specialists in negotiating development projects and recommending solutions to instrumentation and electrical-safety problems
11. Within an organization, his instructions may be limited to general administrative and policy matters, or there may be professional autonomy in relationship with medical personnel regarding instrumentation, etc.
12. Represent the medical center at conferences on biomedical instrumentation and electrical safety and in dealings with engineers from manufacturers and other organizations
13. Safeguard public safety by upholding standards

By virtue of education, training, experience, and ever-increasing skill and knowledge, the clinical engineer is not just another ''machine'' performing a machine task. He is a professional imbued with characteristics that mark the essence of health care and establish the nobility of man caring for man. These characteristics may be inherited, and they may be developed. It is doubtful if they can be learned, and it is probable that they cannot be taught. They include empathy, compassion, mutual understanding, and recognition of man's worth.

The clinical engineer is a generalist in engineering skills and knowledge, and he may be a specialist in one or more technological areas involving electronics, mechanics, hydraulics, fluidics, etc. He is often a teacher. There may be a thin, or very discrete, line separating his activity as a manager and as a technician. He is cognizant of the economic exigencies of health care but never loses sight of the basic value of health care. He implements this by being innovative and persistent. In the course of his professional career, he may at times be a designer, a planner, and an inventor.

The clinical engineer may make known his basic technical qualifications through the submission of academic degrees of relevance, by means of authenticated experience and accomplishment in the field, or both.

He can make known his possession of the very special attributes that mark clinical engineering through personal interviews with his peers and through authenticated references that are highly relevant to his background, personality, and acceptance by those involved in similar responsibilities. The best possible determination must be made that he is willing and capable of accepting the responsibilities inherent in clinical engineering.

Only then can the clinical engineer be recognized by his peers and related professionals and recommended through tangible certification processes to those who need his services.

2

HISTORICAL BACKGROUND OF INTERDISCIPLINARY ENGINEERING

L. A. Geddes

We now live in an era in which physical scientists and, in particular, engineers are applying their education and experience to solve some of the many problems associated with living systems. Various names, such as *biophysics, hospital physics, bionics, bioengineering, biomedical engineering,* and the most recent, *clinical engineering,* have been used to designate such activities. Although it is relatively easy to think of numerous ways in which these new professionals can provide valuable services for the life sciences, it is not easy to define or describe completely these fields of specialization. However, descriptions of these new disciplines are required to inform both the scientific community and lay person.

Biophysics, which is perhaps the oldest of the interdisciplinary specialties, deals primarily with studies of the structure and function of cells, cell membranes, organelles, viruses, and living molecules. The function of receptor and effector organs and the manner in which various types of radiant energy alter this function are also included in the field of biophysics. As a professional specialty, biophysics originated in the mid-1800s when physical instruments began to be applied to the study of life processes. In fact, there existed an informal biophysical society that met at irregular intervals. During these meetings, the members taught each other the principles of physics and sought to identify the physical laws that underlie physiological processes.

Cranefield (1957) elegantly described the origin of biophysics and identified its four founders, Karl Ludwig, Hermann von Helmholtz, Ernst v. Brücke, and Emil du Bois-Reymond, whom he called the "1847 group." Meeting together in Berlin, they issued a credo that Ludwig stated as follows, "We four imagined that we should constitute a physiology on a chemico-physical foundation, and give it an equal scientific rank with physics." They further stated, "The more one advances in knowledge of physiology, the more one will have reasons for ceasing to believe that the phenomena of life are essentially different from physical phenomena.'' To be sure, these strong statements are as true today as in 1847 and constitute a fitting beginning for the various modern fields in which physical and mathematical laws are applied to the study of life processes.

Perhaps a major contribution of these early biophysicists can be traced to modern times in the mathematical models of living systems. Pioneering in this area at the turn of the century were the German physiologists, notably Frank, who developed a theory that describes the energy-storage capability of the aorta; he also was the first to apply, and solve, the second-order differential equation that defines the operation of blood-pressure transducers. Mathematical modeling is now an important part of many interdisciplinary fields. Rashevsky probably was one of the modern leaders in this field.

Although many engineering specialties are being increasingly called into the service of the health sciences, another group consisting of hospital physicists has been providing valuable assistance to clinical medicine for some time. Developing from the introduction of the X-ray to clinical medicine at the turn of the century, hospital physicists became organized in Great Britain in 1943. Long before this time, however, many hospitals had therapeutic X-ray machines and employed hospital physicists to maintain and operate them so that the desired energy dose could be delivered. A prominent radiation physicist in the United States, Otto Glasser, was the editor of one of the best encyclopedias on medical physics, the first volume of which was published in 1944. This three-volume series is still one of the best in dealing with the physical aspects of living processes and in analyzing the various physical techniques used in clinical medicine.

According to Osborn (1964), the first group of hospital physicists was organized in Great Britain in 1943. Their method of identifying their goals and solving their problems commands the attention of all who are forming a new interdisciplinary specialty. For example, from the outset, hospital physicists recognized that they lacked sufficient biological knowledge and medical terminology. Accordingly, they created annual short courses of study designed to eliminate these two defects. The society then held annual scientific meetings that were combined with visits to physics laboratories in hospitals and hospital-related industries. In addition, they set up a training program whereby foreign-hospital physicists could obtain clinical training for about five months in established hospital physics departments in Great Britain. Finally, they created a scientific subcommittee to standardize the measurements of X-ray dosage. Societies of hospital physicists are found today in most large countries. As nuclear medicine develops, there is no doubt that the number and diversity of training of hospital physicists will increase.

An interesting pursuit that began to occupy the physical scientist about a decade ago was identified by the title *bionics*. In this field, studies are made of many of the remarkable feats performed by living organisms with the hope of applying the newly discovered laws or techniques for the benefit of man. An example of one of the many phenomena that merit consideration is the remarkable sensitivity of the sense organs of all living creatures. The amazing night vision of nocturnal animals, the sense of smell in such creatures as the shark, dog, and even man, the ability of the porpoise to communicate over long distances, the sonar object-locating capabilities of the bat, and the myriad transducing functions of the hypothalamus are but a few examples in which exquisitely sensitive and selective biological transducers operate to detect physical and chemical phenomena. Not only are there new facts to be obtained by studying such systems, but it is profitable to consider the manner by which use is made of the information sensed by these biological transducers. For instance, the resolution and dynamic range of human vision is truly remarkable when it is considered in view of the physical system that underlies its function. For example, the retina of each human eye contains 120 million rods (night-vision receptors) and 7 million cones (day and color-vision receptors), all of which send their information to the brain via about 1 million nerve fibers. How human vision is so good in view of the fineness of distribution of retinal receptors and the poverty of the communication channel to the brain remains an unsolved mystery. Although many life scientists now concern themselves with these and other fascinating physiological phenomena, which lend themselves ideally to mathematical modeling, the physical scientist may well discover that the underlying laws and processes are readily adaptable to the purposes of man.

Like hospital physics and bionics, bioengineering and biomedical engineering are of recent origin and appear to have crystallized just after the end of World War II. Bioengineering deals with the application of the tools and analytical techniques of engineering to the investigation of living processes. In most instances, the goal is the discovery of new facts. Of necessity, the design and construction of instruments for investigative tasks constitute an important part of bioengineering. In keeping with the definition of engineering (the application of mathematical and natural sciences to the practical solution of technological problems for man), bioengineering and biomedical engineering provide analytical and building capabilities. Bioengineering activities exist in both engineering and life-science institutions and need not, in general, involve a close contact with human or animal patients.

Biomedical engineering is concerned with the use of engineering principles and practices in the search for new knowledge of life processes that have application to the cure and control of disease and to the support of life if there is a deficit after the disease process has been arrested. Studies of diagnostic, therapeutic, and assistive measures constitute the major activities in this field. An important part of biomedical engineering is concerned with the development of resuscitative patient monitoring and life-support devices. Biomedical engineering activities are therefore linked with and supportive of human and animal medicine and can be found both in a college of engineering and a clinic or hospital.

Clinical engineering, the newest of the interdisciplinary engineering activities, is concerned with the application of engineering tools and theory to all aspects of the diagnosis, care, and cure of disease and life support in general, all of which are embraced by the term "delivery of health-care services." Thus, the clinical engineer is service oriented and is concerned also with personnel and patient safety in all phases of the application of technology in medicine. He also provides a preventive as well as supervisory function in this extremely important area. Since the title includes the term *clinic,* clinical engineers will be found in areas that are closely associated with patients. Inherent in the philosophy of engineering is the goal of efficiency and optimization of services. There is no doubt, then, that the clinical engineer will be involved with communications, the flow of goods and services, and codifying and retrieval of information relative to a patient's progress through his hospital therapeutic regimen and perhaps after discharge.

Perhaps two areas in which clinical engineering will feature prominently will be in the acceptance testing of presently available devices and supervisory assistance with their safe and optimum use on human subjects. Many highly technical devices are now in their research stage and will soon be introduced to clinical medicine. Clinical engineering will certainly feature prominently in speeding the application of, and in training the medical and paramedical personnel in the proper use of these products of research. Thus, it is apparent that the clinical engineer must not only have extensive theoretical training in the life sciences but also extensive training and experience in the medical application of this basic training to such an extent that he will frequently be in appropriate areas a teacher as well as a professional colleague of the clinician who tends the most complex of machines, the chemical engine that we call a living being.

When a technological feat is to be accomplished, regardless of its nature, there is a set of basic requirements that must be met for success to be achieved; this is especially true with interdisciplinary activities. Many have recognized the necessary conditions that must exist for the optimum application of technology for the benefit of man. Jacob Leupold (1674–1727) was an early example whose treatise on mechanics, *Theatrum Machinarum,* as a source book for technology of instruments and machines, listed the educational requirements for engineers (long before they were called such) as follows:

> A mechanic [engineer] ought to be a person who not only understands well and thoroughly all handicrafts, such as wood, steel, iron, brass, silver, gold, glass, and all such materials to be treated according to the arts, and who knows how to judge on physical principles, how far each according to its nature and property is adequate or suitable to withstand and endure this or that, so that everything receives its necessary proportion, strength, and convenience, and neither too much nor too little is done in the matter; but he must also be able to arrange according to mechanical sciences or rules for any required proportion, or effect according to present or proposed force or load; for which purpose he must also have learned from geometry and arithmetic all that is necessary for calculation of the parts of the machine. And when he desires thoroughly to understand his profession, he must have a complete grasp of all the arts and professions for which he will have to make and invent machines; for otherwise he knows not what he is doing, and has also no power to improve anything, or invent anything new, such as is chiefly demanded of a mechanic [engineer]. But above all he has to be a born mechanic [engineer], so that he shall not only be skilled in invention by natural instinct, but shall also grasp with little trouble all arts and sciences, in such a way that it may be said of him: what his eyes see, that also are his hands able to do; and that love of his art lets him avoid no trouble, labour, or cost, because throughout his whole life he has daily to learn something new and to experiment.

Note that Leupold emphasized that an engineer must not only know his own specialty but that "he must have a complete grasp of all of the arts and professions for which he will have to make and invent machines"; clearly, the need for interdisciplinary training for problem solving was never more eloquently stated. Modern engineering education must return to this philosophy and provide engineers who are problem solvers "par excellence" who can apply their specialty in engineering to a wide variety of different fields.

While we anticipate the many contributions to be made by clinical engineering, it is appropriate to look back at some of the discoveries that resulted from interdisciplinary studies. In viewing these, it is important to recognize that from the time of the Renaissance a scientist was considered a natural philosopher who also directed his attention to physical sciences. By the mid-1800s the division of interest was virtually complete, specialization in each field had become well established, and titles such as physicist, chemist, and biologist, were in common use. However, the title *engineer* as we now use it is more recent and derives from the military use of physical scientists, a practice ancient in origin. Engineers who worked on other than military engineering problems became known as civil engineers and began to appear around 1825 with the establishment of colleges of engineering. The graduates of these colleges directed the many construction and building tasks for the benefit of society in general. It was not until the late nineteenth and early twentieth centuries that engineers started to conduct research on a wide variety of problems and became other than civil engineers. Thereafter, those who have conducted interdisciplinary research have borne a variety of titles and have been equipped with very diverse training.

Perhaps the earliest interdisciplinarian who transferred his attention from medicine to physical science was William Gilbert (M.D., 1569, Cambridge), who held the radical belief that theory must stand the test of experiment. From his studies, he distinguished between electrical and magnetic attraction and introduced the terms electrical, electrical attraction, and magnetic pole. He noted the loss of magnetic properties of substances when brought to a red heat. He invented the electroscope and pointed out that the earth behaved as if it contained a magnet. There is no doubt that this tireless physician made contributions above and beyond his major task, which was maintaining the health of Queen Elizabeth of England.

A contemporary of Gilbert was Galileo Galilei (1564–1642), who today could also be called a medical-school "dropout." He anticipated Newton's laws by showing that all bodies fall from the same height in the same time; Newton, of course, generalized the laws relating force mass, acceleration, and velocity. Galileo showed that the path of a projectile was a parabola and that the period of a pendulum is independent of its weight and proportional to the square root of its length. He perfected the telescope and made important astronomical observations from which he concluded that the Earth was not the center of its universe.

The field of thermodynamics derives its origin from studies by the German physician Rober Mayer (M.D., 1838, Tubingen), who investigated the physical aspects of living organisms, which led him to the discovery that heat and mechanical energy were interrelated. He showed that the temperature of water was increased when agitated. Although this concept was strongly rejected by the scientific community, Count Von Rumford (Benjamin Thompson, who started as an American storekeeper's apprentice) provided support for the theory that heat and energy are related by noting that cannon barrels became hot when they were bored. It remained for the physicist James Prescott Joule to quantitate the relationship in 1847.

The dark lines in the solar spectrum, now known as the Fraunhofer lines, were first described by an English physician, William Hyde Wollaston (1766–1828), who practiced medicine for only a few years before turning to research in physics and chemistry. Wollaston carried out extensive studies leading to the discovery of the chemical composition of many of the stones found in internal organs and ducts. In physics, he was the first to discover palladium and rhodium in crude platinum and proved the elementary nature of columbium and titanium.

In 1809, Wollaston devised optical instruments that accurately measured the angles between crystallographic faces. He also noted that the peripheral aberration in the flat lenses of spectacles could be eliminated when a convexoconcave correction was ground into them.

Although Wollaston did not invent photography, he did invent a camera that produced a sharp image. He employed a meniscus lens, stopped down so that the rays of light passed through the center to give an image of amazing sharpness. Previously, light was caused to pass through the whole lens, and only the center of the image was in focus. Wollaston's camera merely awaited the development of the photosensitive surface, which was introduced by Daguerre in 1839. Another optical instrument devised by Wollaston was the camera lucida, consisting of a small four-sided prism mounted on a stand that permitted the observer to view an object and draw an image of it on a sheet of paper.

In the 1820s, Wollaston developed the process for drawing extremely fine wires of platinum and gold. Starting with a hollow silver wire, he put the wire to be drawn inside it and was able by successive drawing of the two wires and etching the silver away with acid, to produce filaments as small as 1/30,000 of an inch in diameter.

Young's modulus is one of the first terms encountered in courses on the strength of materials. Less well known, however, is that Thomas Young was a London physician who for many years held the chair in physics at the Royal Institution. From his researches came proof of the wave theory of light, for it was he who discovered the interference of light waves. He called attention to astigmatism in lenses and was the author of the three-color theory of color vision, later amplified by Helmholtz. In another seemingly unrelated field, he deciphered the meaning of many of the symbols on the Rosetta stone.

Luigi Galvani (1737–1798) was the professor of anatomy and obstetrics at Bologna who made the fundamental observations that started the whole study of current electricity and bioelectricity. One version of the story relates that Galvani was dissecting frogs' legs and chanced to lay them on a table in the vicinity of a static-electricity machine. An assistant happened to pick up a scalpel and touch the spinal nerves, which caused the muscles in the legs to contract whenever sparks were drawn from the electric machine. Galvani wondered if atmospheric electricity would produce the same effect. He therefore hung frog-leg preparations on an iron balustrade with bronze hooks and awaited a thunderstorm. While waiting impatiently during fair weather, the wind blew the legs of the preparations against the iron balustrade (or he accidentally pressed the legs against it), and violent twitching resulted from the contact. He then studied the frog-leg preparation in his laboratory by placing the legs on an iron plate. When the hook inserted into the spinal column touched the iron plate, the legs again twitched. In place of bronze hooks, other metals were observed to give greater or lesser contractions; copper and zinc couples appeared to give the best results. Galvani reasoned that he had discharged the animal electricity present in the muscle, thinking that the muscle and nerve were analogous to the outer and inner conductors of a Leyden jar, the discovery of which had only recently been made (1745–1746). Of course, Galvani's explanation was wrong; instead, he had discovered what is now known as the chemical battery.

Not so ready to accept Galvani's animal-electricity explanation for the discovery was a countryman, Alessandro Volta, the physicist, who showed that current electricity could be produced with dissimilar metals and no frog; hence, the discovery of the voltaic cell. Galvani, for his part, persisted in his idea of an intrinsic animal electricity, and his third experiment, in which muscular contraction was produced without metals, proved the existence of bioelectricity. By laying the nerve of one preparation over a cut and intact surface of another muscle, he obtained muscular contractions at the instant the nerve contacted the cut and intact surfaces, providing the earliest reference to what is now known as the injury potential, the voltage difference between an injured and uninjured area. The study of bioelectric events immediately stimulated the development of sensitive galvanometers to measure this electrical phenomenon in living tissues. As might be suspected, those galvanometers that possessed enough sensitivity to measure the millivolt injury potential were slow to respond and could not reveal the presence of brief electrical events. Galvani's preparation (the rheoscopic frog) did not have this defect and was used by physicists and biologists alike for the detection of brief electrical phenomena. In the hands of Matteucci, the rheoscope revealed the first bioelectric signal accompanying the contraction of skeletal muscles. Koelliker and Mueller later used it to demonstrate the first electrocardiac signal in a frog. It was used even later to record the heart sounds as they were detected by a carbon-button microphone (borrowed from the newly invented telephone). The microphone fed its current changes, proportional to the heart sounds, into an induction coil, the secondary of which stimulated the sciatic nerve of the rheoscopic frog. The muscle was connected to a recording stylus, so that when the heart sounds occurred, the muscle twitched and operated the recording stylus, which did not portray the frequency and amplitude of the sounds but indicated, because of its rapidity of response, when they occurred in the cardiac cycle.

The thermocouple is well known to all; less well known, however, is that its discoverer, Seebeck (1780–1831), was a medical graduate from Berlin. Just after

Oersted's discovery (1820) of the magnetic field surrounding a wire carrying current, Seebeck measured current flow between a couple of copper and bismuth when one metallic junction was held in his hand and the other was at room temperature. He noted that the newly invented galvanometer gave a larger deflection for a greater temperature difference. He also discovered that combinations of different metals gave different thermoelectric currents. An important outcome of Seebeck's discovery was Ohm's finding that a couple of bismuth and copper, one junction maintained at the temperature of ice and water (0°C) and the other at that of boiling water (100°C), gave the most stable source of voltage for his studies on the electric circuit, which gave us Ohm's law. The chemical (galvanic or voltaic) batteries that Ohm had used originally exhibited a change in internal resistance with increasing current, and had Ohm persisted with their use, the discovery of his law may well have been delayed.

After the French physicist Ampère (1775–1836) had shown that a force could be measured between two conductors carrying current, he constructed an apparatus (which is still extant) consisting of two coils, one fixed and one movable. Starting with them at right angles, when current was passed through them in one direction, the movable one would align itself with the fixed one, the initial direction of movement being dependent on the relative direction of the currents in the coils. Thus, the beginnings of the electric motor were at hand. However, it remained for Charles Grafton Page (1812–1868), a physician of Salem, Massachusetts, to develop and patent the split-ring commutator in 1838, which reversed the current in the moving coil at the appropriate moment and thus sustained rotation. Page's device, the first electric motor, differed only slightly from Ampère's apparatus in that Page used a fixed permanent magnet rather than a coil to obtain the stationary field. Page also showed that the eddy-current loss in induction coils could be reduced by using a bundle of iron wires rather than a solid iron core. He also developed self-acting circuit breakers. After these studies, Page became director of the US Patent Office. The introduction of electric power remained his lifelong ambition.

About the same time as Ohm was investigating the electric circuit, a young medical student, Poiseuille (1799–1869) elected to measure the pressure of blood in the aorta of a dog by means of a U-tube manometer filled with mercury; from this study was derived our present-day units of measuring blood pressure (mm Hg). After receiving his medical degree from the École Polythechnique in 1828, Poiseuille became interested in the factors that influence the flow of fluids in tubes. His studies revealed that flow was related to the difference in pressure, the fourth power of the radius and inversely to length and viscosity: he thus gave us Poiseuille's law, the fluid analogue of Ohm's law. Poiseuille later became interested in the flow of all materials, his work in this area originating the field of rheography. His studies on the internal frictional forces in fluids provide the unit for measuring viscosity, the poise.

Hermann von Helmholtz (1821–1894), physician, physiologist, and physicist (in that order), as a child was interested in physics but was persuaded by his father's remarks on the family's slender financial resources to seek training in medicine, which could be obtained without cost by enlisting in the military service. After graduating from the military medical academy, Helmholtz served for a time as a military surgeon, but his scientific abilities attracted the attention of Alexander von Humboldt, who had him released from military duties and appointed as lecturer in anatomy and associate professor of physiology at the Berlin Academy of Arts. The event that stimulated Humboldt to take this action was Helmholtz's publication of his law of conservation of energy, written during his residence in barracks. Although the elements of the law were current in scientific thought at that time and indeed had been proposed by the physician Jean Rey much earlier, it was Helmholtz who collected and unified them. The law was first received as a fantastic speculation.

Proof that Helmholtz was equally at home in the biomedical and physical sciences can be deduced from the list of his appointments: professor of physiology and pathology (Königsberg), anatomy and physiology (Bonn), physiology (Heidelberg), and finally professor of physics in Berlin (1871). After 30 years, he had realized his youthful ambition to become a physicist.

Helmholtz contributed importantly to optics, acoustics, thermodynamics, electrodynamics, and physiology. His study of optics stemmed from his interest in the eye in which he discovered that focusing was accomplished by a change in the curvature of the crystalline lens brought about by contraction of small muscles within the eye itself. He invented the phakoscope to study the changes in the lens and then the ophthalmoscope, which permits viewing the retinal vessels and other structures within the eye. His invention of the ophthalometer made ophthalmology a quantitative study. Then, becoming interested in stereovision, he developed a stereoscope with adjustments for focusing and changing the interpupillary distance; the latter was novel. His continued study of the eye as a receiver of light led to the three-color theory of color vision, which depended on Young's proposal that white light can be made up of three primary colors: red, green, and blue. This theory of color vision still stands and is known as the Young-Helmholtz theory. Helmholtz published these studies in a handbook of physiological optics that still is a landmark in physics and physiology.

Helmholtz's investigations in acoustics derived from his interest in the ear. He first studied the ossicular chain, which translates vibrations of the tympanic membrane (eardrum) to changes in fluid pressure in the inner ear. To account for the perception of sound, he enunciated the resonance or "place" theory, which proposed that the fibers on the basilar membrane in the cochlea constitute a series of tuned resonators, thus arraying the various frequencies in a complex sound wave along the basilar membrane. While the simple resonance aspect of this theory is no longer tenable, the concept of place is still one of the fundamental facts in the mechanism of hearing.

In the appreciation of sound, Helmholtz called attention to the fact that the quality of a tone was determined by the overtones (harmonics) present. His studies on acoustics were published in his *Sensations of Tone,* which is still used in the study of acoustics and the physiology of audition. His researches in sound also led to development of the Helmholtz resonator, a spherical cavity with a circular hole, approximately one-tenth the diameter of the sphere, to which is mounted a short tube. The feature of this device is that it resonates at a single frequency.

In thermodynamics, Helmholtz and Gibbs independently deduced the law describing the energy relationships in reversible chemical reactions. The relationship has since become known as the Gibbs–Helmholtz equation. Its ideal application to the determination of the amount of energy available from the chemical battery established its value. Also, in such batteries the ionic charge distribution that develops at the electrode–electrolyte interface is known as the Helmholtz double layer, which accounts for the unusually large capacitance exhibited by such an interface and forms the basis of the electrolytic capacitor.

Helmholtz's research in electrodynamics led to development of the Helmholtz law, which describes the exponential rise in current when on inductance is connected to a constant voltage. He also found that if current were caused to flow through two identical coils connected in a series-aiding configuration and separated a distance equal to their radii, the magnetic field between them was uniform over a considerable distance. This coil configuration was employed in a variety of instruments for measurement of strength of the earth's magnetic field. From his work on electric circuits, he enunciated his reciprocity law, which states that under specified conditions the same transmission characteristics obtain when the receiver and source are transposed.

His studies of electrical oscillations led him to predict that the velocity of propagation of electromagnetic induction was in excess of 314,000 m/sec. It is interesting to note that it was his pupil, Hertz, who, while working for him at this time, demonstrated the existence of electromagnetic waves, predicted mathematically by Maxwell.

Helmholtz's researches in physiology were by no means secondary in importance. In addition to his contributions to the physiology of vision and audition, he was first to determine the velocity of the nerve impulse. Previous investigators had believed that it traveled with the speed of electric current in a wire. Helmholtz showed that in the sciatic nerve of the frog the velocity was a modest 30 m/sec. Helmholtz also showed that the heat liberated by muscular contraction constituted an important source of animal heat.

It is not generally known that the moving-coil galvanometer, recognized almost universally as the d'Arsonval galvanometer (1882), is an improved model of the Thomson (Lord Kelvin) direct-recording telegraphic recorder (1867). Even less well known is that d'Arsonval (1851–1940), was a physician. d'Arsonval's improvements in Kelvin's galvanometer consisted of placing an iron core within the moving coil, thereby increasing the field strength around the conductors of the coil. He also mounted a mirror to the coil so that its position, which was proportional to the current flowing through it, could be indicated by a light ray reflected on to a screen.

d'Arsonval worked with Claude Bernard as a preparer of his experiments. In particular, he collaborated on the problem of oxygenation of the blood and in amplification of earlier experiments Bernard had discontinued; together with Magendie, they showed conclusively that venous blood was hotter than arterial blood because oxidation had occurred at the periphery. This they proved by passing thermocouples (made by d'Arsonval and connected to his galvanometer) into the right and left ventricles.

d'Arsonval was also active in other areas. Around 1893, when consideration was being given to the choice of a frequency for the distribution of alternating-current energy, he conducted a series of experiments that showed that as the frequency was increased, the threshold current for perception also increased. This he demonstrated in a spectacular way by using a high-frequency (0.5–1 MHz) generator connected to electrodes held in one hand by two subjects; an electrode in each of the other hands of each subject was connected to a 100-W light bulb. Through this series circuit was passed a current of about 1 A, which caused the light bulb to burn brilliantly without the subjects reporting any sensation. He then passed 3 A through his own body. Although these experiments did not affect the choice of frequency for the distribution of electric energy, they did initiate the field of medical diathermy and were among the earliest in the field, which is now called "electrical safety."

d'Arsonval made other important contributions to the life sciences by devising an incubator for bacterial cultures. This device was one of the first water-jacketed thermostatically controlled environmental chambers. He was also interested in the heat liberated by animals and was one of the first to chart and study the factors that affected diurnal temperature changes in man and animals. He measured pulmonary compliance and expired carbon dioxide; he also measured the spectral absorption of hemoglobin and studied the effect of light on microorganisms and the effect of low temperatures on ferments. For all of these scientific achievements, he was elected to the French Academy of Sciences in 1894 and followed his professor to the chair of experimental medicine in the same year.

One of the most fruitful collaborative endeavors between a physicist and a physician was that of Lippmann and Marey in France. Lippmann, a physicist, became interested in the phenomenon of electrocapillarity, the interesting property exhibited by the electrical (Helmholtz) double layer, which exists at a mercury–sulfuric-acid interface. Alteration of the charge distribution at this interface, by passage of a current through it, changes the surface tension of the mercury and consequently alters the contour of the meniscus. Although Lippmann believed that the phenomenon could be used to create an electric motor, Marey, the physician and physiologist, thought that it could be used to display rapidly changing bioelectric events for which there was no recorder. Accordingly, Marey and Lippmann used the phenomena to develop the first rapidly responding bioelectric recorder (the capillary electrometer) and obtained the first electrocardiogram of a spontaneously beating heart.

Lippmann and Marey's capillary-electrometer electrocardiograph consisted of a glass capillary tube that contained the mercury–sulfuric-acid interface. One electrode dipped into the sulfuric acid, and the other dipped into the mercury. These electrodes were connected to electrodes placed in direct contact with the beating heart of a tortoise. The bioelectric currents produced by the beating heart rhythmically altered the contour of the mercury meniscus. By transilluminating the meniscus with a strong light beam and projecting the image on a moving photosensitive surface, a record of the amplitude and time changes representing the electrocardiogram were obtained with this device.

The capillary electrometer thus initiated electrocardiography. In Great Britain, a physicist (George J. Burch) and physician (Burdon-Sanderson) teamed up to make and use capillary electrometers for the investigation of bioelectric phenomena. Together they recorded the action potentials that accompany the contraction of the leaves of several types of plants. They also recorded frog cardiac electrograms and developed the interference theory that accounts for the R and T waves of the electrocardiogram. Bayliss and Starling used one of Burch's capillary electrometers to record the first mammalian electrocardiograms, and Waller employed one to record the first human electrocardiograms. In this study, he investigated the effect of electrode location and likened the ventricles to a dipole within the chest. Successful as this instrument was in the hands of its developers, it was inadequate to Einthoven, who openly criticized it. The erratic behavior of the capillary electrometers he made so frustrated him that he set about designing a string galvanometer for medical use, fashioning it after Ader's string telegraphic recorder.

Einthoven abstracted from the technology and science of the day and adopted as well the same recording surface speed as was advocated by Marey and Lippmann (25 mm/sec). Although it is now well known that clinical electrocardiography derives its origin from Einthoven's work, it is less well known that the very first electrocardiograms were obtained by a physicist and a physician working together.

Another of the fruitful interdisciplinary collaborations was between Burch and the team of Gotch and Horsley, physicians and physiologists. With Burch's capillary electrometer, Gotch and Horsley were the first to record the waveform of the action potential of nerve in response to a single stimulus; they also recorded action potentials from the spinal cord.

Burch also had a fruitful association with Burdon-Sanderson in relation to the latent period of muscular contraction, that time between the action potential and the initial development of muscular force. Many had thought that the action potential was synchronous with muscular contraction; others thought it followed the development of tension. Burdon-Sanderson, with Burch's assistance, presented two-channel capillary electrometer photographic recordings of the time course of the action potential and the development of muscular tension, which clearly showed that the action potential preceded the twitch and hence proved the existence of the latent period.

An interesting physicist, engineer, and physician is Craib, who, in 1929, showed theoretically and experimentally that the propagation of excitation in the heart can be equated to a dipole. (He used the term doublet.) He also showed that recovery is also equatable to a traveling dipole. This theory forms the basis of much in modern-day electrocardiography.

One of the most interesting recent interdisciplinary contributions to science is that of von Békésy, the physicist who won the Nobel Prize in medicine in 1961. Von Békésy received his Ph.D. in physics from the University of Budapest in 1923. Using his training in this area, he showed, by the use of delicate and elegant instrumentation of his own design, that the elastic properties of the basilar membrane determined the region in which the maximum amplitude of vibration occurs for a given frequency. Although he also showed that the maximum amplitude of vibration was broadly distributed, not sharply resonant, as was previously believed, his work established the role of the place theory in the mechanism of hearing and gave it new meaning.

It is interesting to contemplate the factors that are responsible for a scientist's making a contribution to knowledge in a field in which he did not obtain his primary training. There is no doubt that the first-hand view and experience of a foreign field by a person with an entirely different specialty results in a refreshingly different view and the evaluation of evidence with a different frame of reference. Although it is still possible for a few to become fully qualified in both the life and physical sciences, progress in all branches of science has accelerated to such an extent that it is now almost impossible to acquire mastery over one. As a result, many who are qualified in one field seek enough training in another in order to obtain adequate working knowledge of that subject so that they can use it for their own ends. This practice is not new. James Clark Maxwell, the mathematical physicist who predicted electromagnetic radiation (the existence of which was proved by Hertz, a pupil of Helmholtz), stated (1878):

> I have said that the telephone is an instance of the benefit to be derived from the cross fertilization of the sciences. Now this is an operation which cannot be performed by merely collecting treatises on the different sciences and binding them up into an encyclopedia. Science exists only in the mind, and the union of the sciences can take place only in a living person. Professor Graham Bell, the inventor of the telephone, is not an electrician who has found out how to make a tin-plate speak, but a speaker (orator and speech teacher) who, to gain his private ends has become an electrician.

From these brief glimpses of human endeavor, it is amply apparent that there has been a considerable interplay between the physical and life sciences. Recognition comes to scientists because of their discoveries, and central to the process of discovery is the development of a theory, then its experimental proof; the latter usually requires the creation and use of specialized instrumentation. Although the creation of instruments has been labeled by some as an unscientific pursuit, the critical role that instruments play cannot be overlooked. For example, receipt of the Nobel Prize has traditionally been the recognition awarded to a scientist for a new discovery.

Of the 138 Nobel laureates in physics and chemistry from 1901 through 1960, 112 were honored for research in which instruments were dominant. The application of old knowledge to new problems through the use of instruments is clearly a scholarly and honorable pursuit and a fundamental premise in clinical engineering.

This review has shown that there have been physicians who have made discoveries in the physical sciences and physical scientists who have made discoveries in the biomedical sciences; there have even been some who made discoveries in both fields. Important discoveries have also been made by teams of physical and biomedical scientists. There has been no standard path.

Since clinical engineering is in its infancy, we can anticipate with eagerness the contributions and discoveries it will make. Perhaps perspective can be gained here by defining a discovery as merely an event after which things are done differently or new things are done. For clinical engineering there are no hindering precedents to be broken and few guidelines for future direction. Thus, there is a golden opportunity to create something new that can be of lasting value to society. In this connection, it is important to recognize that since clinical engineering is designed to serve the patient, it is necessary for clinical engineers to recognize the goal of medicine, which has remained the same since the time of Hippocrates (400 B.C.), namely, healing the sick and injured and providing symptomatic relief when healing is not possible. Traditionally, physicians have been trained to know what to do when a set of symptoms or signs is present. All preclinical and clinical training is dedicated toward attainment of this goal. To nonphysicians, the procedures taken to attain this goal are not always obvious and seemingly indirect at times. Interestingly, only two processes are carried out by the physician in reaching this goal: diagnosis and the application of therapy. The former involves detective work, and the latter requires encyclopedic knowledge of the measures that have proved successful in restoring physiological function. Clinical engineers can assist in both processes.

It is appropriate to make several observations that may optimize the application of clinical engineering talent. Perhaps a clue for optimization can be obtained by examining the various acts of the physician.

The unaided senses of the physician provide a tremendous amount of information via the history and physical examination. Carefully selected laboratory tests, appropriate for the suspected disease and usually employing instruments, then narrow the possible diagnoses to a few. Careful consideration of the symptoms and signs, plus the results of the laboratory tests, provide the consistency necessary to establish the correct diagnosis; if not, more refined laboratory tests are performed, and the cycle is repeated to gain more precision. It is usually the instrumental phase of these processes that attracts the engineer's attention, and some remarks are perhaps appropriate regarding the type of information provided by clinical instruments. In 1885, Morey, the French physiologist, called attention to an important aspect of all instrumentation by stating: "In effect, in the field of rigorous experimentation, all the sciences give a hand. Whatever is the object of these studies, that which measures a force or movement, or electrical state or a temperature, whether he be a physician, chemist or physiologist, he has recourse to the same method and employs the same instruments.'' Thus, the feature that distinguishes biomedical instruments from physical instruments is the manner of application for the special requirements presented by the living organism.

Engineers are, by training, preoccupied with accuracy of measurement. When they view the data provided by clinical instruments, they naturally concern themselves with accuracy and follow Lord Kelvin's belief (1910):

> I often say that when you can measure what you are speaking about, and express it in numbers, you know something about it; but when you can not measure it, when you can not express it in numbers, your knowledge is of a meager and unsatisfactory kind; it may be the beginning of knowledge, but you have scarcely, in your thoughts, advanced to the stage of science, whatever the matter may be.

Important as this aspect of measurement is, its application in biology and medicine often has to be tempered, in fact, by an admonition also given by Kelvin, who said that the addition of the measuring instrument must not alter the quantity being measured. Very often in the biomedical application of instruments, indirect measures are the result of the trade-off between Kelvin's two recommendations.

With regard to accepting semiquantitative measurements of living processes, examples serve best to illustrate the basic clinical goal. A diagnosis is often made by noting the presence or absence of a quantity that carries the essential diagnostic information, and the amount present contains only secondary information. Depression or rise in the S–T segment of the electrocardiogram or a characteristic in the QRS wave tell of an inadequate supply of blood to the myocardium or a disturbance in the system controlling the spread of excitation to the main pumping chambers of the heart. Note that in each of these examples attention is directed toward only a small part of the whole waveform, and from the observation a decision for the type of therapy is made. Adding super high fidelity in reproduction of the waveform will contribute little additional information of value. Noteworthy, however, is that the diagnostic instrument plays an important role in initiating and guiding the intensity of therapy.

Another example can be presented to illustrate the relative value of diagnostic information. Years ago, heroic efforts went into the development of plethysmographs to quantitate the blood flow in the body extremities. Successful instruments were indeed created, but they were so cumbersome to use that they were abandoned because the clinician could obtain the information needed about the circulation in an extremity by merely palpating an artery serving the extremity and feeling whether the member it served was warm or cold. The conclusion to be drawn is that it is unwise to expend a large amount of effort on instrumentation that provides information obtainable by an easier method.

Jacob Leupold's remarks about ''inventing something new'' is interesting to note. Many papers presented by physical scientists working in the life sciences have shown a considerable disregard for work previously carried out. There is often undue pleasure taken in the glamour of the modern method rather than concern for the value of the information produced. Although earlier studies may not have the benefit of the sophisticated instrumentation of the present, they nonetheless may have defined the parameters of the problem. To review the history of a problem is really scientific detective work that provides tremendous psychological as well as scientific rewards. It will come as a pleasant surprise to see how much the ancients used brainpower to compensate for the absence of scientific tools. Just as a physician is expected to know the past and latest therapies, and the attorney is required to know the old and newly passed laws, so the physical scientist, working in medicine, must be aware of the prior and recent studies of the problem with which he is engaged.

3

TECHNOLOGY AND PEOPLE

J. C. Aller, G. B. Devey, M. Ridgway, A. Schwan, S. Aronow, G. Webb, and G. T. Grisner

Throughout our society, technology has modified the way in which we commute to work, the procedures and type of work we do, and the products we buy. It has also changed the character of health care. Technology, however, is not just a simple black box that can run unattended. It is not even a complex system that, once installed, can operate with little attention. Technology is sterile without its component of people who are responsible for its continuous, reliable operation and adaptation to new possibilities.

The professionals associated with technology in clinical care are appropriately termed clinical engineers. Sometimes, when one is close to a process, it is difficult to see the total picture. Perhaps this has been the case of engineering in medicine. For example, periodicals, technical meetings, and talks emphasize the new and the different but give short shrift to reports that are a repeat of previous work.

In an attempt to distinguish the differences between two emerging professional groups working in the medical field, the engineering community has accepted the following definitions:

> **Biomedical engineering:** the application of the tools of mathematics and physical sciences to biological and medical problems
>
> **Clinical engineering:** the application of the art and science of industry, that is, technology, to health care delivery and clinical problems in medicine

The clinical engineer practices his vocation for, or within, a clinic, hospital, medical center, or other health-care delivery institution. The function of the clinical engineer depends on the health-care setting. However, the broad technical sphere of the clinical engineer includes not only all aspects of the hardware, from initial specification to responsibility for continued safe, reliable operation, but also the correlated activities of training and consultation.

Biomedical engineers and medical engineers, on the other hand, typically would conduct research in a university or medical school or could be employed in an industrial activity. For these activities, one can think of the engineer as being remote from the patient. Clinical engineers, on the other hand, must deal with the medical staff and the administrator and be prepared to interact with patients. Clinical engineers must be knowledgeable technologists, for they are the essential ingredient that ensures that technology will function.

As in any new specialty, there are problems of definition of duties, questions of organization methods, and the fundamental question as to why older groupings are not sufficient. Nearly 300 years before the advent of the first graduate engineer in the United States (1835), there were researchers who might fit the title of biomedical engineer. The definition of biomedical engineer that seems to be generally accepted emphasizes the importance of discovery and does not include the problems involved in reduction to practice. The sector devoted to biomedical research grew logarithmically for nearly 25 years but has recently tended to level off.

Productive programs depend on resources that a nation allocates for research. The level of activity spawns a continuous stream of new research findings and possible uses for technology. But it is in the follow-up phases, that is, application, that one should expect continued growth in engineering opportunities. The cumulative impact of most research has not yet been fully felt. The foregoing points, however, reinforce the need to scrutinize carefully what impact a continuous flow of new developments implies in the way of people support in locations of use.

A perfectly feasible alternative is the insistence that the M.D. acquire skill in two different disciplines. A few gifted individuals can achieve this, but the training of any substantial number would imply even longer periods than now required. Such a solution should be rejected as uneconomical as well as unnecessary. The alternative solution involves subdividing duties so that members of a team can perform individual tasks contributing to overall accomplishment, which leads directly to organizational questions. Review of what can be done shows that there are three general avenues. If the hospital or activity is of sufficient size, it can justify its own department. A number of examples of this type can be found in the large teaching hospitals as well as in the smaller hospitals.

Organization

In 1969, the first clinical engineering department was established at George Washington University to provide for the combined needs of service, research, and education, which suggested that smaller teaching hospitals might consider separate departments using functional support very much more than just service activity alone. In the smaller institution, one can consolidate the activity with an existing group of hospital engineers or separate the function into a new group to keep hospital engineers as an administrative department.

A smaller institution can share services in some sort of regional grouping or consortium. A number of examples of this type can be found even in an institution large enough to justify its own department. Certain economies of scale or subspecialization can be achieved.

Finally, a small institution can turn to external specialized support. Some companies provide elaborate service organizations for their products. Where systems composed of many products are concerned, there have been developed specialized firms that provide services in a competitive market. There is difficulty in separating the engineer function from the technician function in this area. Both are needed, and the borderline between the two is gray and hard to define.

A point often overlooked in staffing or discussion of needs is the long-term flow. Many individuals have presented their estimates that, overall, somewhere between 8000 and 50,000 clinical engineers are required in the United States. While this may be a small fraction of the million engineers available, it is sufficiently large to raise some sharp questions as to how these individuals should be recruited, trained, motivated, and offered the potential for a rewarding lifetime career. The United Kingdom examined these questions in a 1968 study, *The Zuckerman Report*. What are some of the questions to be asked? Dominating is the question of magnitude. If 50,000 engineers are required for this new field in the United States alone, nearly 1000 new entrants a year are required once steady state is reached, or about the number needed for electrical-utility support. If 50,000 are needed now or in the next 3 years, a crash one-time effort would be necessary. The transient and steady-state solutions are different problems and require different solutions. A mixture of solutions is probably the best answer. Steps are under way in several universities to train clinical engineers. One alternative suggests, too, that upward mobility should be provided for the technicians so that formal education need not be the only mode of entry, but it may not be suitable to most areas. Exit or advancement into governmental, administrative, and planning groups is also an essential so that opportunities are not limited for the gifted or ambitious.

One of the most striking impressions from watching the evolution of engineering in medicine during the past two decades has been the unchanging nature of the issues that have concerned professional groups. Professional recognition has always been a primary concern. One reaction to a lack of recognition could be self-aggrandizement, resulting in a serious misrepresentation of the potential career situation for highly trained clinical engineers and technicians, especially in the hospital sector. It would be more helpful if serious attempts were made to gather together and disseminate statistics and descriptions of the true job situation in the hospitals and other institutions. The rationale for optimistic employment projections should be explained carefully and realistically and the difficulties emphasized.

Professional certification programs can be useful aids to better public relations and increased professional recognition. Because clinical engineering is a particular, technically diverse profession, clinical engineer certification programs may not advance in a desirable direction unless implemented very carefully. It should be very clear as to just how these programs will serve the hospital community, and careful considerations should be given to safeguards against any negative consequences that could result. For example, clinical engineers could become an additional direct cost burden to the hospitals at a time when they are under considerable pressure to reduce costs. Clinical engineers or biomedical equipment technicians without adequate equipment and facilities are additionally not good investments. There is also the handicap of carving out a new type of job and trying to introduce new ways of doing things within the established patterns of the hospital. This may tend to impede the engineer's attempt to prove his cost effectiveness.

Clinical engineering is a newly recognized, interdisciplinary practice of art and science, for it addresses itself to both technology and people in a health-care environment. Included in this spectrum is an understanding of the many and variable dimensions associated with diverse human and organizational interrelationships and a comprehensive grasp on the technical support resources available and required to assure that "quality of patient care" is not merely a slogan but a responsible commitment of substance and meaning to the patient.

Goal Orientation

This discipline is primarily concerned with the application of engineering principles, analysis, and understanding to a very broad range of interfaces between a patient and his physical and instrumented environment through a firsthand knowledge of the needs for and problems with these interfaces. It is this firsthand knowledge of the day-to-day needs of the patient environment interface that permits the term "clinical" to be used. "Engineer" denotes that the individual is involved at the decision-making and creative level. The two go together when a number of interface situations are encompassed in the responsibilities and experience of the individual.

An engineer can perform medical engineering tasks without being a clinical engineer. To design an ECG monitor, taking into account the many scientific requirements and the interaction of the instrument with the patient, medical staff, and environment, is engineering; however, the person doing this is not necessarily a clinical engineer.

The broad range of interfaces within clinical engineering can be described as a three-dimensional space. The operations' axis starts with the definition of the functional clinical requirements and includes specifications, research and development (R & D) or selection evaluation, acceptance testing, training, maintenance, and discard. The category axis includes diagnostic and therapeutic devices, the immediate environment of patient-care areas, and support functions directly affecting the patient both through services and the general environment. The third axis identifies the particular device, service, or environment, such as ECG monitor, delivery of food, or quality of air. The clinical engineer must be familiar with all of this clinical engineering space and be actively involved in a number of intersections from points on the three axes.

Few activities escape the present and potential contributions that can and are being made by the clinical engineer in the health care facility to include reinforcement of the traditional hospital engineering function as a cooperative partner in the delivery of responsible care amidst an ever-increasing aura of complexity. Perhaps the greatest challenge ahead lies in the all-encompassing management of external, technological, and related political changes being imposed on health-care facilities. Those who are certified should be engineers whose professional competence through training and experience entitles them to make responsible decisions affecting the safety and treatment of patients. Subject, of course, to substitutions in individual cases, a certain minimum of education and responsible work experience would be implied. It is not intended that ''clinical engineer'' be an initial title when entering the field, no more so than others in the field of medicine who, on entering, go by other names, for example, medical student, and intern.

While clinical engineers will, on occasion, repair apparatus, they are not technicians. They may establish protocols and supervise the technicians who carry them out. The technicians may be far more skilled in the execution than is the engineer; however, he does not carry the same responsibility.

One concept of the clinical engineer as a partner copracticing hands-on with the physician is largely unrealistic. The engineer may more often be a professional who uses engineering to provide the materials for the physician, to teach him how to use them, and to assist occasionally in their use.

The clinical engineer is called on to solve a myriad of perplexing problems involved in improving health-care delivery, which implies that recognition is being given to the fact that engineers will bring new devices and methodologies into medicine. Thus, there will be through legislation, accreditation, and litigation a demand that these persons be qualified and responsible.

Interfaces with Physicians

Medical devices form an important base for the delivery of optimum health care. The number of medical devices and the growth of this industry have been almost exponential. Technological applications in health services have emphasized problems of patient safety, standardization, data, zooming costs, and proper definition of the plethora of new electronic technical job functions. The physician is implicitly and explicitly involved in a new, sometimes bewildering, health-care domain. The interface between the medical and technical worlds remains indistinct.

Concerned individuals in medicine and industry have sought answers to these problems and have to address, for example, problems of standards, functions of technical staff, and, lately, the legislative aspects of medical devices. In addition, many professional medical societies are establishing an interface with engineering societies, in order to further improvement in patient care.

This interface has not been totally defined nor developed. As expected, there are levels of communication necessitated in the interface. Formal communications exist between the liaison officials of some various societies attending specific committee functions and involved in specific administrative goals, that is, preparation of legislative presentation. Informal, productive associations have existed between physician and manufacturer. However, what is lacking is a meaningful interface between the broad membership of the involved societies, disciplines, and industry.

The lack resides in identification of mutual areas of interest as well as the role of the physician, technical personnel, and the medical device in health services. It is a complex problem influenced by factors of hospital relationships (where most instruments are purchased and reside), the changing role of other allied health staff in patient care, and the foment within the ranks of the electronic instrumentation industry and engineering and medicine seeking identification and position in the health-services format. In addition, the technical language for communication suffers a replica of the Tower of Babel.

Mechanics for communication are needed. Examples of means to do this can be suggested:

1. A better level of communication between disciplines could result from an in-depth study of the medical needs by joint task groups of individuals representing the various interested professional—and industrial, where appropriate—groups.
2. Workshops in terminology, pathology, physiology, instrument standards, reliability, use, and abuse, must be developed. The physician, nurse, administrator, and paramedic might better understand the role of a clinical engineer or a biomedical engineering technician if examples are demonstrated. With such output, science, as well, would be able to grasp required social goals.
3. Of utmost importance is the study of programs to provide (*a*) clinical training to engineers in conjunction with basic scholastic work; and (*b*) follow-up internship and specialization programs.
4. Exchange of publications as a result of workshops, etc., in the journals of both medical and engineering disciplines and in areas of science would also be most beneficial.

4

A FORWARD LOOK

J. A. Rippel

In order to provide increasingly satisfactory medical diagnosis and treatment to more people, further development, extension, and improvement will be needed in the acute general hospital system. The medical system will also need more and better facilities, personnel, and means to deliver extensive primary screening, diagnostic testing, and first-stage medical treatment outside the larger, more sophisticated hospitals and medical centers. In addition, we must develop and expand a system that will encourage and assist in the maintenance and improvement of existing health practices so that many more persons can attempt to prevent or avoid serious sickness. These systems for medical care and for preventive medicine will merge at various points, and they will require various types of medical instrumentation and the services of qualified clinical engineers and technicians.

The development and improvement of medical instrumentation has become a worldwide objective. The instruments are already of a wide variety; they range from simple and inexpensive to complex and expensive. Those engaged in this work need to cooperate and exchange information with their counterparts in other countries. Even the most knowledgeable in this field are able to learn from others; also, they have some professional duty to impart their knowledge to others who need, sometimes urgently, to learn what they can do to help their own countrymen. Governments, foundations, and private interests should assist in these efforts.

The function of clinical engineers in hospitals goes beyond the use and maintenance of medical instrumentation that can be performed by M.D.s, nurses, and technicians. Although the concept of clinical engineers in hospitals is not entirely new, there is too little detailed knowledge about competent clinical engineering, its function in hospitals, and its value to patient treatment and care. This lack of knowledge exists among the general public, hospital trustees, the various government groups now being given certain controls over hospitals, and perhaps even among hospital administrators and medical professionals as well. Some medical personnel may tend to resist merging clinical engineers into medical teams in hospitals. Because lack of knowledge and understanding about clinical engineers could partly account for this resistance, medical personnel and the lay public must be educated as to the contributions that can be made by clinical engineers.

There may be other reasons for resistance by hospital medical personnel to clinical engineering. Physicians, surgeons, and other medical specialists may also become successful businessmen. Overzealous protection of their professional status and business interests may lead some medical professionals to resist the addition of nonmedical personnel to the broad medical team. Furthermore, medical professionals or administrative personnel may understandably prefer to maintain control over the purchase, maintenance, and use of medical instrumentation in their hospitals even though they are not trained or professionally qualified for this supervision. It seems inevitable that this situation must change. Today's social, political, and legal climate is quite different from that of 10 to 20 years ago. Personal and organizational risks in this specialized field may become a factor leading to change. How much could just one lost malpractice suit cost a hospital?

A forward look suggests that hospital-related government agencies, hospital trustees, administrators, and third-party insurers will eventually become convinced that competent and qualified clinical engineers are needed on many hospital medical teams; the more aware medical people will advocate adding clinical engineers to their hospital staffs. This has already occurred in some hospitals and is in progress in others. However, will this proceed fast enough, and will enough clinical engineers be available who are sufficiently qualified, flexible, and motivated to live up to the promise of clinical engineering once they have joined the hospital team?

Our medical system is not going to accept or retain a person just because he has adopted a clinical engineering title to go along with some nonhospital engineering experience. Hospitals will have to be convinced that this man is a trained, experienced biomedical engineer, that he is flexible enough to adapt productively to the particular hospital involved and that he can and will be cooperative, creative, firm when necessary, and receptive to good ideas in his field from those who are not qualified clinical engineers but who are knowledgeable in certain areas of that field. It has sometimes been said there are many technologists now available for clinical engineering positions. However, technologists are not qualified to be clinical engineers, and they would need special training and experience to become qualified.

Efforts should be encouraged to find those with the abilities needed to become good, well-rounded clinical engineers. Does this lead directly to the idea of certification of clinical engineers? Does it suggest the need for training engineers to understand biomedicine, to become familiar with today's complex, complicated hospitals, and to become proficient in all the various clinical engineering abilities needed by hospital staffs? There will be a continuing need for some constructive way to bring the right engineer and the right hospital together to consider these aspects.

A forward look can perceive that more hospitals must soon demonstrate, through practical operating experience, the value of incorporating clinical engineering into their working medical structures. "Nothing succeeds like success" is an old adage, and it retains validity. Medical instrumentation is now used in many different hospital departments and will be used increasingly as time and instrument development progress. Clinical engineering functions will not be static and narrow. Quite the opposite!

Regarding certification of clinical engineers, who will certify whom, and to whom? Has the time yet arrived when certification will be accepted and relied on by pertinent government departments and the health and medical system? Is there a need to have many more clinical engineers in the system? Should there exist a national organization of recognized, outstanding, proven clinical engineers as the foundation for a certifying procedure? Has the process of determining curricula for bachelor's, master's, and doctor's degrees been completed? Have enough good colleges and universities shown genuine interest in providing proper training for degree programs in clinical or biomedical engineering?

It is realistic to suspect that profit-oriented, medical-instrument manufacturers and their sales staff prefer to deal only with hospital administrators and department heads rather than to have competent, knowledgeable clinical engineers included on the hospital buying team. The many hundreds of millions of dollars that are spent on health and medical systems are the potential bonanza that once led Wall Street to consider medical-supply companies as "growth industries."

These huge sums should not be fair game in a perpetual "open season" for instrument companies. The money will come almost entirely from hospital operations, newly borrowed funds, and scarce government grants. Because its supply is meager to the hospital, this money must be used wisely and constructively. Certainly, it must not be wasted by hospitals in buying products that are inefficient, dangerous, defective, or obsolescent. There is evidence that some hospitals are becoming aware of their legal rights, are seeking competent technical guidance, and are demanding more from manufacturers than they have often received.

Many companies are fighting to survive. Not all are doing so. A forward look indicates that the best will survive, but better quality and greater availability of service are important needs. It may be expected that high-quality, socially well-motivated manufacturers will welcome the most competent and knowledgeable buying ability possible on the part of hospitals. One can foresee the development of new medical instruments and the improvement of those now in use. It is believed that instrumentation will be better constructed, more efficient and effective, and safer for both patients and those handling the instruments. Competent clinical engineers, qualified in this field through training and experience, can be major factors in these developments.

Medical instrumentation is bought to be used, hopefully regularly and often. Ownership and use of biomedical instrumentation require the capabilities required to maintain, service, repair, and calibrate. Otherwise, assets and opportunities are wasted. There is a tremendous amount of costly medical equipment lying about unused because it has failed from lack of maintenance or from incomplete maintenance. Clinical engineering is needed to cut down to the lowest minimum this type of waste.

One basis for a forward look is that every facet of buying, using, and maintaining medical instrumentation in hospitals should be directed toward benefiting medical systems and patients. The goal is to have only excellent equipment that will work effectively, that will be available at all times for proper use, and that will provide the patient with accurate, prompt results at reasonable cost.

The total effort of medical systems is to supply better care to more people for longer periods of time per day and per week. Further progress in medical instrumentation is one of several factors involved in how close this goal can be achieved—and how soon.

Changes in medical systems are now progressing that will steadily increase the numbers of persons who will be given regular testing or multiphasic screening and, if indicated, will be sent on to more extensive diagnosis, treatment, care, and rehabilitation. Hospital emergency and clinical outpatient facilities have recently been expanded. More expansion is under way. Much more will come. Widely prevalent is the conviction that acute-care hospitals can and will serve, in essence, as the doctor for many people within their areas. Some are now doing so. If more of the public's needs are going to be met, more medical instrumentation will be needed to make up for the shortage of medical personnel and to perform various functions more readily, more quickly, more accurately, more productively, and more economically. Instrumentation will be necessary to store routinely detailed medical records of patients on a quickly retrievable basis. If these views are accurate, and there is considerable evidence that they are, health, medical, and hospital teams will require the services of clinical or biomedical engineers and technicians.

Against this background, the concepts of hospital clinical engineering departments are now under determined development somewhat too late rather than too early. The advancement of these cannot afford wasted time or many false moves or mistakes. If sound, steady progress toward this development is to be made, important segments of the hospital and medical systems, of related health and government agencies, and of medical instrumentation manufacturers must devote serious, unselfish, cooperative efforts to the task.

There are various patterns for clinical engineering in hospitals. The term "hospitals" involves widely differing institutions. Some will require departments of clinical engineering, with clinical technicians and perhaps more than one clinical engineer. Others will need only one full-time engineer and perhaps one technician. Some will be served adequately by joining with other hospitals to employ a clinical engineer to serve each hospital part time or by working with independent service people. The number, ability, competence, flexibility, and motivation of available clinical engineers will be a continuing major factor in their employment by hospitals. Although most hospitals are nonprofit, they are nevertheless complex, difficult businesses to administer and manage. Municipal, county, state, and federal departments know this only too well from their own experience in running their hospitals. Our hospitals are now involved in improving their business operations to accomplish more at less cost; avoid waste of time, manpower, and space; and increase productivity. New, sophisticated electronic systems, machines, and instruments are becoming increasingly involved in these business operations. Here, too, is an important area requiring trained, competent engineers and technicians.

The details of just what a competent clinical engineer should be must be put together by those who will be involved with clinical engineers on hospital staffs. The clinical engineer is not to be thought of as either a high-class tube changer or repairman or as a second-class citizen on the hospital staff. He, like the physician, should enter the hospital system at a top level. To deserve such a status, he must, of course, have the knowledge to qualify him and be capable of exercising the responsibility involved at his staff level. His minimum responsibility is the use of medical instrumentation that helps the process of delivering medicine in its fullest sense to individual patients, usually in hospitals. This process should involve electronics, physiology, nuclear physics, and biochemistry and will require increasing competence in various computer techniques. There will be a need for the clinical engineer to have some knowledge of the law as it applies to the purchasing of equipment and the type of performance this equipment delivers after purchase. He will have to work closely with medical professionals, and, hopefully, each will deserve the respect of the other. He will need fundamental training and subsequent experience in a variety of pertinent areas. As a technical person entering the professional and sophisticated working area of medicine, he cannot be naïve.

It seems clear that setting a code of current standards covering this new profession cannot be avoided. The code should be periodically examined, expanded, and perhaps revised. The potentials of clinical engineers will be of indispensable importance. The broad medical system, related government agencies, and the public must be thoroughly informed about these potentials. The potentials must become actualities.

5

TECHNOLOGY AND CLINICAL MEDICINE

J. H. U. Brown

Affluence in a country dictates that its citizens should be provided with three essentials of a good health-care system: *easy access* by everyone to *high-quality* care at a *reasonable cost*. If efforts must be bent toward these ends, a major input will be technology.

Today's health-care system is under many strains. The complexity of modern medicine places a premium on the exchange of information and the handling of data. The physician is faced with increasing pressures toward group practice, the advent of a variety of paramedical personnel who may pose as great a threat as a help to him, and the many problems of a system that is not designed to handle the number of cases it receives.

Each of these problems demands immediate solution, and most of the solutions are in the area of technology. Most of the needed technology is state-of-the-art; vast new instrumentation and theorectical studies are not needed. What is needed is to apply the knowledge now present in engineering to the often mundane problems of everyday medicine. Many of these problems are not glamorous, but they are worthy of solution. Before the health-care-delivery system can progress, they must be solved.

A classic example is the records system. The present health-care system is based on patient records. In the large majority of cases, these are numerous documents related only in a time sequence and with no detectable relationship between the problems of the patient and the records of progress. The patient who transfers from one part of the system to another is at a great disadvantage. His records are difficult to transfer, the numbering systems do not coincide, and the new unit to which he transfers may use a different record format.

The theoretical solution is simple. What is desperately needed is a standardized admissions form, discharge abstract, and also some form of problem-oriented patient record. These records must be computer based and should be tied to the billing and bookkeeping systems in the hospital, an engineering problem pure and simple. But like so many facets of health care, it has a strong sociological base. The system must be used by doctors and nurses, so it must be acceptable to them.

Many other such problems are related to the hospital as a system. Hospitals have not taken advantage of the savings in time and money resulting from proper use of technology. For example, through efficient use of computers, diets can be planned, nurses' schedules can be arranged, purchases can be coordinated, and procedures can be scheduled. The operating costs of the hospital can be reduced.

There are many problems relating more directly to the patient and his needs. The laboratory in a hospital may perform hundreds of thousands of tests per year. These tests are often archaic—performed in the same manner as the same test of 50 years ago. They have been mechanized, not automated. Tests are inaccurate and often must be repeated many times. There is no real process control and no real operations research on the procedures and the arrangements in the laboratory. True automation of the hospital laboratory, new tests that are more specific, and new approaches to the design of health-delivery systems are needed.

There is now more and more development of multiphasic health testing based on the premise that repeated tests on an individual can record changes in health status. Difficulties may arise if such tests may not be reliable unless they are repeated at regular intervals. Also, the tests can be useless unless the results are tied closely to a follow-up and treatment regime. Finally, the tests may not be valid for the purpose for which they are intended because many of the tests used are designed to measure overt illness, not incipient disease. Technology must produce new tests, determine the frequency, provide the automation, and provide data-handling methodology to reveal results and permit follow-up.

Other problems occur in handling the critically ill. Invasive techniques are used that actually may be measuring the wrong parameters—and this on a critically ill patient who needs as little interference with his life processes as possible. Again, technology may help solve the problem. The newer magnetic flowmeters, for example, can be used to measure blood flow without arterial puncture. Consider that trauma and emergency illness is the third largest "disease" in the United States. Each year hundreds of thousands of people die, and millions are hospitalized from injury, heart attacks, and other major sudden illnesses. It has been estimated that 25% of all these deaths could be prevented with an adequate emergency-care system. Such a system could be a miracle of technology: Communications involving ECGs and other vital signs, if necessary, transportation of the most modern kind, trained personnel, resuscitative devices, planned and equipped emergency suites, and critical-care monitoring are all badly needed.

The problem is enormous when it is considered that no city has a totally adequate emergency system at the present time, and only a few of the approximately 7000 hospitals in the United States can meet the standards of a Class I emergency facility. More than one-third of all the ambulance pickups in the country are made by hearses with untrained drivers, and the patient, in the vast majority of cases, is delivered to an emergency room inadequately equipped and without a trained emergency physician in attendance.

Most of the discussion so far has centered on the hospital and its problems, but the hospital is only a small part of the system. For every 1 million people in the hospital beds of the United States, there are 20 times as many in outpatient clinics, in doctors' offices, or receiving no care at all. Attention must be turned from the care of the sick in the hospital to preventive medicine and health care of the citizens as a whole. Here again, technology plays a critical part.

To supply care to all people and to provide them with access to the system means that another kind of care must be emphasized. The physicians in the rural area must be provided with advice, assistance, and back-up. It is now possible to connect the rural practitioner with a medical center through terminals that can help him bill his patients, read his ECGs, process laboratory data, and keep patient records.

Each paramedic in remote areas can be in communication with a physician through a satellite or microwave link. Each of these methods is now in use, and their use is expanding. As an example, a private physician in central Missouri is connected by telephone to the medical center of the University of Missouri 100 miles away. The center computer provides information, maintains records, reads ECGs and other tests, and in general acts as a "physician's assistant" to the practitioner. There appears to be no reason why this system could not be expanded to reach the many isolated physicians in the country.

Another way to promote access to the system is to develop units that can provide comprehensive medical care to an enrolled population. These large health-maintenance organizations can depend on testing, education, and immediate treatment to reduce hospital stay and therefore costs in the system. Each unit could serve tens of thousands of subscribers and would require a healthy technical back-up in computers, laboratories, transportation, etc.

One of the major problems in applying technology to health care is the lack of a clearly definable subject. It is true that the health-care industry at $80 billion per year total expenditure is one of the largest United States industries. It employs millions of people in thousands of locations. It should be ripe for technology and the advantages of mass production that come with technology. Unfortunately, this is not a true picture. In reality, the system consists of 250,000 private entrepreneurs—the practicing physicians—backed up by 6000 independent hospitals, 75% of which have fewer than 200 beds. Resistance to mass production arises not only from this complex but also from other less definable factors. The practice of medicine is ultimately a personal service, and people do not like regimentation. Second, the private physician "does his own thing" and may resist the development of a uniform technology, which is reflected in the thousands of small companies that produce the medical equipment. The diverse patent policies of the federal government and its impact on the system do not help to resolve problems.

Any development in the medical market is expensive. A product to be used on humans requires thorough testing and high development costs and may not command a large market. The feedback is all negative. Without a firm patent policy, a manufacturer hesitates to incur heavy development costs with risk of not recovering funds. This chain must be broken, and the government may eventually undertake some of the development costs with return based on profits. As large-scale health organizations develop with greater demands for uniform equipment, the standardization of products will occur more readily, and the market will be stabilized.

Obviously, the previous statements are aimed largely at the problems of consumer access to the system through communication and containment of costs through more efficient operation and mass production. Each of these is technically oriented. Improving quality is more nebulous. A health-maintenance organization may improve access and decrease costs, but it may not improve overall quality. Here again, technology may help. The development of programs and methods of visual instructions and the provision of materials to aid in diagnosis and treatment are in their infancy.

In summary, technology is playing a part in the delivery of health services. This role can only increase. The real market, however, is not in the development of intensive instrumentation for the modern hospital. Rather, it is the development of state-of the-art projects that will provide the input, the communications, and the physician back-up to provide health services to the vast number of ambulatory patients and the advice and education to turn our thoughts toward prevention as opposed to sick care. The surface of technological needs has barely been touched. So far, attention has been concentrated on the hospital. Now attention must be focused on the people—the consumer in the system.

PART II

EDUCATION

6

THE OBJECTIVES OF CLINICAL ENGINEERS

H. H. Sun

Various approaches to the objectives of clinical engineers from the viewpoint of curriculum development in academic institutions have been given careful consideration. Many universities have graduate engineering programs at the MS level with emphasis on training toward engineering and the technological side of the clinical problem, usually coupled with a hospital internship for the student. Other universities have developed undergraduate programs directed at students working either as engineers in a clinical environment or as premedical students preparing for clinical medicine. There is also a third program that trains clinical doctors with the necessary background in engineering and computer knowledge to enable them to perform some functions of the clinical engineer.

The role of the clinical engineer in relation to his contribution to the solution of the many problems in the health-care-delivery system has been well established. There are several basic hypotheses in the development of clinical engineers.

1. There is a great demand for clinical engineers in hospitals and clinical laboratories.
2. The clinical engineer is application oriented, as opposed to the research-oriented biomedical engineer.
3. Universities and hospitals should both play major roles in graduating the proper type of clinical engineer

Many universities have already developed a number of programs aimed at training students based on the above hypotheses. These programs should be analyzed from a critical viewpoint with the objective being to improve the present programs rather than to make a judgment on the relative standings among the existing programs.

Hypotheses

It must first be assumed that there is a need for clinical engineers at the present time or in the foreseeable future. A committee of the National Academy of Engineering (NAE) has defined three broad areas of biomedical engineering. The third area applies to the definition of a clinical engineer.

> The application of engineering concepts, methodology, and technology to the improvement of health-service-delivery systems in the broad context of interrelated institutions (hospitals, clinics, governmental units, universities, industry, etc.) as well as within the specific confines of individual components of the health-care systems.

In a recently published NIH report, this was further exemplified as an area including

> Not only most of the multitude of ways in which computers and automation are coming to be used in hospitals, such as automated clinical laboratories, data collection and management systems, patient monitoring systems, multiphasic health testing, etc., but also the communication systems and devices necessary to link together various parts of the health-care-delivery system to provide emergency services, health care in rural areas, etc.

These statements clearly define the need for clinical engineers and the importance of their contributions to the area of health-care delivery. However, the demand for service from clinical engineers has not yet been quantitated, and the projected number of clinical engineers that will be needed in the next 5 years cannot be clearly predicted at this time. This question can also be asked about other types of engineers. However, with the introduction and heavy emphasis on the sociological and human approach in the engineering profession, slow development of employment opportunities for biomedical and clinical engineers raises some concern from an educator's point of view. Several questions can be raised at this point. Are biomedical and clinical engineers being trained, and could the law of supply and demand be working against them? Are we training a type of engineer who is not suitable for this specific purpose? Has there been a failure in overall objectives in the training of clinical engineers?

The second hypothesis deals with the question of whether we need application-oriented or research-oriented engineers. Many schools have prematurely initiated new programs such as urban engineer, transportation engineer, commerce engineer, and so forth. Some have advocated the development of "software engineering" as opposed to traditional "hardware engineering." There is no question that the educational programs of most colleges have been extensively disciplinary oriented. About 40–50% of the engineering graduates continue on to graduate schools; consequently, the number in advance-degree brackets has been greatly increased. What is now happening is that Ph.D.s have a more difficult time finding proper positions than a college graduate having a BS degree. There is a gradual swing of the educational pendulum toward the other direction. However, most of the engineering schools are highly concerned with the sudden evolvement of new name programs with no proper substance and quality.

There is a prevailing feeling among educators that too many borderline schools have produced low-level engineers, some even at the advanced degree level, and the change of name alone cannot solve the problem. Some have predicted that the number of engineering schools will be greatly decreased, with most of the marginal schools disappearing within the next decade. The engineering schools accrediting agency (ECPD) has introduced new standards requiring at least 1 year of design, synthesis, and system for the 4-year engineering colleges. It is evident that the trend is in the direction of application-oriented engineering programs.

The third hypothesis is meaningful if this can be done with proper care and arrangements. Hospitals are adequate for the training of professional persons, M.D.s, and nurses, most of this training being almost entirely self-taught. An engineer is thus qualified if he is problem oriented and also if he can learn from the job with very little supervision. The majority of work in the hospital at present cannot be considered overly challenging for the engineer; therefore, a major investment in equipment and administrative orientation is needed to change the environment. Otherwise, hospitals will only be served by a group of underpaid, second-rate technicians because a slight turn around of our economy will immediately return the qualified engineers to industry, working in areas other than clinical engineering. Therefore, a study of the objectives of clinical engineers must also include the availability of hospitals with large investments in equipment and teaching facilities and a willingness to accept this type of training program.

Because of the three basic conditions as outlined, at the present time, the training of clinical engineers should proceed with great caution, and only programs with highly qualified faculties, facilities, and environment will survive.

Objectives

During the past 10 years, new programs have suddenly evolved at both the graduate and undergraduate levels in the interdisciplinary field of biomedical engineering, and several of them have recently turned toward the training of clinical engineers. Many of them are training true "hybrid engineers," a person who is not only strong in one area but is also versatile in others. Evidently, a good electronic engineer will have a better chance to become a successful biomedical engineer or clinical engineer than a weak and deficient one. The same applies to mechanical engineers, chemical engineers, or computer operators. Similarly, a competent life scientist can be trained to be a biomedical or clinical engineer if he is a good life scientist and is versatile enough to become a "hybrid."

The problem as it is seen today is a combination of low-level engineering and life-sciences courses such as those given for the training of nurses or paramedical personnel. High-quality programs are the only answer to successful training, especially in this crucial period of development and evolvement of new programs.

Standards must not be compromised, and, if necessary, an additional amount of time and course requirements for this new hybrid type of training must be required. It is only through the evolvement of first-rate, high-quality programs that industries, hospitals, and government agencies will be convinced that it will be worth their money to hire this new breed of engineer.

It has been stated that the reasons why the actual growth of the demand for biomedical engineers is smaller than projected may be a result of the following.

1. Industries have not been interested in research programs and have been dependent on other laboratories to conduct them. This reduces the need for biomedical engineers and also slows down the development of new products.
2. The development of the medical instrumentation market, such as monitoring equipment, has failed to materialize and therefore decreased the demand for the utilization of application engineers.

Others have suggested that the lack of innovation in medical electronic industries as compared to the efforts of the aviation and color television industries is the major blame for the failure of their development and expansion. All these reasons point to the fact that qualified biomedical and clinical engineers must continue to initiate new ideas so that new programs can be developed. They must bear the responsibility to speed up the expansion of medical instrumentation industries and, most of all, must make the hospital and clinician accept their services with enthusiasm. This again means the development of a first-rate, truly hybrid clinical engineer who will not be taken over by second-rate programs that have not received any respect from the consumer. Only qualified engineering and medical faculties and research and clinical facilities must be used to accomplish this purpose. It must be insisted that engineering and medical programs be taught by highly qualified instructors. Accordingly, only qualified students must be selected for this purpose. Only after these individuals have become qualified and are accepted by industries, governmental agencies, and hospitals can it be said that the objectives have been fulfilled in the training of clinical engineers.

Analysis of Existing Programs

From a brief survey taken of the existing programs in clinical engineering, there are three types that merit some description.

1. Graduate program leading to MS with internship in the hospital. The entrance students must have a designated degree of engineering, for example, a BS in electrical engineering. The program can therefore be considered a good hybrid, with a total duration of about two academic years. Usually, it is 1 year of course work emphasizing the engineering and medical areas and a definite period of internship in a contracted hospital.

2. Undergraduate program in an engineering college. This may be classified into two categories.

a. A program leading to a BS in (designated) biomedical engineering. The details of an undergraduate, biomedical engineering program are still uncertain, although many universities have already offered this program for several years. Many of the graduates have found places in industry, graduate schools, and medical schools. This program provides a hybrid curriculum by which the student may enter his career at an earlier date. The length of and the details of curriculum times are still under active discussion.

b. A program leading toward a BS in engineering (undesignated). This is a general engineering program with great flexibility, allowing the student to enter areas other than those of a regular engineering major for his future career of medicine, law, or management.

3. Life-scientist program. This is usually a special training program for life scientists (M.D., D.V.M., or Ph.D.) in the area of engineering, mathematics, and computers. It is a graduate program and usually leads to an MS degree. It is also a truly hybrid type of training and thus produces very good results.

The objectives of clinical engineers must be clearly identified with good-quality training programs both at universities and hospitals. Because of his newly acquired title, the clinical engineer is under constant surveillance by all parties concerned. He therefore must be aware of his background and always conscious of his quality. He must not only be a good engineer in his own area of competence (e.g., E.E., Chem. E., etc.) but must also be knowledgeable in medical and clinical areas. He must be constantly improving himself, learning all the new ideas, and keeping abreast of the latest developments in engineering and the life sciences at all times. Only with all the above objectives will a clinical engineer be fully accepted in a hospital as a colleague to a clinician and be rewarded according to his services.

7

EDUCATION FOR THE CLINICAL ENGINEER

C. A. Caceres

There is no disagreement that the engineer entering the field of medicine should first be proficient and earn a degree in one of the basic engineering disciplines, preferably in electrical, mechanical, or chemical engineering. Thus, a basic recommendation is that the student take standard engineering courses and supplement his education with courses in areas that apply to medicine without compromising the basic engineering degree.

Do basic engineering school courses have sufficient breadth to allow development of a *clinical* engineer? Studies have shown that they do. Consider a school of engineering's current electrical engineering and computer science courses. All that seems to be required, on review of their course catalogues, are examples of applications and problems that deal with medicine. Network courses are an example. The methodology for integration of a multiplicity of instruments that must be related to patient care on a simultaneous basis, not just within the hospital but also out of the hospital, conveying information back and forth throughout the course of the patient care in a sample real-life problem. Design and function problems in the network courses could orient the student to the medical needs.

Courses dealing with electromagnetic waves are of extreme significance. Certainly, much of the misunderstanding of medical signals that currently exists among physicians is due to a lack of knowledge about pulses and waveshapes and their true significance in an engineering sense. An engineer's sound background is necessary for needed improvements in the usage of these signals in medicine.

Communications will drastically change the mode of health-service delivery and should be a basic in engineering. We are still roughly in the beginning of the Alexander Graham Bell era in medicine and do not take advantage of telemetric science. Additionally, many of our medical signal problems could be solved on an economic basis if appropriate analogue and hybrid computer systems were used for processing, storage, and retrieval. Computer science, laboratories and measurements, control systems—all of these areas are already ideal for clinical engineering programs.

Operations research is ideally suited for the clinical engineer entering administrative areas and management. The lack of engineers in medicine with this background is primarily responsible for the failure of the current group of physician-administrators to solve national health-care needs. Certainly, some of the principles of materials science, mechanics of solids, the metal structures, and hydraulics warrant inclusion in the field of medicine. The application of the principles of fluid mechanics is certainly lacking in cardiovascular research. One can conclude that what is required is orientation of the engineering *faculty* to the medical area. If the faculty will incorporate the problems that orient the student to the medical field as one in need of his services, much of the current curricula can do the basic job.

But once an engineer elects to work in the medical field, he must decide in which area his interests lie. There are two approaches he can take.

Biomedical Engineering—An Opportunistic Educational Approach

Presently, this area has the largest number of engineers working in medicine. The term *biomedical* does not directly imply *medical* (indeed, concise medical dictionaries such as Dorland's Pocket Edition do not include the term *biomedical*) but instead infers a combination of biology and medicine. In this field, engineering is concerned mainly with basic research. There does not have to be any necessary extension into applied research. Generally, the research that the biomedical engineer performs will reach fruition in the future, that is, years. He must be prepared for that length of time to see results.

The education of the biomedical engineer must be based on an opportunistic approach. This is necessary, as requirements for an engineer in research are highly variable, dependent on the faculty that is available, the geographical environment, the state of the economy, and the individual engineer. Faculty interests will generally be overriding. A close, almost one-to-one relationship is needed to develop and produce a good researcher in any field.

There is little reason to formulate a well-defined program for this area. Engineering programs developed in this discipline should be similar to those for any of the other doctorate degrees and must be individualized. A doctorate is mandatory in this area to guarantee the prospective employer or support source that the individual can deal with new and novel problems that require ingenious thought, comprehension, and new and different results.

Clinical Engineering—A Deterministic Educational Approach

The engineer in the clinical area should be clearly differentiated from the biomedical research engineer. That is not to say that there could not be free flow of knowledge between the two groups. A specific individual might best produce for himself and his community by going from one to another of the two areas at different times.

The term *clinical engineering* was coined to describe the area of major engineering impact needed in health-care delivery today. The field encompasses such immediate needs as:

1. Patient-oriented services such as (*a*) health testing in community health-care centers; (*b*) automated monitoring for interpretation of status change in surgery, obstetrics, medicine, and other areas of intensive care, particularly to aid nurses and staff; and (*c*) operation of special facilities such as pacemaker clinics and hemodialysis centers
2. Communication of advances in comprehensive health care made possible by electronics, computers, and health systems analysis to the medical staff
3. Implementation of systems such as integrated medical records and hospital information systems with appropriate interface with the community
4. Analysis of community medical services supplied through hospitals to determine the interfacing mechanisms with other disciplines in order to use combined talents for medicine, for example, statistical techniques of diagnostic and prognostic simulations
5. Hospital and health-center safety implementation in regard to all phases of equipment
6. Research into technology utilization to produce less expensive and more effective management of patients and better use of medical manpower, instrumentation, and systems

The clinical engineer should be capable of passing his professional engineering examinations early in his career. Scholastically, this suggests a general approach requirement to his background course work. The clinical engineer could have a master's degree heavily dependent on courses in engineering, wherein clinical application as stated previously is readily apparent. The clinical engineer might, however, have only a bachelor's degree, accompanied by background obtained through specialized short courses, apprenticeship, or refresher courses in engineering, wherein clinical application problems are used. Clinical training during school years and internship thereafter would be the ideal.

In any event, education for the clinical engineer should, in contrast to the biomedical engineer, be deterministic. The needs of patient care are known, so the development of the professional engineering assistance required can be planned. It is in this deterministic area that a school of engineering can and should play its greatest role.

Overview of Requirements of Clinical Engineering

As a result of several years and numerous conferences, one can state that there is consensus that the clinical engineer should not be simply a generally capable engineer. Instead, he should (*a*) be an engineer with emphasis in a defined engineering field; (*b*) be oriented toward solving everyday problems; (*c*) be ready at a moment's notice to carry out, with or without staff, the suggestions that he himself has proposed to solve the problems in his field; and (*d*) have the knowledge of consultants immediately available to solve problems out of his field.

Training is required to orient oneself toward the goal of working in the current medical environment. It is a system that currently exists in the real world, which cannot, for the benefit of the patient, sustain much change at any one time. Working daily in the current system is not usually palatable to the research-oriented individual.

Specialization Requirements

Usually, the clinical engineer will have specific interests, for example, facilities or perhaps specific functional areas, for example, anesthesia. These examples of general areas suggest advanced areas for engineering course work required and represent different programs that the master's student could undertake. These same areas could produce courses that could also be offered as special or audit courses for others who wish to seek certification in major areas without a master's degree. Combined, such areas can be envisioned as forming the foundation for a doctorate program in clinical engineering.

Interface Courses

There are obviously introductory courses, transition courses, and courses that have to be developed for items of unique need and because of new developments.

Interface courses should utilize seminar and symposia techniques. Faculty in such courses should acquaint engineers to the health field with the differing points of view of the researcher, community, consumer, industrial concern, and "middlemen" or overviewer groups that coexist in the field.

A basic philosophical approach in such courses is relevance to today's needs. The concept of hospitals as institutions in flux and not as monuments, for example, must be considered and understood. Mobility, flexibility, and responsiveness to current needs must be a consideration. The international role of United States hospitals as training media for developing areas must be considered. The faculty constantly study the results of its teaching sessions as the input for new material to be up-to-date and revelant to health-care delivery is mandatory.

Apprenticeship, Clinical Training, and Internship

By additionally providing supervised service projects in clinics and hospitals, students would be in a better position to acquire the needed creditable experience.

This is the area that must develop by use of the university or nearby hospitals with or without other teaching programs.

The basic facility of provision of care is the clinic. The hospital is its logical extension. It is there that the mechanism for delivery of health services (due to volume) can be studied and perfected, but the student must be aware of the core as only the core and not the full system. Today, the engineer usually works out of the hospital. The utilization of a single structure is, however, not suitable for the real world. Numerous entities are the key to delivery of health services appropriate for the current decade. After obtaining a thorough engineering background with clinical training, "internship" programs should be made available.

Faculty for Clinical Engineering

The faculty for clinical engineering should encompass physicists, statisticians, analysts, and programmers, as well as physicians, nurses, and engineers. In general, the faculty should be comprised of persons experienced in clinical systems in order to effect the general purposes of clinical engineering by: (*a*) design, adaptation, and application of new technology and methods to achieve modern health care at determined quality and cost objectives; (*b*) promotion of acceptance and routine use of quality control; (*c*) education for community responsibilities in care and health-services research; (*d*) evaluation of old as well as new methodologies and techniques; (*e*) supervision of the facilities required in these efforts; and (*f*) consultative services to serve national, regional, local, and other institutional groups.

The clinical engineer is at the heart of the formal means by which our national and world health problems can be solved. The growth of health services has increased the demand on the people capable of delivering services. Thus, the cost has risen. The quality will tend to decrease unless we can educate all those concerned with health to focus appropriately on the community's most urgent and solvable health problems. This includes the engineer (student and principally the teacher). The methods of service delivery, manpower utilization, and better tools must be the background from which engineering teachers consider their courses.

To utilize engineering capability, the educational role of the academician must be oriented to stimulate the development of practical service systems. To make this possible, the school should provide academic background as well as guide and oversee the practical training needed and being received.

Educational programs for clinical engineering can be implemented with alacrity. Effort is, however, needed as a basic step by the faculty in determining which of the current courses could most easily have examples of medical and clinical applications incorporated in their standard format.

8

THE UNIVERSITY'S ROLE IN THE DEVELOPMENT OF THE CLINICAL ENGINEERING PROFESSION

V. L. Newhouse and P. E. Stanley

The history of the clinical engineer as well as his current and expected employment opportunities are being carefully reviewed. Under-utilization of clinical engineers may be interpreted as a result of the lack of an adequate pool of such engineers. The university could be a key element in breaking this deadlock.

The existence of the subspecialty of engineering called bioengineering, which may be defined as the application of engineering techniques to the problems of biology and medicine, goes back to at least 1948 when the Joint Executive Committee on Medicine and Biology was established by the American Institute of Electrical Engineering (AIEE), the Instrument Society of America (ISA), and the Institute of Radio Engineers (IRE). Until recently, the primary interest in this field and the closely allied field of biophysics has been the fundamental research into biological mechanisms as opposed to engineering development aimed at problems of instrumentation. This tendency is well illustrated by the fact that the Biomedical Engineering Society, formed in 1968, requires a Ph.D. for membership.

This same philosophy has been demonstrated by government support in the form of training grants that have been limited almost totally to students studying for the Ph.D. degree or beyond. However, since instrumentation and automation have begun to play increasing roles in health-care delivery and health maintenance, the emphasis in biomedical engineering has begun to shift from the previous almost exclusive preoccupation with research on biological mechanisms to increased efforts in the field of systems and instrumentation research and development applied to health-care delivery. A typical example of this tendency in the United States is the initiation by the National Institute of General Medical Services at (NIH) of a program of research aimed at automating the clinical laboratory. This movement toward clinical engineering may be said to have started with the formation of the Association for the Advancement of Medical Instrumentation (AAMI) in 1965. It is quite evident that more attention has been paid to defining the job market for clinical engineers than to their education. Attention to defining an educational program for clinical engineers is, however, basic.

The role of the clinical engineer in the hospital is different from the research role with which the bioengineer has been identified. New engineering tasks in hospitals involve the supervision of the proper operation and safety of instruments, the design of engineering systems and those components of such systems that are not commercially available, the introduction of industrial or management engineering techniques to optimize information handling, and cooperation with the clinical team in the long-term management of life-support systems. The functions of such an individual in a hospital may also include the training of nurses and medical technicians in the operation of various clinical instruments and the management tasks currently associated with the function of the hospital engineer. The clinical engineer will also play a vital role in the organizations to service and advise groups of hospitals. He will also be active in a number of government agencies, particularly those concerned with certification and the setting of standards in clinical instrumentation. The above tasks are engineering and development functions rather than research and therefore do not require a degree higher than the MS. Many of these tasks will be conducted in conjunction with biomedical equipment technicians. In addition, just as solid-state-device research in industry is gradually being shifted from physicists to engineers, the hospital tasks associated with radiation therapy (currently described as medical physics) will probably be carried out in the future by clinical engineers possessing a Ph.D. degree.

Finally, it seems probable that clinical instrument manufacturers will gradually introduce clinical engineers into their engineering positions in design, development, manufacturing, sales, service, and management. The maturation of this new engineering specialty of clinical engineering was emphasized with the publication of Clinical Engineering News by AAMI, beginning in May 1973.

The number of biomedical engineers employed in hospitals, universities, and industry has been studied recently by an NAE committee and an NIH committee and has been found to be somewhat smaller than would be anticipated when considering the hospital and industrial-engineering functions we have listed. The NIH study just mentioned estimates that the number of professionals who have a major involvement with biomedical engineering in the United States is approximately 7500. Of these, 3000 are estimated to be in industry, mostly at the MS or BS level. The National Academy of Engineering study estimated that 3000–4000 companies are active in the field of biomedical engineering. This is a surprisingly low number even though most of these companies are known to be small. The number of engineers employed in hospitals is estimated at about 3000, also a surprisingly low number since there are approximately 7000 hospitals in the United States with an average of 227 beds, and it has been estimated that a BS in clinical engineering could "pay for itself" in a hospital having no more than 150 beds.

Before analyzing the reasons for the relatively low employment level of biomedical engineers in health-care engineering and delivery, it is pertinent to ask how the various organizations involved in the manufacture or use of clinical instrumentation do in fact fulfill those needs that medical or clinical engineers are intended to fulfill.

As far as system design is concerned, hospitals without a clinical engineer tend to rely on manufacturer's representatives even though this often leads to inadequate and unnecessarily expensive purchases. To cope with the problem of equipment breakdown, these hospitals employ redundancy, purchasing two or three times as many instruments as are required at any one time. For routine servicing and maintenance, hospitals use manufacturer's representatives, service organizations, or even local television repairmen. It is suspected that this system leads to increased breakdowns and malpractice suits. Thus, in the absence of adequate safety and maintenance, the hospital with a clinical engineer tends to make up for this lack by increasing its expenditures on legal fees and malpractice insurance. Finally, when the hospital requires engineering design information, for example, in connection with the construction of new facilities, it will use outside engineering consultants often associated with hospital architects. In summary, all the engineering needs of the hospital are being faced and met in some fashion, even by hospitals that do not employ clinical engineers. However, when these needs are dealt with by methods not involving clinical engineers, they are presumably satisfied in a vastly less effective and more expensive manner than would result using specialized engineers.

At least four reasons can explain the current under-utilization of bioengineers in hospitals. It has been pointed out that a way needs to be found to certify that an engineer or technician is capable of operating effectively in the clinical environment. Such certification would be similar to that provided by state boards in the medical and legal professions and would serve to ensure the individual's competency to assume his assigned responsibilities, which can directly or indirectly affect patient care, and to signal to the medical staff the professional nature of engineering. The second reason for the lack of interest in bioengineers shown by organizations involved in health-care delivery rather than research is that the conventional bioengineer produced by the universities in the past is too research oriented and not sufficiently interested in the design and service aspects of engineering. A third reason is the well-known communication gap existing between the physician and the engineer. As a fourth reason for the lack of as strong a current interest in bioengineers as would be expected, it has been suggested that hospital administrators are simply not knowledgeable in respect to the functions and capabilities of clinical engineers.

The reasons for the lack of biomedical engineers in industry have been attributed to the feeling that managers believe a bioengineer might have a less than adequate background in either engineering or biomedicine and would therefore be less competent than a team composed of conventional engineers using physicians as consultants and to the fact that the biomedical industry is made up predominately of small companies that employ fewer engineers per dollar of sales than are employed in the more concentrated type of electronic industry serving the nonmedical market. Specifically, in the electronic industry, one engineer is employed per approximately $200,000 of sales, whereas in the biomedical engineering industry, only one engineer per $500,000 of sales is employed.

To cope with the previously mentioned difficulties, it has been suggested that adequate licensing procedures for clinical engineers be established; that universities produce more bachelor's and master's degree medical engineers, as opposed to the Ph.D. bioengineer; and that more management engineering studies be performed and publicized in the right quarters. Finally, it has been shown that specific curricula adapted to clinical engineering and differing from the curricula appropriate for bioengineering should be developed in the universities.

Without underestimating the importance of the various problem areas and their solutions, it has been suggested that the primary cause for the lack of available clinical engineering positions in today's hospitals may simply be the lack of qualified clinical engineers to fill such positions. As pointed out above, the current hospital administration is forced to cope with the problems a clinical engineer would handle by a number of *ad hoc* methods involving the purchase of redundant equipment, the use of outside consultants, the use of inadequate service personnel, and possibly the need of extra malpractice insurance to cope with the consequences of engineering malfunction. For the hospital administrator to reorganize his spending and working procedures in order to employ a clinical engineer would be a major task that would lead to disaster if he then found that not enough clinical engineers were available to fill the positions in his hypothetical, newly optimized organization. One cannot expect the hospital administrator to tamper with his current system, even if he feels it to be unsatisfactory, unless he is assured that an ample supply of legally qualified clinical engineers is available. Thus, one cannot expect a large number of clinical engineering positions to be formed in the health-care system until the clinical engineering profession has become well established and an ample supply of qualified clinical engineers is known to be available.

From the standpoint of the student considering specialization in the field of clinical engineering, however, the shoe is on the other foot. He cannot be expected, however great his altruism, to specialize in a field unless he is assured that an ample number of employment opportunities exist in that profession. How can the university help to break this vicious circle?

Our suggested solution is to train fully qualified clinical engineers with a background in one of the older engineering specialties. These engineers will be available to fill medical engineering positions, yet their employment will not be solely dependent on the existence of unfilled medical engineering positions. They will always be able to work in their "alternate" professions if necessary. Thus, once an adequate pool of clinical engineers has been formed in this way, the hospital administrator will have the confidence, as regards the availability of these trained specialists, he needs to realign working procedures to open up clinical engineering positions.

The engineering background of the medical or clinical engineer may be concentrated in electrical or mechanical engineering, chemical engineering, or industrial engineering. In addition,the clinical engineer will have taken extra courses in chemistry and the life sciences and will have become familiar *by actual experience* with the language and *modus operandi* of the hospital.

Although the clinical engineer will, in the main, be active in fields other than research, his university training will be organized by holders of the Ph.D., as is the training of all other engineers at present. These Ph.D.s will probably engage in research involving the application of engineering principles to clinical instrumentation and the organization and operation of clinical systems in general. Although the emphasis of university departments producing clinical engineers will no doubt be on the production of the BS and MS, one may assume that enough Ph.D.s will be produced automatically since the production of Ph.D. students is nowadays an inevitable by-product of the university education process.

The engineer produced from this type of program will be a hybrid between clinical engineering and some other specialty, such as electrical engineering. Other programs might appropriately be devised to produce what one might refer to as clinical (chemical) engineers, clinical (industrial) engineers, or clinical (mechanical) engineers. Since the role of clinical engineers is in service rather than research, most of them will finish with the MS or BS degree.

Since the language and concept structure of medicine is very different from that of engineering, it is vital that the clinical engineering student obtain practical experience in the hospital. In Purdue University's clinical engineering program, there are four different ways of obtaining this hospital experience. The first is as a cooperative student in a program similar to conventional cooperative programs in which the student spends every alternate semester, including summers, working in a hospital or in an industry serving the hospital. With this system, the engineering student can complete his BS program in only 5 years, in addition to which he earns most or all of the money required for living expenses. The second method for obtaining practical experience is by means of summer jobs. The third technique, which we call an engineering internship, is a scheme in which the student spends 6 months just before or just after his graduation in a hospital position. The fourth technique for obtaining practical hospital experience is to work for several years as a technician. Although this procedure is not recommended for students who already know that they wish to attend college, retraining experienced hospital technicians into engineers may serve as a valuable way of avoiding the inevitable bottleneck to the production of clinical engineers caused by the shortage of engineering training positions in hospitals.

This bottleneck is a result of the fact that engineering students can only receive their practical hospital training under the supervision of hospital engineers who, although they need not necessarily have a degree, must at least have ample practical experience. Since there are not very many medical engineers in hospitals at the present time, the lack of available hospital training positions will inevitably act as a brake on the rapid expansion of medical engineers in somewhat the same manner as the lack of medical intern positions in teaching hospitals acts as a brake on any rapid increase in the number of physicians.

The curriculum of the clinical (electrical) engineer will be somewhat different from that of either the conventional electrical engineer or the bioengineer. In addition to the basic electrical engineering courses, the clinical engineer will require additional education in clinical chemistry and chemical analysis, statistics, physics of fluids, mechanical design, anatomy, physiology, biochemistry, and possibly industrial engineering and law. He will also need a certain amount of information on clinical medicine. To compress all this extra material into the 130 hours of a bachelor's degree is clearly impossible without dropping some of the electrical engineering topics presently taught. To economize the time of the student as much as possible, it is necessary to develop special control, computer, and field courses that are replete with medical and biological applications.

Since medicine is becoming more and more automated, there is a need for physicians who have an engineering undergraduate background. Curricula are therefore made available to the medical engineering students at Purdue that will allow them to fulfill the premedical requirements of chemistry, life sciences, etc. Students of this type, who plan to apply to medical school after their bachelor's degree, are not encouraged to spend time getting practical experience in the hospital since it is felt that they will have ample opportunity for this at a later stage in their education.

In conclusion, hospitals will only restructure themselves to set up clinical engineering positions when an ample supply of qualified and certified clinical engineers is available. Since it would be irresponsible to encourage students to specialize in this area until it is clear that a sufficient number of positions are available, it is felt that the university has the opportunity of breaking this impasse by training clinical engineering students who are equally qualified in one of the older engineering fields. These clinical (electrical) engineers will be motivated to move into whatever clinical engineering positions exist and will take up other positions in electrical engineering until other positions become available. The university can play a decisive role in the fastest possible creation of this important new profession. It is also pointed out that since opportunities for the practical training of clinical engineers are limited by the rather small number of clinical engineers already practicing, the number of qualified clinical engineers can only grow slowly, so that no oversupply can be expected for many years.

9

THE CLINICAL ENGINEER AS AN INTERFACE

H. R. Weed

A report on industrial activity in biomedical engineering by the National Academy of Engineering Committee on the Interplay of engineering with biology and medicine listed four factors as dominant in the interaction of industry and the community with biomedical engineering: communication between those who must interact in the field; the nature of the marketplace; government involvement; and product efficacy and safety. The clinical engineer, emphasizing one important aspect of the general field of biomedical engineering, is directly and vitally involved with many of the specific elements of these four factors.

Communication Exchange

Meaningful communication is a two-way process involving mutual acceptance and understanding of concepts and abilities as well as identification of appropriate rolls before effective interaction between engineering and the medical profession or clinical engineering and industry can take place. The report further points out that the major element in support of this essential communication exchange is the development of a larger common ground of knowledge and understanding than found in the usual engineer–industry–life-science situation. This will require major alteration of the educational process for all those involved in health care—the engineer and the physician, the technician and nurse, the hospital administrator and the industrial manager. In short, each must be given opportunity to learn about the other, their needs, abilities, and constraints. The interface of the biomedical–clinical engineer with industry as well as with medicine and health-care delivery must be a working, on-the-job experience combined with the theoretical educational background necessary to permit application of the latest advances of technology to the problems of the moment.

Both in his education and work situations, the engineer must be given opportunity to interact directly with the life or death problems and decisions of medicine, the make-a-profit or go-broke economics of industry, and the determined confidence of the theoretical engineer that a better way does exist. While pointing to the joint responsibility of engineering colleges, medical schools, industry, government, and the community to provide this interactive opportunity, the report emphasizes specifically the unused potential of large-scale educational programs to provide this vital hands-on experience along with a theoretical base.

The biomedical–clinical engineer must have direct practical, applied experience with both the health-care-delivery system and the industrial complex that produces the technology in order to carry on their part of the vital communication transfer between those who must interact in the biomedical–industrial field. No less important, industry and the health-care professional must have direct knowledge of and experience with the engineer and each other to carry on their part of the three-way communication exchange.

The Biomedical Engineering Marketplace

The nature of the marketplace involves a realization and understanding of how industry operates and how it must utilize and optimize its capabilities and assets. The biomedical–clinical engineer must operate between the real work of mass production, practical capability, and cost and the idealistic hopes of the medical world that some technology dropout can develop his earth-shaking but absolutely dependable technological advance in his garage over the weekend.

Thus again, the clinical engineer, along with the industrialist and the health-care community, must come to know enough of each other's problems and, in particular, the need for a viable, predictable market in order for industry to devote major capital and manpower assets to the development of a practical and dependable product. Experience again seems to be the best teacher and should be a part of the educational process.

Government Involvement

The biomedical–clinical engineer must have direct practical, applied experience ernment patent problems, possible technology transfer possibilities from government agencies, as well as the many other involvements of government in the support and direction of the development of a new field such as biomedical engineering. His interaction with the government biomedical engineering community must be as carefully planned as that with industry or health-care practitioners.

Product Safety

Whether it is called safety, consumer protection, or product efficacy, the biomedical–clinical engineer will be at the interface between industry, the health-care delivery system, and government protection agencies. As the complexity of health-care instrumentation increases, it is quite likely that the biomedical–clinical engineer will be given direct responsibility for the safety and proper functioning of medical instruments. The medical practitioner will no longer be able nor wish to take personal responsibility for every piece of mechanical and electronic gear used in health care. The heart pacer installation will be the responsibility of the surgeon, but its functioning, insensitiveness to stray signals, life expectancy, and leakage currents will be the joint responsibility of industry and the biomedical–clinical engineer.

The Biomedical–Clinical Engineer

The biomedical–clinical engineer, both in his education and practice, must interact directly with the health-care community and the industrial-research-development organizations. His training and experience must reflect the practical world of economics, personal preference and credibility, as well as engineering theory, medical physiology, and qualified teaching.

The training and work experience of the biomedical–clinical engineer must be carefully planned and implemented. Most important, perhaps, is the recognition that these interface actions must take place both during the educational phase and during the after degree working period of the clinical engineer. He must be a practical, design-development engineer with experience and capability in meeting real work problems rather than the more common research-biophysics type of biomedical engineer.

NAE Recommendations

Several of the NAE recommendations relate directly to the biomedical–clinical engineer interface with industry and the community. These include the following:

> Involve industry in the formulation of biomedical engineering problems admitting to technological solutions, stimulate means of attacking important problems not currently being pursued, foster adequate protection of industrial investments in research and development, and provide for uniform clinical evaluation procedures and facilities.
>
> Identify more precisely the appropriate role of engineering in the life sciences and investigate the means of providing engineers specifically for this role.
>
> Involve industry at the earliest stages of prototype design, be able to issue exclusive, finite term licenses for production when required, and be able to subsidize needed production when the market potential is too limited for profits to be realized.

Encourage industrial organizations to provide systems engineering, logistical studies, failure analyses, patent and material flow studies, and so on for the health care delivery system.

Require realistic engineering involvement in government grants and contracts. Allowing engineers a greater opportunity to serve as principal investigators (in lieu of medical researchers) would be consistent with this objective.

In addition to maintaining the current Ph.D. training programs, support university trainee programs for design- and product-oriented biomedical engineers at the B.S. and M.Sc. levels.

Provide for engineering internships of NIH and other medical centers (both government and civilian) for practicing engineers from industry and for participants in the biomedical engineering programs of universities.

Provide for internships in industry to better identify the value and deficiencies of biomedical engineers in industrial situations.

Develop closer relationships between industry and the medical profession during the specification of product needs by expanded use of medical consultants in industry and collaborative industry-hospital and industry-clinical programs.

Create greater employment opportunities within industry to permit the demonstration by competent biomedical engineers of the contributions that they can provide.

Recognize the uniqueness of the biomedical engineering marketplace and develop the specific managerial techniques and personnel required to operate effectively within it.

Develop means to properly train the users of biomedical engineering instruments and provide for adequate maintenance, calibration, and repair services.

Whether considered in detail or in overview, the message is the same—cooperation and interaction. The biomedical–clinical engineer will be the critical link in this exchange and must be trained and have experience in the real work of engineering design and problem solving, the real world of industry economics, and the practical day-to-day delivery of health care. Whether this is viewed as a new type of engineer, the clinical engineer, or a rational objective of biomedical engineering that does real work on real problems with real money for real results is not terribly important.

Biomedical–Clinical Engineering University Programs

Several educational facilities across the country are attempting to develop or redirect their biomedical engineering program toward this practical, experience, work-on-real-problems type of curriculum. Some early programs with major emphasis on the Ph.D.–research–biophysics type of curriculum find this direction sufficiently incompatible to suggest a new name as necessary, admitting their inability to include the original problem-solving, real-world engineer in their present version. Industry, government, and now the health-care system are finding the practical do-a-job engineer more and more desirable compared to the mathematical theorist. While the research-idealist is vital to our continued national technological advance, somewhere we must have some braves and not all chiefs.

A number of schools, including Ohio State's Biomedical Engineering Center, are attempting to provide this practical, experience-oriented background as a part of a broad general program of biomedical engineering. While a few Ph.D. graduates from Ohio State would qualify as research-biophysics-type scientists, the majority are practically oriented with up to several years experience in real health-care problem solving and technology application. Essentially, no Ph.D. or MS is granted his degree without having had one to several years experience working directly with medical practitioners in clinic and hospital situations, life-science researchers wanting results from their technology, industrial-development organizations, or research-development groups.

The Ohio program possibilities can be viewed as a model and include

1. Biomedical option of 10–20% in BS curricula of electrical, mechanical, aeronautical, chemical, ceramic, industrial, agricultural engineering, and computer science
2. Premed in engineering–a 4-year BS leading to vet school, dentistry, or medical school entrance with 10–20% biomedical option
3. Biomedical option of 20–50% in MS and Ph.D. in electrical, aeronautical, mechanical, chemical, ceramic, industrial, agricultural engineering, biophysics, and physiology
4. Combined M.D.-Ph.D. programs between engineering and medicine
5. Engineering programs for majors in physiology, biophysics, pharmacology, veterinary medicine, dentistry, or other life-science areas
6. Specialized technological programs in allied medical professions for the highly trained medical equipment specialist.

At all levels, the emphasis is to provide competence in the basic field and experiences at the interface in solving real problems.

The program is broadened and supported to include the industrial-community health-research-development aspects by ties with many community facilities:

1. COBECC—The Central Ohio Biomedical Engineering Community Council, with over 100 members representing community hospitals, industry, research-development organizations, physicians, professional engineers, and educators
2. Battelle Memorial Institute, providing employment and experience support for students and close support of COBECC
3. Workshops, seminars, and special problem situations for engineers and life scientists, students and professionals at Children's, Riverside, Mt. Carmel, and University Hospitals
4. Industrial support of students, providing financial and experience situations such as Western Electric, Bell Laboratories, Industrial Nucleonics, Sensotec, Dytronics, and others
5. Facilities, experience, and student support by Aeromed Laboratory, Wright Patterson Air Force Base, coordinated with the part-time OSU graduate programs using closed-circuit television and live class presentations

These and other facilities serve to provide the breadth and experience of the extensive and varied OSU Biomedical Engineering Center program, involving over 90 faculty from 20 departments and 7 colleges and over 135 students working on projects and programs totaling more than $600,000 per year. These include such programs as: Cardiovascular-Clinical Research Division of University Hospital; Spinal Shock Treatment Center; Center for Education of the Handicapped; Hospital Safety Programs; Prosthetic Rehabilitation Center; Vestibular Research–Anatomy; Speech Therapy for Hearing Handicapped–State School for the Deaf; Simulation Studies; Physiological Blood and Respiratory Flow Studies; Institute of Vision; Neurological-Biophysics Research; Cell Membrane Studies; Cerebrovisceral Physiology Simulation and Data Analysis; Heart Pacer Function Tester; Cardiac Catheter Development; Agricultural Animal Growth; and Hospital Data Analysis.

The lessons learned in the operating room or cardiac catheter laboratory may be much more meaningful than the blackboard tracings of conventional education. The OSU graduate is an experienced practitioner—a true biomedical–clinical engineer at his respective level with explicit and meaningful experience at the interface.

The clinical engineer, perhaps even more than in other engineering applications, must be trained to interact directly and productively with the industrial–life-science community with which he will work. While the engineering industry is well known for its ability to concentrate on the practical problems of putting ideas into production, there is the haunting question of whether or not the present type of engineering college graduate, particularly the graduate MS and Ph.D., are optimally trained or motivated for such positions. Perhaps even more critically, the work of the biomedical–clinical engineer involves both industry and the practical life-science clinician, who is primarily interested in results, performance, and dependability. The emphasis on Ph.D. research-oriented biomedical engineers has been largely the result of theoretical university professors and directed government agency support. While perhaps justified during the development period of university faculties in this new field, the marketability of the graduates to industry was at best inaccurately estimated.

The present emphasis, whether through new programs such as clinical engineering or by biomedical engineering curricula with design-development objectives, is toward an engineer with cooperative industry-health interaction during both his training and practice.

10

CLINICAL ENGINEERING INTERNSHIPS

H. Laufman

It has become apparent that one weak link in the chain of training and useful employment of clinical engineers can be unavailability of a period of training in the hospital environment. Another is the lack of a specific job definition. Although the need for clinical engineers in hospitals is beginning to be felt, their precise roles are ill-defined, and there is therefore, little or no budgetary provision for the clinical engineer in the hospital. When or if a clinical engineer is hired, he must come to the hospital with medical background or hospital training. He cannot fulfill his potential until he acquires a certain amount of on-the-job training.

Communication barriers between medical and engineering personnel are well known. These barriers tend to disappear as experience is gained by both physician and engineer working together. Thus, internship for engineers will not only accomplish this goal but will prepare engineers for participation in other important health-care goals, such as improvement of the quality of patient care in hospitals of all sizes and types, improvement of hospital safety, and improvement of efficiency and economy of procedural activities in virtually all departments of a hospital, from primary care to administration.

Biomedical and clinical engineering requires the expertise of various engineering and scientific disciplines, such as chemical, electrical, electronic, engineering; mechanical engineering; systems engineering, operations research, managerial science; computer science; biostatistics, data processing, and materials science.

Modern medical practice provides many areas in which the engineer can find a place to suit his own particular interests; all of these fields can be explored during his internship. If he settles on a chosen field early in his internship, he would benefit from exposure to other clinical fields, nonetheless. Thus, the clinical engineering internship serves essentially the same purpose as a clinical internship does for medical school graduates, that of acquainting them with patient care and hospital practices and preparing them for their future professional work.

The need to encourage more engineers to enter the "field" is paramount. Hospital exposure is indispensable to the proper training of bioengineers or biomedical equipment technicians (BMETs). From the standpoint of the hospital, their training represents an additional load and expense initially, but experience has shown that this liability is converted into an asset because of the technology and training the clinical bioengineering student brings to the hospital.

At the technician level, there is an entirely different approach to the education and job description for BMETs as opposed to engineers. Technicians are necessary and essential to the running of a hospital but must not be confused with the qualifications or the job description of the engineers. The clinical engineers in the hospital setting are to be considered coprofessionals with physicians and nurses, whereas the technicians serve an important but separate role of providing technical aid to the professional staff.

By the time a clinical engineering intern reaches the hospital, he will have completed at least a baccalaureate program or its equivalent in engineering and perhaps one of the biological sciences. The BMET will have completed a course of study at an appropriate technical school or its equivalent. Some are run by industry, others by private as well as the military in the United States.

The development of a training program for clinical bioengineers and BMETs at a hospital requires an examination of what the hospital can and should supply. The program should provide an exposure to real problems and their solutions, a laboratory environment to develop concepts, and training for those who will apply these concepts. The hospital is not well equipped, however, to deliver basic fundamental education in the physical and biological sciences along with the ancillary education necessary to the engineer or BMET. This role should be left to a cooperating school or university.

The school or university, conversely, cannot supply the practical laboratory environment needed for proper training. It is obvious that a cooperative program between hospital and school is the best arrangement for training engineers or BMETs. It is readily apparent that hospital-based training or background is a *sine qua non* to qualifying for certification either as a professional clinical engineer or as a BMET.

As an intern, the clinical engineer is assigned to one or more clinical departments, in which he becomes acquainted with various facets of patient care (blood bank, cardiac catheterization laboratory, clinical cardiology, bacteriology department, radiology department, operating room, special-care units, anesthesiology, and rehabilitation). He may become involved in a project in a particular department but must rotate through all other departments. He should attend seminars and lectures to broaden his medical base.

Counseling during the internship is a joint responsibility of the chiefs of the clinical departments concerned, as well as the heads of the concerned university. Periodic meetings among all clinical engineering interns and advisers must be held for the purpose of reporting on work in progress, discussion of problems of common interest, and reports of specialty meetings.

Examples of hospital departments in which clinical engineers require training and exert an important influence on the quality of medical care are given below under various departmental headings. The roles of the engineer in the hospital setting seem to be divisible into four main headings, all applicable to direct patient care:

1. Problem-solving
2. Application of technology
3. Analysis of information
4. Methodologic advances

Engineering in Immunohematology

Blood Bank

Engineers have participated in the introduction of new principles of detecting red-cell antibody reactions. This method provides far greater sensitivity in the detection of antibodies that may exist in the recipient's blood. As a result, many recipients of blood transfusion in whom previous techniques failed to detect antibodies may now be successfully transfused after rapid automatic detection of red-cell antibodies.

Study on Autoimmune Diseases

The automated techniques developed in the laboratory have been applied extensively to the study of autoimmunologic diseases. Data obtained thus far indicate that it is now possible, in a significant number of cases, to make positive diagnoses, determine the etiology of the disease and prognosis of the disorder, and, finally, obtain guidelines for therapy solely by analysis of information obtained from study of red-cell immunology characteristics.

The immunology laboratory can provide continuous consultation to all physicians who treat patients with these immunologic diseases.

Cardiac ICU

Preventive maintenance programs for the testing of new equipment, the organization of specifications, and other duties aimed toward device safety and electrical and mechanical hazard prevention can be under the direction of the clinical engineer and BMETs. The clinical engineer in charge is more knowledgeable than the medical resident or the nurse about evaluation of patient-monitoring devices and their operation. The clinical engineer instructs residents and nurses in the use of equipment. In turn, he has been taught to screen chest X-rays, clinical electrocardiograms, and to understand diagnosis.

Pacemaker Clinic

A clinical engineer is a consultant to the pacemaker clinic and on call for any problem in interpretation of electronic data used and measured in following the battery depletion of patients with artificial-heart pacemakers or in diagnosing electrode malfunction. Patient data collection is conducted by practical nurses or operating-room (OR) technicians trained in the use of oscilloscopic instrumentation by the clinical engineer who monitors their performance, checks patients using such instrumentation, keeps their equipment standardized, and consults with them daily on problem patients. A clinical engineer is present during the operative procedure of any pacemaker insertion or pulse generator change of a nonroutine character or when problems are exhibited in order to perform the tests and advise the physician as to whether he is at a safe performance level for the patient.

Cardiac and Life-Support Systems

The entire concept of cardiac support is applied engineering. At some hospitals, laboratory research programs involve the construction and design of cardiac-assist equipment, including triggering from natural cardiac activity, determination of the optimum synchronization to spontaneous cardiac output, cardiac work parameters, intracardiac pressures, and epicardial and limb lead electrocardiograms.

The collection and analysis of these data and patient monitoring are, in themselves, major clinical engineering efforts requiring significant theoretical and practical input. A clinical engineer involved in the study of materials for fabrication of assistive devices and design and construction of drive units to achieve the maximum physiological benefit, as well as measurement, computerization, and analysis of cardiac-assist parameters.

Rehabilitation Medicine

The work of clinical engineers in rehabilitation medicine is spread over two broad areas: instrumentation and physiological research. Instrumentation in this field includes therapeutic devices such as limb prostheses and the entire area of orthotics. Several of these fields of activities include structural and fabrication improvements; measurement of forces such as weight bearing; application of external power; and application of control systems to powered devices such as myoelectric control. Engineers have made additional contributions with the paralyzed patient. This includes advances in electrical wheelchair controls, reading machines, television controls, etc., as well as improvements in hearing aids, talking devices for laryngectomies, and teaching devices for the deaf and dumb.

Ongoing research deals with cutaneous communication channels as a feedback path in myoelectric control devices, external chronic skeletal muscle stimulation as a motor nerve bypass, and application of correlation and averaging techniques for multichannel electromyographic analysis.

Measuring physiological work in ambulatory patients and developing telemetric and other monitoring techniques require engineering input in many phases, such as continued improvements in the measurement of oxygen consumption, electrocardiographic recordings, cardiac work, blood pressure, heat production, and respiration in various tasks of ambulatory patients. New instrumentation includes such devices as electrical impedance plethysmography to measure cardiac contractility, and devices to correlate bodily functions, such as heat production, oxygen consumption, and cardiac stress, require engineering background for full utilization capability.

Surgical Studies

The evaluation of technological advances relating to the delivery of hospital care and derivation of the most meaningful advances in the design of surgical-care facilities involve the collaborative efforts of architects, environmental engineers, bioengineers, clinical investigators, basic scientists, and specialists in allied fields. Other collaborative activities include new product research and development, clinical testing cost analysis of systems and products, conceptual design of facilities, and architectural and engineering requirements of surgical facilities and equipment. Some of the projects include the design and performance specifications for new surgical centers, concepts and products in surgical illumination, materials handling, and air conditioning. Some other projects include working in collaboration with other research groups.

One particular hospital has a prototype OR which was designed for surgical studies. This OR was added to the surgical suite and, since its addition, has carried on a regular schedule of surgical operations, especially open-heart surgery. The room is unique in that it is equipped with a variety of modular and trial systems such as illumination, air systems, surface materials, cabinetry, etc. A broad array of tests are constantly being carried out in the fields of microbiology, visual task evaluation, air-movement physics, cleaning methods, electronic monitoring, and materials research engineers who serve the internship at this hospital are deployed to work in various facets of the activities.

Applied Biomedical Engineering

Bioelectronics and biomechanical laboratories serve as a "home base" of bioengineers who are not engaged in a specific department of a hospital. Here, models are built, and equipment is tested and rebuilt.

Among the devices built in prototype or model form in these laboratories are cardiac-assist devices, electrical and electronic safety testing equipment, and advanced monitoring systems of several types. These laboratories prove invaluable to interns in clinical engineering.

The Manpower Market for Clinical Engineering

Concern has been voiced repeatedly as to whether the job market for clinical engineers is broad enough to absorb an annual crop of trained clinical bioengineers. One of the chief reasons for this position is the lack of a clear definition of exactly what the clinically trained engineer can offer. Up to this point, a bioengineer has been typically an engineer who has found employment or interest in a biologically oriented field. Rarely has an engineer with specific health-care training been available for employment. It is not a simple matter to convert an engineer into a clinical engineer. He must undergo a period of retraining in the health-care field within a health-care institution in order to appreciate the requirements and the scope of the field and its many subspecialties. Internships exist that serve not only to provide in-hospital training for bioengineers but should serve to define better the field of clinical engineering and clarify job definitions in the hospital.

Hospital Employment for Clinical Engineers

Of the approximately 7000 hospitals in the United States, about 700 have a capacity of 300 or more beds. Another 600 hospitals have over 200 beds. Hopefully, every hospital over 200 beds (1300 hospitals) will ultimately employ at least one clinical engineer. Larger hospitals, specialty hospitals, and university centers will undoubtedly employ more. Several such institutions already have formal departments with up to 15 clinical engineers, in addition to the bioengineers already working in specific clinical departments.

Many hospital administrators still look on an engineer as one whose activities are confined to electrical safety. Once clinical engineers with actual hospital training in a large number of clinical-care fields as well as in hospital administration itself become available, their contributions to efficient, economical, and safe health-care delivery will set a precedent. It is in the broad area of health-care delivery that many of the acute needs lie today. Therefore, it is appropriate to examine the role of the clinical engineer in these areas in more detail.

The clinical engineer is equipped to bring the technologies of the physical sciences to bear on the problems of health-care delivery. These problems are multiple; however, one of the most significant problems deals with the logistics and communication of making a hospital run more efficiently at less cost, with the delivery of better care to more people. That the expenses are so high and the services relatively poor in these areas are indications that traditional approaches are inadequate. The clinical engineer, who has a background in operations research and man–machine interface, is ideally qualified to help solve some of these problems.

He is ideal because he serves as the necessary interface between the administration, which has insufficient knowledge of operations research, and the systems engineer, who needs to know something about the nuances of hospital operations and patient care. Indeed, a good point can be made that the hospital administrator of the future will have a clinical engineer assistant.

In the interface of man and machine, there is a need for clinical engineers and BMETs at all levels. Machines are indispensable to good medical care and will become more so in the future. Proper selection and application of these machines requires the engineer. Proper maintenance and operation of these machines requires the BMET. These needs are particularly obvious today in the OR and ICU but will extend (even more than at present) throughout the hospital in the future. If computers are to be used to serve the hospital, their proper care and feeding will rest with the clinical engineer, but, more importantly, the man–machine interface with the patient, medical staff, and administration will require the participation of the clinical engineer.

There is good reason to expect that the clinical bioengineer will become a member of the medical team involved in the diagnostic and therapeutic aspects of patient care. Sophistication in data acquisition and processing will open new vistas in medical care. An appreciation of the dynamics of physiological systems and their relationship to external control systems, especially when the concept of closed-loop control is instituted, will demand of the physician a technological competence he is not likely to acquire soon or maintain long. Good care requires a team approach. A clinical engineer will be a part of that team.

Inappropriate use is often made of doctors and nurses, who spend time better devoted to other activities than on performing tasks that could be done by others or automated systems. The concept of the paramedic properly trained to relieve doctors and nurses of some of these unnecessary activities has become very popular in recent times and appropriately so.

Industry Employment of Engineers

There is evidence to support the contention that industry prefers to hire hospital trained engineers over those without a hospital background. The real value of this type of background to many types of industrial organizations is realized in the more pragmatic approach to research and development and a greater realization of clinical problems by hospital-trained engineers. This value is eventually reflected in financial gain to the company not only in terms of actual sales but in savings on on-the-job training and more rapid solution of conceptual problems. Clinical engineering input is required in all types of hospital hazard control, solid-waste handling, food service, air control, maintenance, and repair. A well-defined clinical engineering internship would provide exposure to practical problems in most of the fields.

In short, as technology develops in virtually every facet of the health-service field, both in and out of the hospital, the need for the expertise of the clinical engineer is readily apparent. Therefore, the future demand for clinical bioengineers in the medical-care and device market may be anticipated with much optimism.

Internships for clinical engineers in suitable hospitals will help in the delineation of these markets. Having served an internship, clinical engineers will find job opportunities in hospitals as well as industry.

11

INTERDISCIPLINARY EDUCATION

P. Klatell and I. M. Meth

The major objectives of interdisciplinary programs should be

1. To formulate and implement an interdisciplinary educational framework to be used for teaching varied groups at undergraduate levels such as nursing, engineering, and the basic sciences the principles and applications of technology used in the delivery of health care
2. To introduce students to the patient-care environment as well as the interdisciplinary team approach necessary for the delivery of health care. This can be accomplished by providing laboratory experience. The laboratory should simulate the hospital patient-care area equipped with current biomedical instrumentation as well as mannequins to simulate human physiological signals
3. To establish a series of continuing education offerings for graduate levels such as registered nurses and engineers to assist them in maintaining a workable level of knowledge of contemporary health-care technology
4. To offer a series of interdisciplinary lectures for the faculty on current topics related to health-care technology

Since World War II, there have been marked advances in the development of biomedical instrumentation and technology. These changes are clearly reflected in the sophistication of monitoring devices and other instrumentation currently in use in hospitals and clinical laboratories. However, across the country, the introduction of technology into the health-care environment has been piecemeal, and the full effectiveness of improvement of health care has not been realized. In addition, the response of health professionals to these innovations has been haphazard, with little anticipation of the educational needs created by the new technology.

What happens to the deliverer and to the recipient of health-care services when they are surrounded by technology? Clearly, machines and technology are not a replacement for people. Rather, their impact is in the change they generate, in the kind of jobs that must be done, and in the knowledge base required to function in this new environment. Nursing and engineering educators have tended to react to change rather than to anticipate and plan innovatively. Unless constructive action is undertaken by the educational institutions responsible for the training and development of health-care professionals and technicians, confusion and obsolescence will permeate the academic and service fields.

It can be stated that nursing students do not understand and consequently fear the technology they are expected to use in the delivery of health care and that engineering and technology students are not aware of the functions of biomedical instrumentation in the health-care environment.

The focus of part of the education required must then be to provide hands-on laboratory experience in the use of oscilloscopes and chart recorders for nursing students in conjunction with their clinical work. The focus must also be to introduce technology students to the hospital environment and the biomedical instrumentation in common use.

To formulate the academic framework, multidisciplinary seminars on "Technology and Its Implications for Health Care" are a good first step.

As a result of these seminars, a working committee can be organized to formulate the program in health-care technology, ranging from undergraduate through postbaccalaureate instruction. For the initial effort, an interdisciplinary laboratory-oriented undergraduate course for nursing, engineering, and science students is needed. A modern health-care technology laboratory, designed to simulate a hospital environment and equipped with mannequins and other equipment to simulate human physiological parameters, appears to be a fundamental need of such programs. The laboratory should contain three major sections: a simulated hospital environment, including a critical-care area and a central nursing station; a basic introductory instrumentation section; and a shielded section for housing nuclear medicine and X-ray studies.

Program Components

Course Offerings for Undergraduate and Graduate Students

"An Introduction to Health-Care Technology" should be offered to undergraduate nursing, engineering, and basic-science students for the second consecutive semester. A second undergraduate course, "Bioengineering Systems for Patient Care," can be offered as a follow-up.

Continuing Education Courses for Professional Nurses and Engineers

The content of the introductory courses as well as the laboratory facility should offer the opportunity to provide knowledge of contemporary health-care technology to professional nurses and engineers already in practice.

Faculty Seminars on Selected Topics in Health-Care Technology.

Development of the field of health-care technology has been so recent and rapid that is is generally necessary to offer a seminar series to the faculty each year on selected topics in health-care technology.

Preparation of Audiovisual Material

Illustration of the principles and applications of biomedical instrumentation by the use of tools such as video tape to demonstrate the difference between volume and pressure ventilators and their application in respiratory care, etc., should be taught. There must be an evaluation of students' competence in the use of health-care technology through their response to a situation as shown on videotape. There exists a vast potential use for these tools for both course testing and evaluation of professional practitioner competency.

Interdisciplinary research

The laboratory facility offers the ideal environment for research, encompassing a broad spectrum of disciplines, to study not only aspects of health-care technology and human reactions to health-care technology but also the short-term and long-range effectiveness of this type of multidisciplinary program on different groups of students.

Introduction to Health-Care Technology

To illustrate the interdisciplinary aspect of the required program, as well as the course content covered, the following is a description of an introductory course:

The basic course should teach the principles underlying the most commonly used biomedical instrumentation and illustrate the commonalities between various types of equipment. It should foster an interdisciplinary team approach for the solution of health-care problems by providing practice in an environment that illustrates the multidisciplinary aspects of health-care technology.

All teaching and instruction should be conducted by a team of engineering and health-care faculty. Laboratory sections should be divided into groups consisting of students from a number of different disciplines. All major pieces of laboratory equipment illustrate applications of technology for solving health-care problems.

A laboratory outline is shown in Table I. It illustrates the multidisciplinary development of the subject by a mixture of topics from various disciplines. Equipment that is impractical to house or unable to be simulated in our laboratory can be demonstrated on field trips to local medical centers.

TABLE I
Developmental Aspects

Experiment	Topic
1.	Review of background material (anatomy, physiology, electrical circuits)
2.	Field trip 1: hospital patient-care unit, including critical-care areas
3.	Measurement of vital signs: physiographs, sphygmomanometers, digital thermometers, pulse-rate meters, plethysmographs
4.	Spirometry: measurement of respiratory volume and the use of ventilators
5.	Cardiopulmonary resuscitation
6.	Oscilloscopes, physiological and patient monitors, chart recorders
7.	Cardiac pacemakers and defibrillators
8.	A simulated coronary-care unit in operation
9.	Field trip 2: extracorporeal circulation: heart-lung machines, artificial lungs, hemodialysis machines
10.	Pumps and drainage systems
11.	Electrical safety: macro- and microshock hazards
12.	Ultrasonics
13.	Field trip 3: nuclear medicine and X-rays

Description of Laboratory

A health-care technology laboratory can be a unique educational facility designed to simulate accurately the clinical environment and technological complexity of a unit such as an ICU typically found in a hospital.

The immediate use of a multifunction laboratory is to educate nursing, engineering, technology, and science students in the general operating principles and use of the electronic and mechanical instrumentation involved in patient care. The laboratory can also be used to update professional nursing skills or to train paramedical personnel. The laboratory can also be used as a research and development complex for investigations in biomedical and clinical engineering and for nursing research.

A laboratory can occupy a floor space of approximately 3000 square feet and be divided into three sections. The largest subsection should be designed to simulate the spatial atmosphere of an actual ICU. Hospital beds, furniture, lighting, flooring, service connections for vacuum, oxygen, electrical power, and other bedside facilities will be grouped to form four patient-care islands. A nurse's station and storage area, consistent with accepted hospital architecture, should be located adjacent to the bed areas. Development of a monitoring station should be planned for.

The basic objective in the design of the simulated patient-care complex will be to reproduce, as closely as possible, the spatial, technological, and psychological environment perceived by both the patient and the clinical worker. The latter is an important component for accurately simulating the atmosphere of apprehension experienced by critically ill ICU patients. This is especially so when they are surrounded by and connected to a variety of strange and incomprehensible equipment that emits sound and light in an already frightening environment.

The laboratory must be equipped with a wide spectrum of monitoring, diagnostic, and therapeutic medical equipment as well as physiological simulators and mannequins to simulate the hospital setting. The equipment inventory should include dual-channel patient monitors, blood-pressure transducers, ECG recorders, external and implantable pacemakers, defibrillators, stethoscopes, sphygmomanometers, Bird respirators, spirometers, ultrasound monitors, electronic thermometers, drainage and infusion pumps, syringe pumps, and a fully equipped crash cart. The beds can be occupied by mannequins such as the Recording Resusci Anni with a cardiac simulator or the arrhythmia Torso Trainer (with tape player system for generating cardiac rhythms).

The second subsection of the laboratory can be developed as a conventional classroom-laboratory for equipment demonstration and instruction. This section can be furnished with electrical laboratory benches and equipped with basic oscilloscopes, chart recorders, analogue and digital electrical meters, pressure gauges and manometers, physiographs with a full complement of biological transducers, cannister-type spirometers, and a full complement of leakage meters, ground quality testers, receptacle analyzers, and hospital safety inspection kits.

The third and smallest section should be shielded and intended for the nuclear medicine, X-ray, and ultrasonic scanning instrumentation. The teaching module must all focus on the fundamentals of electrical safety.

12

TRAINING OF BIOMEDICAL EQUIPMENT TECHNICIANS (BMETS)

J. K. Cywinski, P. DeSalvo, and R. Reder

There is a need to provide upward career mobility for persons employed in medical engineering. The specific objectives are to broaden the BMET's knowledge in the theory of operation, the underlying medical principles, and the practical and safe clinical applications of biomedical equipment.

A program to accomplish the above objectives could consist of four sections to include

1. Background program
2. Practice workshop
3. Rotating internship
4. Examination

A model for such a program has been developed at the Massachusetts General Hospital (MGH) in Boston.

Background Program Section

This section of the program is to prepare the student to understand the practice workshops and to provide the necessary basic academic background in mathematics, mechanics, electronics, and medicine to allow the individual to function in a BMET capacity.

The background section is based mainly on the courses and curricula available outside of a medical engineering department in the institutions of academic training. This academic training at MGH provides a total of 48 quarter hours (Q.H.) of formal college credit. It is felt that this is adequate to form a solid foundation for a BMET to operate in this field. When coupled with the other sections of the program, it will produce highly trained BMETs capable of working on a broad range of hospital equipment. Furthermore, the accumulated credits can and will be used by some participants toward obtaining higher academic degrees (BS). The section consists of four categories:

Mathematics

Consists of algebra, trigonometry, and calculus and provides 14 Q.H. of college credit. It will enable a BMET to handle the majority of math-related problems to be encountered in further studies or activities as a BMET.

Mechanical

Provides 6 Q.H. of college credit and enables a BMET to develop a basic understanding of mechanical problems in terms of properties of material, theories of stress and failure, lubrication, and mechanical power transmission.

Electronics

Provides 20 Q.H. of college credit. It is designed to look at electronics from a functional level and will, with workshop sessions, enable the student to become adept at circuit analysis and circuit trouble-shooting.

Medical

Provides a general overview of hospital operation, allowing the student to understand and be able to communicate effectively with the hospital staff. It will also build the vocabulary required to understand problems and to offer meaningful help (8 college credits).

Practice Workshop Section

An introduction to the hospital environment and biomedical equipment practice is an integral part of BMET education in order to bridge the gap between theoretical studies and actual performance. A series of workshops can provide this introduction organized to cover the two basic fields.

The first type of workshop should familiarize the student with the physical and sociological structure of the hospital and the type of patient care offered by various specialty areas. For example, familiarization with the OR can consist of a lecture on the history of surgery and anesthesia, a description of the OR team and the asks that each member performs, peculiar environmental problems, such as maintaining a sterile field and handling flammable anesthetic agents, and a walk-around tour of the OR, which should be conducted by the OR staff.

The second type of workshop can consist of a detailed familiarization with the actual equipment. These equipment workshops can consist of three parts: the theory behind the operation of the instrument, the normal operating characteristics of the instrument, and maintenance procedures and trouble-shooting techniques. These workshops give the BMET trainee background in the underlying medical engineering principles and practical and safe clinical use of the equipment and impart knowledge of the normal functioning of the equipment to the extent that the abnormal functioning can be readily recognized. Finally, the trainee must gain knowledge of the preventive maintenance procedures and of general principles as well as of particular cases of trouble-shooting and repair procedures. The list of workshops at MGH is given in Table II.

Rotating Internship Section

The purpose of an internship is to allow students to apply their knowledge in a practical way by working for two months in each of four different shops of a medical engineering department. The areas covered can include: instruments and anesthesia systems, cardiac monitors and life-support systems, general electronic instrumentation, mechanical systems, and fabrication.

TABLE II
Workshop Sequence and Subjects

1. Algebra review (1.5 sessions)
2. Plane geometry, trigonometry, and solid geometry (1.5 sessions)
3. Ohms law (1.5 sessions)
4. Electrical metrology (1.5 sessions)
5. Materials
6. Mechanical metrology, layout, sketches
7. Grinding, brazing, machining, soldering, tapping
8. Parts, fasteners, gears, pulleys, bearings
9. Electrical parts, schematics, circuits, electrical motors
10. Basic circuits, amplifiers, oscillators, etc.
11. Graphics (schematics, blueprints)
12. Hospital organization and function: MED organization and function; patient rights and hospital ethics
13. Sterilization techniques and purposes
14. Cardiovascular anatomy
15. Area orientation: Emergency, Ward, ICU, OR, Catheter Lab., etc. (4 sessions)
16. Hospital electrical power systems, fire safety (hospital's programs), NFPA standards
17. Preventive maintenance program, record keeping, and procedures
18. Corrective maintenance, trouble-shooting and repair, records and procedures
19. Cardiac pacemakers
20. Chart recorders
21. Fluid-injection pumps
22. Defibrillators
23. Electrosurgical instruments
24. Electrocardiography and ECG recorders
25. ECG monitors
26. Monitoring of blood pressure
27. Circulatory assist devices, intra-aortic balloon pumps
28. Analytic chemistry laboratory equipment
29. Mass spectrometers, spectrophotometers, pH meters
30. Anesthesia machines, ventilators
31. Respirators and respiratory therapy
32. Vacuum pumps, thermal blankets, centrifuges, balances
33. Review of radiation physics
34. Nuclear-medicine instruments and X-rays

Each participant must complete all three internships outside of the primary job responsibility.

Examination

The successful completion of previous sections constitutes the criteria for eligibility for examination. Successful completion means: (*a*) accumulation of at least 48 Q.H. academic credits at a qualified university; (*b*) attendance and passing grade on an intermediate test of at least 75% practice workshop sessions; and (*c*) completion of at least three 2-month internships, each in a field of specialization other than the individual's own. The examination, in turn, can have two parts: written, multiple-choice test and practical oral task to be performed in the presence of an educational committee.

PART III

ACCREDITATION

13

PROFESSIONAL ACCREDITATION

H. S. Bennett

In trying to arrive at an understanding of what a professional is, it is important to consider the matter from the viewpoint of the layman. From his viewpoint, the professional is someone who is to be admired and scorned at one and the same time, much like Freud's hate–love duality. This ambivalent feeling on the part of the layman can even be seen among world leaders. For example, George Clemenceau said: "War is too serious a matter to be entrusted to the military." However, at the same time, he was busily rewarding his generals with medals and other honors.

An anonymous report writer within the US General Accounting Office said, in commenting on the C5A Transport situation: "Contracts with incentive clauses are too important to be left to lawyers." So we see it is not just the anonymous John Doe or John Q. Public who must rely on the professional and nevertheless distrusts that which he cannot clearly understand.

However, when the public forsakes the role of blind acceptance and takes over control of professional matters, things can go awry in the opposite direction. For example, in Georgia, professional photographers were required to take Wassermann tests (and, of course, pass them, whatever passing means) before they could roam the streets with a camera. One could easily visualize a requirement for a township engineer who must vote properly to determine whether or not he is a competent engineer. We can, of course, go on with many other hypothetical as well as real or believable examples of control of professional activities strictly by nonprofessional standards.

Professional societies have therefore evolved a philosophy stating that because the profession springs from the exercise of the specialist's skills, which the public is not competent to judge but on which, nevertheless, a judgment must be made, this judgment should be exercised by the professional practitioner's peers in the field. As civilization gets more complicated, however, there tends to spring up an important segment of society, "the professional class," and sociologists have shown that such a tendency is being exhibited more and more, at least in highly industrialized Western civilizations. The activities of such a sociologically distinct class tends to extend into political and other nontechnical aspects of daily living. One must be careful to guard against peer-group control of an individual's actions when such are not germane to the practice of one's profession. Sometimes, even in professional matters, peer-group control fails miserably. For example, in the 1720s, the leaders for a cure of smallpox by means of inoculation were Cotton Mather and other clergy, whereas the leading opponents were physicians. An even more interesting aberration of the concept of professionalism occurs when two distinct sets of professionals claim jurisdiction over the same area, for example, the clinical psychologist and the psychiatrist.

The psychiatrist may say that the clinical psychologist who does not have an M.D. degree is not competent to administer to the ills of human beings, to which the psychologist retorts, "How dare the psychiatrist practice psychotherapy without a Ph.D. on his shingle." The practice of parochialism is not the exclusive property of John Q. Public but can extend into the sacred halls of professionalism as well.

Therefore, what is a professional? Among other things, he is a human being who suffers from many of the mental abberrations, prejudices, and neuroses common to our present-day society. However, a member of a learned profession does have certain distinguishing characteristics; among these are the need to accumulate a large number of "know-how" viewpoints and techniques before he can presume to be a qualified practitioner of his particular profession. Once he becomes a member of a profession, the professional is interested in maintaining a high quality of service to the recipients of his activities. He also nourishes a desire for continuing his education and maintaining his initial equipage at a continuing high level of relevance and modernity.

Professional Utilization

In discussing how a professional should be utilized, it is well to go back for a moment to gather historical perspective on this subject. This is instructive not only for the purpose of tracing the roots of the concept involved but also for instructing one in the pitfalls and disabilities of the professional concept. As in any case of historical current, there are many false starts, blind alleys, and circular routes through which the level of time flows. Being aware of these makes one abler to realize the failings and shortcomings of the modern, evolved concept of utilization of professional services.

In London, guildsmen had organized tight companies at least as early as the twelfth century. In more widely separated areas, one can trace the roots of the guild movement to somewhere in the fourteenth century when cities began to proliferate and the more skilled serfs escaped their vassalages and flocked to these new cities to apply their special skills.

The wax candlers, for example, protested to King Edward III in 1371: "There still is great scandal . . . because they have not Masters chosen of the said trade, and sworn before you, as other trades have, to oversee the defaults that are committed in their said trade, and to present them to the Mayor and Aldermen." Again in 1322, the armorers petitioned Edward II to grant them autonomy and monoply of their trade, with the result that it "was ordained for the common profit and assented to that from thenceforth arms made in the City for sale should be good and befitting according to the form which follows." Four armorers were appointed to "observe and supervise." Thus was established the first "professional" ethics committee. One of the most successful tactics for limiting the number of tradesmen was the establishment of overlong apprenticeship periods, the most common of which was the 7-year custom of the London guilds. The Bristol barber's guild sought aid in 1420, and for the next 140 years, Parliment acted in special cases until finally the Statute of Apprentices of 1562 prescribed the 7-year system for all "sciences, crafts, mysteries, or arts." Many unscrupulous guildsmen took on apprentices only to dismiss them shortly before the end of their training period. This malpractice was finally condemned by Queen Elizabeth in 1562. In fact, the Statute of Apprentices provided that the master be fined unless a justice of the peace gave prior consent to the dismissal, which had to be "for some reasonable and sufficient cause."

The United States devotes an impressive percentage of its gross national product to the training of professionals. In fact, the "knowledge industry" occupies the same key role in the present economy as the railroad industry did a hundred years ago, and the fashion is becoming evermore prevalent. For example, 83% of the graduating class at Harvard College in 1962 planned to do graduate work of some sort. At Yale, it was 74%.

As previously mentioned, to individuals, organizations, governments, or even to whole classes or groups of people and the public at large, the nature of the knowledge on which the advice and action are based is very often a mixture of both the practical and the theoretical. In other words, professionals profess that they know better than others the nature of certain matters, and they profess to know better than their clients what ails them or their affairs. From this flow many consequences. They claim the exclusive right to practice the arts that they profess to know and to give advice derived from their special lines of knowledge. This is the basis of the licensing and accreditation procedures both in the narrow sense of legal permission (by the state licensing boards) and in the broader sense that the public allows those in a profession the privilege of setting their own peer-group standards for an accreditation over and above the basic legal licensure.

This accreditation involves several subtle moral aspects. The professional asks that he be entrusted by the client, who is not a true judge of the value of the services he receives, and furthermore, that some problems and affairs of man are in such a state of disrepair that the best professional service and action will not always correct them. Thus, a central motto of all professionals may well be taken, *credat emptor,* in contrast to the well-known *caveat emptor*. This philosophy leads to the next proposition, namely, that only the professional man knows when his colleague makes a mistake. In other words, ethical or unethical conduct, information or misinformation, and ept or inept behavior are to be judged by the professional's peer group rather than by the public at large.

This kind of prerogative requires a relatively close solidarity to be maintained by the members of the profession, which in turn implies a deep and lifelong commitment to the practice of a particular profession. Peer-group regulation of professional activities cannot work properly in a profession whose members or membership are constantly in a state of flux. That is, "masters" of the calling are one day "in" and the next day "out" of the profession. The peer group must be relatively stable, and its standards must also be stable enough to permit initiates to plan a lifelong commitment. On the other hand, it must not be so "stable" as to cause stagnation.

Many of the institutions of a modern society depend on an adequate supply of professionals: people to plan and build water systems, communications, roads, and industrial plants, and people to train others to perform these self-same tasks. The sociologists have "entered the act" (in addition to their own private status as a profession) in the sense that they are studying the sociological phenomenology of the profession. The sociological definition of the profession limits itself so far as possible to the specifics of professional behavior, which differ from those of the nonprofessional. For example, concepts such as a like style of life, corporate solidarity, and socialization structures and processes, insofar as these differ significantly from those of the nonprofessional, would enter into the formal definition. There are three such essential attributes: (*a*) a high degree of generalized and systematic knowledge, primarily oriented to the community interest rather than to individual self-interest; (*b*) a high degree of self-control of behavior through codes of ethics via voluntary associations organized and operated by the specialists themselves; and (*c*) a system of rewards (monetary and honorary) that is primarily a set of symbols of work achievement and is thus an end in itself rather than the means to some end of individual self-interest.

What is the distinction between an "intern professional" and a "professional intern?" Besides being a play on words, it has a serious intent. It involves the concept of achieving true professional status only after a period of practice or internship in the field of one's choice. In other words, an "intern professional" is one who is preparing himself by actual practice to become a true professional. This is in contrast to the individual who, because he is not able to discern or because he is unwilling to work toward the professional goal, remains a "professional intern." The latter will always remain in a subordinate role—a dilettante, so to speak, in the professional field of his choice.

In the field of science and engineering, this institutionalization or professionalization concept has taken place essentially in the past 50 to 100 years and has been of the nature of a second scientific revolution. Its effect has been the fusion of rapidly maturing scientific and engineering disciplines with simultaneously maturing management and administration techniques and philosophies. The lone practitioner of science of the early nineteenth century, who neither had to worry about his peers nor, in some cases, be even aware of them, is a thing of the past. He must now fit into a relatively tight sociological structure involving peer-group relationships and controls.

While the use of the term "professional intern" is not recommended, the concept of a group of practitioners who are engaged in activities tangential to but concerned with the basic professional field in question is to be encouraged; and the present trend in engineering toward a 2-year (and even 4-year) course in engineering technology is an indicator of the popularity of this trend. The engineering sciences will still be emphasized in the basic 4-year engineering program, with the view that graduates from this program are proceeding along the professional engineering route, whereas graduates from the technological programs would be unlikely to proceed with graduate and other continuing education inherent in the true professional philosophy.

Relationship between a Professional Engineer and Management

The practice of the profession of engineering is rather unique among professions, at least in the following point. A relatively small percentage of engineers are self-employed. Most contribute their services on a salaried rather than a fee basis. This situation is inherent in the historical development of engineering. The first organized activity arose in connection with architecture, roads, waterways, bridges, fortifications, heating, and sanitation. Supporting these activities was a growing need for metals, hence the importance of mining with associated activities of pumping, hoists, ventilation, and purification and smelting of ores. In this role—namely, that of an engineer directly employed by a larger more diversified organization—we find engineering performed in the ancient world, particularly in Egypt. Also, at the height of the Roman civilization, there had developed the image of the professional engineer, perhaps best illustrated by Marcus Vitruvius, the famous architect and engineer. The slow transition from the Roman to the Western system was not wholly a "dark age." There was a steady advance in technology even during the medieval ages. As early as the fourteenth century, one can detect the birth and emergence of a Western technology. Lewis Mumford has suggested that technology evolved through three overlapping epochs: the "eotechnic phase," to about 1750, the "paleotechnic," to the period after World War I, and the present "neotechnic phase," from World War II until the present. The first phase he describes represents the first thrust by modern man toward control of his environment. Of course, Leonardo da Vinci (1452–1519) is the greatest exemplar of this period. Others in this period are Simon Stevin (1548–1620), who generalized his expertise with machinery into the beginnings of modern science, and, of course, Galileo (1564–1642), who may be called the founder of modern science. Even the origins of the English word "engineer" go back to this epoch. In the time of Edward III, in the fourteenth century, the officer who was responsible for firearms was referred to as "artilator" or "ingeniator." Also, the men who ran the ballista, a large crossbow missile launcher (sometimes called gins), were referred to as "engyners." The modern name *engineer* undoubtedly sprang from these origins.

It is now customary to think of engineering as the application of science to the fulfillment of human needs, but it is also important to remember that the early engineers played another important role: They made science respectable. They provided the transition from intuition to knowledge, facts, and data. For example, Simon Stevin, the early Dutch engineer, said, "A miracle is no miracle." In other words, in our physical world, all happenings are based on natural laws.

Even though many inventions of decisive importance, for example, the steam engine, belong to the eotechnic phase, the engineering profession as we know it was born out of the paleotechnic phase. In this period, a greater and greater dependency on the steam engine was born. JamesWatt and Matthew Bolton began one of the first modern enterprises in mechanical engineering. In fact, the spirit of the paleotechnic phase, with its great dependence on the steam engine, patent system, machine tools, and industrial organizations, may be said to be the "age of mechanical engineering." Of course, the later phases of this epoch saw the development of both chemical and electrical engineering and such new prime movers as the internal combustion engine, the steam turbine, and the diesel engine. Also, professional organizations and publications, together with formal educational programs in engineering and science, were developed during this epoch. In England, engineering societies having some of the characteristics and idealistic motivations of the Royal Society were begun. The first was the Society of Civil Engineers (later called the Smeatonian Society), which was organized in 1771. In 1818, the venerable Institution of Civil Engineers was organized in England.

In general, early Americans seemed to concentrate more on invention and amateur engineering than on the natural sciences. The greatest advance into technology and engineering was triggered by the Civil War; from then to World War I the engineer contributed fundamentally to the progress of the United States as a nation. During this paleotechnic phase, a detailed history of the steam engine, the railroad, the textile mill, and the iron ship could be written without more than a passing reference to the scientific work of the period. With the neotechnic phase, however, this is no longer so. The scientific method now rules engineering and far outweighs in importance the previously used empirical approach. However, it is interesting to note that with the advance of the large-scale computer, a new type of empiricism may be gaining a foothold. The need for closed-form quantitative expressions is diminishing, and a type of quantitative trial-and-error procedure is gaining importance.

A second characteristic of the neotechnic phase is the rise of theoretical and quantitative methods in biology and other life sciences. It is this trend that, when married to quantitative engineering approaches, has given us the field of biomedical engineering. As Lewis Mumford states, "The concepts of science . . . were now applied to every phase of human experience and every manifestation of life."

Thus, we see that throughout the development of the profession of engineering, the engineer has always worked as a specialist and as a part of the larger team, carrying out the mission of bringing the fruits of technology and science to our civilization. It is true that in the eotechnic phase the projects were less complex and involved smaller teams, so that in many cases it seemed as if the engineer were operating independently of the rest of the team; however, even then, the roots of the engineer-management relationship were already present. They became more evident in the paleotechnic phase, and, in our present neotechnic phase, there are very few engineering activities that allow the engineer to act independently of the rest of the team. For example, in 1960, when there were a total of 840,000 engineers in the United States, 77% were employed in industry, 7% in government, and only about 100,000 were either self-employed or were teachers of engineering. A large portion of these 100,000 were not ''independent'' operators; however, even if we attribute a nonmanagement orientation to all of these, we come up with approximately a nine-to-one ratio.

The position of the engineer in the overall industry team, however, is somewhat unique. Since the project team working on the engineering aspects of a problem is usually sizable, the professional engineer (i.e., the one with a minimum of 5 years of experience) is usually a supervisor or manager in his own right. Simultaneously, however, his engineering activities are part of a plant-wide or company-wide effort to produce an end product.

This dual role complicates the engineer-management relationship. In a broad sense, the engineers' activities govern in large measure major company policies. Thus, they are often considered to be a part of the management team. On the other hand, they are just one unit in a more complex project team and as such must submit to the same type of management controls as other employees.

For the engineer in particular, the ''dual-track'' philosophy of career development is important—especially in view of his often ambiguous role in management. The dual-track philosophy states that there are two ways for an engineer to advance in his career. One way is by becoming more and more involved in the management aspects of the company's activities. This track often leads away from the practice of engineering, or at least the kind of engineering that presumably attracted management to the individual being advanced along the track. The other track for advancement is for the engineer to become more expert in the practice of engineering. This may mean more specialized or more generalized, depending on the type of engineering involved. For example, systems engineering requires a more generalized background, whereas specialization in the design of megawatt electrical generators might well require a sharper focus on a particular aspect of engineering.

Examples of Professional Engineering Activity

At this point, it might be useful to illustrate the preceding generalizations concerning the practice of a profession by some examples taken from the general area of clinical engineering and man–machine interfacing problems in communications-systems engineering.

The hallmark of professionalism is the attitude of responsibility—a responsibility to the client to give him a competent and conscientious product or service. In many cases, the client may be looked on as the physician in charge of the activity to which clinical engineering services or instrumentation are contributing. In other situations, the client may be regarded as the patient himself. The latter situation may become more prevalent as the practice of preventive medicine becomes more widespread. While somewhere in the chain the physician is still the final contact with the patient, the acquisition of physiological data from the individual may involve such geographically distributed locations and timing as to make it impractical for the attending physician to participate directly. This would leave the technicians at a given testing location under the supervision of the professional clinical engineer in charge. Here, the responsibility of the clinical engineer would be not just to the physician receiving the data but also to the individual yielding the data.

Another interesting set of responsibilities occurs in the field of communications-systems engineering, in which the broad aim is to send a message originated by one human being to another human being, with the assistance of a whole conglomeration of machinery. One way of looking at this problem is that the engineer is only responsible for the inanimate portion of the entire communications link. This attitude, however, usually does not lead to the design of an optimum communications system. To be optimum, the system must consider that the message initiation is in the brain of the originator and that the destination of the message is the brain of the human receptor. Thus, the entire system has both animate and inanimate elements, along with the acompanying men/machine interfaces. The responsibility of the engineer, therefore, includes an understanding of the physiological aspects of the total system as well as the physics of the inanimate portions. Since a professional engineer is responsible for preparing himself to properly discharge his duties, he must learn a great deal about the functioning of a human being.

One illustration of this situation occurs in the cutaneous communications system. Here, instead of entering the animate portion of the system through the agency of sight or sound, we enter by the electrical of mechanical stimulation of the nerve endings in the skin of the receiver of the message. In this case, there is no physician to fall back on.

In considering this new way of crossing the man–machine interface at the receiver end of the communications link, many new problems face the engineer, who is primarily trained to consider inanimate circuits. The safety of the animate receptors is, of course, a primary concern. In this connection, it is not enough to seek the advice of the physician or physiologist. There are many aspects of the detailed electrical operation of the system that are not appreciated by the medically trained specialist.

A simple example of this concerns the electrodes to be used. At first glance, it would seem that the electrodes used to pick up the signals from the body (such as the

ECG and the EEG) would suffice to reverse the process. However, a closer engineering study of the problem reveals that the two processes are not reciprocal. The nerve endings to be stimulated (basically by a disturbance of their associated electric double layers) are not the sources of the signals picked up by ECG and EEG electrodes. It turns out, in this case, that a pin type of electrode is a much more efficient vehicle for providing the necessary electrical stimulation of the cutaneous nerve endings. Even the very concept of skin resistance or impedance as commonly used in lie-detection apparatus and other psychological testing methods (i.e., the GSR, galvanic skin response) is not a significant contributor to the overall impedance at the electrode skin interface. The GSR is primarily an indicator of the activity of the sweat glands on the surface of the skin, whereas the skin impedance factor in cutaneous communications includes both the surface effects and the electrochemical ionic conduction effects occurring in the stratum corneum, the epidermis, and even the derma sections of the skin. Here, therefore, it becomes the responsibility of the engineer to learn the details of electrical conduction within the human physiology before proceeding with the design of the system.

Another example from the communications field involves the modeling or characterization of the human production of intelligible sound. Here it is necessary to isolate those factors contributing to the "sameness" or intelligence conveyed by the sounds coming from a wide variety of speakers and those factors that contribute to the individuality or "accent" of the speaker, enabling one to distinguish between two speakers who are delivering identical messages. Again in this case, a fusion of electrical, mechanical, and physiological knowledge is required. The key to the process is in the upper vocal tract (the lips-mouth-tongue-pharynx combination). The three major organs of articulation are the lips, the tongue (a major nonlinear impedance element), and the soft palate. The resonators include the mouth, the nose, the associated nasal sinuses, the pharynx, and the chest itself. Voice quality or accent may best be studied by utilizing methods of engineering to formulate a physical and mathematical model of the vocal tract as a series of acoustic horns, each section matched to the succeeding one, each having a nonlinear, acoustic impedance characteristic.

Here again, the responsibility of the engineer engaged in such studies is to delve deeply enough into myographic and other physiological phenomena to be able to formulate an adequate physical and mathematical model of the physiological process of speech formulation. This example could be carried even further into the realm of human physiology by considering the psychological and cerebral origins of speech formulation. The point, however, is already made. The professional biomedical engineer has the primary responsibility of preparing himself with all the tools and techniques he deems necessary to do a conscientious and adequate job of solving the problem he has accepted. It is also his responsibility not to accept problems or assignments for which the tools and techniques at his command are not adequate.

How Should a Profession Police Itself?

The engineering profession in the United States has been in transition for many years, but most of the important changes can be traced to the period after the 1920s. The American Society for the Promotion of Engineering Education was formed in 1893 and changed its name soon after that to the present one, the American Society for Engineering Education. In a series of studies and reports, this society has exerted a strong influence on the destiny of the profession. Two landmark reports are one issued in 1967 entitled "Engineering Education Goals" and one issued in 1929 entitled "The Wickender Report." On the direct initiative of this latter report, the Engineers' Council for Professional Development (ECPD) was formed in 1932. This organization is supported by all the leading technical societies and has as one of its main functions the policing of engineering education. It accredits engineering curricula at institutions of higher learning that are already accredited by state and regional accreditation groups as proper academic organizations. The purpose of this organization is to see that incoming intern professionals have been properly prepared to begin the experience phase of their career development.

Another organization that attempts to police the profession in a subtle manner is the Engineers Joint Council (EJC), which was formed in 1946 and is a federation of engineering societies. (Individual engineers are not directly members of the EJC.) Officials of these societies meet regularly to consider problems of public policy that affect the profession of engineering. Approximately 26 societies are presently affiliated with the EJC. The National Council of State Boards of Engineering Examiners is also a member of EJC. In its own right, the NCSBEE performs a policing function for the professional by attempting to secure uniformity among the various state boards of engineering registration. This is accomplished by the drafting of a model registration law and lobbying in the various state legislatures for its adoption. Its activities have resulted in a moderate degree of uniformity among various state engineering registration or licensing laws.

Another organization that acts as a spokesman for the profession is the National Society of Professional Engineers (NSPE). It has recently opened up its membership to nonregistered engineers who are qualified but have not gone through the formal registration procedure. This society, by actively attending hearings on pertinent matters in both the national and state legislatures and executive bodies, is attempting to keep the engineering profession attuned to the vital issues of the day as they may be affected by engineering and vice versa. Also, by drawing up a code of ethics covering the professional behavior of engineers, an attempt has been made to establish standards for the guidance of practitioners in the engineering profession.

It can be seen that many efforts are being exerted by the profession to police itself, at least on an aggregate basis, if not by efforts to judge each individual's performance. However, in this latter respect, most organizations and state boards have clauses in their membership applications permitting expulsion for unprofessional conduct. Regretfully, these are rarely enforced.

Certification or Accreditation Program

Many efforts are under way to raise and assure the quality of the services offered by the profession of engineering. State licensing laws are prime examples of this effort. One must now take into account the explosive growth of science, engineering, and the supporting technologies. Entirely new disciplines are springing up almost overnight. Whereas in the eotechnic and paleotechnic phases of our technological development the four major branches of engineering (chemical, civil, electrical, and mechanical) were sufficient to blanket adequately all existing specialties, during the present neotechnic phase, this is hardly the case. Aeronautics and electronics started the ball rolling early in the neotechnic period, and now we would need a sizable pamphlet just to list the new engineering variations of the standard engineering and scientific disciplines.

Of course, clinical engineering is a prime example of a multidisciplinary specialty. It involves all four of the standard or founder engineering disciplines plus a goodly number of the life and behavioral sciences. Past experience has shown that legislatures and registration laws have very large time constants associated with change. This is not necessarily a fault. If one realizes that an ideal professional structure is one with solid foundations adorned by a flexible superstructure, a case can be made for keeping legal registration on as general a basis as possible.

Broadly speaking, the registration examinations involve the basic engineering sciences and the four engineering disciplines. The flexible superstructure would consist of a series of certification or accreditation bodies, each specializing in an appropriate sector of the total field and supported by the interested technical and professional societies.

Accreditation or certification boards provide a service to the individual engineer, so he can have available, for use in conjunction with his career development, an evaluation of his qualifications by an impartial group of experts in the particular specialty in which he feels qualified to participate. These procedures serve further as an aid to individual engineers who would like to train and qualify themselves for entry into a new area of specialization by giving them a concrete set of requirements to assist them in planning their self-improvement programs. Since accreditations are voluntary rather than mandatory for individual practicing engineers, the degree of their utilization is a measure of the usefulness to them of the accreditation procedures.

An accreditation procedure is also useful to prospective utilizers of engineering services. Here again, the fact of certification need not be a hard and fast requirement for employment but merely an additional indicator of the quality and extent of the qualifications of a prospective purveyor of engineering services. Since many utilizers of specialized engineering services may not themselves be expert in the specialty for which they are engaging the engineer, accreditation boards could mean the difference between a poor and a good performance.

In the clinical engineering specialty, there are especially large advantages.

Clinical engineering is basically the practice of engineering in a clinical setting. This would include hospitals and other health-care-delivery organizations and locations. For the discipline of clinical engineering, accreditation systems offer a balanced service to at least three parties—the purveyor of the services (i.e., the engineer himself), the utilizer or employer of the services (i.e., the health-care-delivery organization or physician), and the patient (for whose benefit the entire process of health-care delivery is carried on). Also, if a profession has as its main aim service to society, then in the aggregate, these accreditation boards must also serve the entire engineering profession.

In particular, let us examine how accreditation can operate for clinical engineering. The primary aim of accreditation for this specialty is to properly identify that subset of all engineers who are qualified to practice in the field. For this purpose, it is only important to identify the broad or macrostructure of the discipline. These may be listed as follows:

1. Those activities directly associated with patient care (including use of specialized instrumentation and devices)
2. The design and development of biomedical instrumentation and devices
3. Those research activities associated with an application of engineering principles to the life sciences and vice versa
4. A general or catch-all category for individuals who participate in some degree in more than one of the above categories.

Clinical engineering may be said, roughly, to be comprised of at least the patient-care category and most often performed in a hospital setting. In addition, of course, the clinical engineer interfaces very closely with the engineers performing design and development of biomedical instrumentation and devices. In fact, in many large health-care-delivery organizations, the clinical engineer will perform design and development functions for specialized gear. He almost always will be performing the systems engineering required to meld and weld into one series of noninterfering subsystems all the instrumentation and devices directly associated with patient care. Looking in more detail at the clinical engineer's functions, it becomes immediately obvious that his activities require liaison and coordination with many other specialists within the health-care organization. Some of these people are themselves oriented in some field of engineering, while others are specialized in the life sciences, and still others are in the administrative field.

The industrial suppliers of patient-care instrumentation and devices and the hospital engineer are both technically oriented, and the level of communication between them and the clinical engineer would be in the terminology and conventions of engineering. The medical staff of the hospital and the staffs of preventive-medicine units will most likely be oriented toward medical practice. Therefore, communication between this type of personnel and the clinical engineer will involve a complex intermixture of medical and engineering jargon, with the consequent danger of serious misinterpretation of meaning.

The situation concerning communication with the research faculty of the hospital is a little less precarious, although misunderstanding may still occur frequently. The research faculty is generally more science and mathematics oriented than the regular medical staff (albeit still basically oriented in the life sciences), and their problems and requirements can be more adequately met by the clinical engineer using the terminology and modes of presentation standard in the engineering sciences.

Finally, there are the relationships between the clinical engineer and hospital administrator. These mirror most closely the professional-client relationships mentioned previously. The administrator is usually nontechnically oriented and must accept much of the advice and opinion of the clinical engineer on faith—just as he must do when communicating with the medical staff. Therefore, the more professional basis clinical engineering can assume in its function and duty, the smoother the interactions with the hospital administrator. If the latter can be convinced that the clinical engineer in his sphere of expertise has the same creeds, code of ethics, and philosophy of service as the physicians in their sphere of expertise, then a like *modus vivendi* will exist.

What should be the mechanics of an accreditation system? The initial certification should not be a permanent action. A written examination must be required for initial certification, testing the applicant's knowledge in both the engineering and life sciences. The applicant could be able to choose either of the two as a major test unit, and the other could then become the minor. The duration of the initial certification may be 5 years or more, with a reaccreditation procedure to be made available to those whose initial certification has expired. Also, reaccreditation should be on a periodic basis.

The basis for instituting a reaccreditation procedure concerns the freshness of the accredited individual's experience. In a technical specialty, one quickly loses one's expertise if the skills are not used and expanded by that use. Thus, if accreditation is to be a useful process for the engineer and his employers or clients, it must be timely. Legal registration is an indicator of general professional qualification, at one point in time, while the accreditation certificate is an indicator of the present possession of certain specialized qualifications.

The cost of maintaining the entire accreditation system (including the cost of designing, validating, administering, and grading any necessary written examinations) should be defrayed partially by fees charged to the applying engineers and partly by grants from the participating professional and technical societies. Grants should also be accepted from employing organizations on a general basis, that is, not identified with any particular applicant.

14

CURRENT CONCEPTS

A. Zara

The surge in technology after World War II led to new programs encompassing engineering and medicine that, in turn, required new types of engineers such as clinical engineers. Practicing this technology requires a complete and coordinated system of training and employment.

Many of the participants in the system will, of course, see only the subsystems or their individual interfaces. The system, however, involves three major steps. One step, education, has immediate feedback control requiring the supplier institution to be "accredited." The other two steps are registration (licensure) by legal authorities and certification by professional societies. Through the concept of feedback theory, the overall system may be viewed as one of coupled feedback with different response times and instabilities.

A wealth of material on the accreditation process and its interaction with other steps of registration and certification has already been developed and translated into clearly identifiable health/manpower categories. But clinical engineering, with its various subspecialties, has not been fully identified. So the efforts to use certification as a quick response to the challenge of technological change and as a corrective remedy for inadequacies in other parts of the system must be seen in perspective. The engineering programs aimed at clinical work are scattered in several hundred institutions and must be thought of as part of the overall process leading to the creation of a new human resource. The need to assure accreditation of educational institutions is clear. Coupling mechanisms to other parts of the overall system are also necessary so that developments in any part of the system are not isolated but kept in proper view.

Clinical engineering is an evolving field whose practitioners should now be widely recognized and their work certified by a peer group. Certification is a necessary process in a chain that includes education, internship, and training, registration and licensure, as well as experience.

Licensure is the responsibility of state and local governments. Certification can be the responsibility of professional organizations. Certification should be viewed not as a minimum standard for qualification but as a mark of excellence. This view has developed with input from, and the concurrence of, a variety of concerned groups and individuals.

This implies that all the needs and interests of clinical engineers, along with all other disciplines involved in the field of medical instrumentation, must be considered. An appropriate group to implement initially must be one whose objective is to further the application of technology to medicine and increase communication among all the disciplines involved in clinical engineering; it should be composed of engineers, physicians, administrators, others in health delivery, educators, and government and industry representatives. Such a directorial grouping can directly reflect not just engineers but, properly, the users of their services and all types of ultimate consumers of medical electronic equipment. A multidisciplinary organization is needed to undertake the significant and difficult task of initial development and implementation of a program like a clinical engineering certification program from a user's viewpoint as required in today's world.

The ultimate objectives of a certification program are (*a*) to define the emerging role of the clinical engineer as an integral member of the health-care community; (*b*) to provide a method of assuring and improving the competence of clinical engineers; and (*c*) to help develop a competent specialty that can improve health-care delivery at reduced costs. The end result of certification will thus (*a*) elevate, recognize, and optimize the quality of the professional services offered in the interdisciplinary field of clinical engineering; (*b*) provide a useful service to health-care institutions by providing unbiased peer-group review; (*c*) provide evaluation of personnel qualifications for those in clinical engineering; and, most important; (*d*) assure safe patient care in those areas that are affected by technology.

Background for Modern Certification

1. There is ample precedent among the learned professions for peer-group evaluation of a practitioner's professional qualifications in a particular professional specialty over and above any legal registration or licensing requirements.
2. In view of the interdisciplinary nature of clinical engineering, there is a need for the establishment of professional certification procedures that serve both as a service to the individual practicing biomedical engineering and to the organizations seeking the services of such an engineer.
3. The establishment of professional certification procedures tends to increase public confidence in the profession.

4. There is a need for both an initial certification procedure and for a periodic follow-up or revalidation procedure designed to evaluate the current professional qualifications of the individual practitioner.
5. The certification procedure (particularly for practitioners presenting the minimum acceptable level of qualifications) should, at an appropriate time, include a written examination.

Considerations for Certification

The qualifications for certification can include one of the following:

1. A bachelor's degree in engineering or physical sciences with practice years or the equivalent, initially without examination
2. A degree in clinical engineering or life sciences and/or equivalent relevant experience and practice, initially without examination
3. Practicing clinical eningeers who have years of relevant experience (with a reasonable number of years of experience directly involving clinical engineering) can be certified without examination if recognized by their peers as "eminent"

But a certification program primarily is organized to help in the future and not solve past problems, so individuals who do not fall directly into the above but wish to be certified should be required to pass an examination.

There are two aspects to the technical content of any certification interview or examination: (*a*) consideration of the criteria that people have used or may currently use to consider themselves members of a group; and (*b*) the requirements to test whether newcomers are like those in the group. Thus, the initial consideration has been the establishment of those qualifications that people currently have or think should be had by those that practice clinical engineering. These initial qualifications are the basis for professional interviews that determine and recognize the validity of the criteria in the specific individual. Establishment, through interviews and written examinations, that such qualifications are fulfilled by an individual serve as the basis for certification. Such an approach is commonly followed in the medical area.

Various clinical engineers have studied qualifications they believe essential for clinical engineers. The underlying factor that they express is that a clinical engineer must use concepts, techniques, and methods of engineering science that are applied to clinical health-service-delivery problems.

Objectives of Certification

Two objectives are prominent:

1. To elevate, recognize, and optimize the quality of the professional services offered in the interdisciplinary field of clinical engineering
2. To provide a useful service to health-care institutions by proving unbiased peer-group review and evaluation of qualifications in clinical engineering

The objectives of a certification program are (*a*) to define the emerging role of the clinical engineer as a member of the health-care community; (*b*) to provide a method of assuring and improving the competence of clinical engineers; and (*c*) to help develop a competent specialty that can improve health-care delivery at reduced costs.

To effect these objectives a certification board must initially appoint a group of clinical engineers that will expand as needed to act as an examining Board. That board will (*a*) interview applicants and prepare written examinations in specific geographical areas to attest to qualifications; (*b*) consider if there are any further qualifications that might be suitable or examinations that could be considered for future applicants; and (*c*) provide feedback to the certification board on relevant matters.

Why become certified? What advantages are there to certification? The principal advantage of certification is that it recognizes ability to meet a certain set of standards related to one or more of the many aspects of modern clinical engineering. These standards pertain to the academic requirements needed, but, more important, they pertain to the practical experience and achievements required of a clinical engineer.

Many currently employed can successfully measure themselves against standards, but they cannot provide documentation concerning their ability. Certification provides successful candidates with documentary evidence of their abilities. Philosophically, the purpose of engineering certification is to improve and thus gain increased acceptance of clinical engineering as a profession. Peers, of course, establish the basic standards.

The Certification Process

Initially, one of two routes can be followed, depending on the applicant's educational background and work experience. These routes are: (*a*) the certification interview and written examination; or (*b*) the "grandfather" provision. Any applicant having a record of employment in responsible charge of important clinical engineering methods, design and use of clinical equipment and systems, and administration related to the use of clinical engineering techniques should be eligible for the interview and examination.

Academic training in accredited technical, science, or engineering schools should be acceptable for partial experience. A candidate may qualify (*a*) with a degree in science or engineering/technology from an accredited school; (*b*) evidence of professional engineer's registration; or (*c*) appropriate experience. The applicant must submit references from persons whose standing and ability are recognized.

What does a certification interview and written examination involve? Usually, the interview involves two parts: (*a*) a basic interview given to all candidates covering the fundamentals; and (*b*) a specialized interview or written examination in an area of specialty chosen by the applicant if that area is relevant to clinical engineering.

The Grandfather Clause

What is a grandfather clause, and how does one qualify for certification under this clause? As is the case in professional registration, certification can be conferred on candidates who satisfy certain professional requirements. More specifically, "grandfathering" means the granting of certification without benefit of formal methods.

To qualify for certification under a grandfather clause, the applicant must provide documentary evidence of years of employment in responsible charge of important clinical engineering projects of a character satisfactory to the certification committee and furnish the names and addresses of satisfactory references who are accepted as clinical engineers or individuals whose standing and engineering ability are generally recognized.

How does one apply for certification? After filling out an application form, the applicant should submit it for review. A fee for certification must accompany the application. The form and fee must be submitted prior to announced dates. Assuming approval of the application, the applicant will be advised as to when and where to appear for the interview. Should he agree to take the interview but fail to appear at the appointed time and place, he is usually permitted to take the interview at the next scheduled date for an additional fee. If an applicant fails, he must wait usually one year before being examined again and must pay an additional fee.

Each candidate is notified after the interview. This and all results are always confidential. If he passes, he will be so advised and issued a certificate that is valid for a prescribed period. The certification may be revoked for failure to recertify, falsifying information on the application for certification, malpractice, or unethical behavior.

Preparation

Is the interview or examination especially difficult? How much preparation is necessary? The interview is difficult only to the extent that it presupposes knowledge of fundamentals and a good working knowledge of the applicant's field of specialization. The amount of preparation needed will, of course, vary with the individual. This can best be determined by a review and study related to the applicant's field of specialization.

Recertification. An applicant who passes should not become certified for life. Recertification should be accomplished in either of two ways: (*a*) professional credits; or (*b*) reexamination.

Professional credits. Recertification requires the accumulation of professional credits. These credits can be obtained by participating in recognized conferences, seminars, clinics, workshops, forums, or symposia. Other ways of obtaining professional credits include successful completion of courses from accredited institutions of higher learning, in-house training, approved home-study courses, technical-paper presentations, teaching of accredited courses, and other appropriate technological activities. These activities must be approved by the commission on certification for credit to be given.

One "model" proposal on certification of medical engineers is presented in detail for review here.

The Canadian Medical and Biological Engineering Society (CMBES) is a professional organization that has set up a procedure for the certification of its medical engineers. The following describes the concepts used in considering the certification and is useful to review as a model.

Rationale

Introducing, developing, and maintaining a certification procedure should have the following advantages:

1. It should provide governments and hospital administrations with a guideline for assessing the qualifications of medical engineering consultants or employees. At present, there is no way of assuring that a television repairman or a plant supervisor is not performing medical engineering duties.
2. It should serve to increase the level of expertise, hence the safety of techniques and technology that are applied to patients. Certification should serve as a screening process to assure that only qualified individuals enter the field. (Only those individuals directly involved with the health-care-delivery system would be likely to seek certification.)
3. It should give medical engineering recognition as an integral part of health care.

Role of the Medical Engineer

The application of engineering techniques, technology, and theory to the solution of medical problems is, by definition, medical engineering. This, therefore, includes the application of whatever traditional branch of engineering is necessary to solve a particular medical problem.

The medical engineer's function is to provide education for nursing, medical, and paramedical staff so that present technology and future trends will be fully understood by them. He must provide consultation for medical and administrative staff in order to provide assurance that equipment purchases and hospital designs are optimal. He must engage in research and development at all levels to improve patient care. He must make provisions for the safe and efficient operation of all patient-care equipment.

Accordingly, the following functions can be taken as legitimate medical engineering activities:

Equipment Management

1. Consultation with medical and paramedical staff in the planning and purchase of equipment
2. Prime responsibility for maintenance and modification of the equipment

Hospital and Patient Safety

1. Prime responsibility for the integrity of the power systems to patient-care areas
2. Prime responsibility for the safety of electromedical monitoring equipment
3. Prime responsibility for safety of mechanical equipment, especially technical aids used in life support and rehabilitation

Systems Management. Design and evaluation of highly technical systems, such as ICUs, cardiac investigation systems, telecommunication systems, transportation systems, etc. Professional skills required here include industrial engineering (systems engineering) as well as the normal skills of electrical and mechanical engineering.

Technically Assistive Devices for the Disabled

1. Design, development, and, in some cases, fitting of pacemakers and stimulators
2. Rehabilitation aids (prosthetics, orthotics, and technical aids)
3. Orthopedic implants
4. Sensory aids, and communication devices

Clinical R & D

1. Interdisciplinary research directed toward the development of new diagnostic and clinical procedures
2. Design of new equipment and patient aids

Computer Applications

1. Development and management of hospital patient information systems involving admissions, patient records, medical statistics, etc.
2. Diagnostic computing involving long-term patient monitoring and computer-controlled alarm systems

Education

1. Education of medical and nursing staff in fields of science required to adequately cope with present and future technology in medicine

2. Education of paramedical and medical staff on the operation and safety of equipment
3. Education of medical engineering students
4. Advising administration on matters related to the influence of technological advances on the delivery of health care

Consulting/Liaison

The medical engineer often consults directly on a technical problem or more often acts as the intermediary between the clinical setting (doctors plus patient problems) and technical resources outside his facility. This role of consulting/liaison is an activity that takes place throughout most of the previously listed functions.

Name

The name for the certified individual in Canada is *certified medical engineer,* as contrasted to the United States functional designation *clinical engineer.*

Qualification for Certification

It should be recognized that the qualifications proposed herein are meant to be guidelines. There are people within the field at present who do not fit this mold and yet would be certified under a grandfather clause.

A certification is recommended based on education and experience, but in the long run it may be desirable to include special examinations. The following criteria must be met before consideration for certification will be granted.

1. The candidate must be a professional engineer in good standing.
2. The candidate must be an individual whose principal occupation is medical engineering or consulting involved significantly in medical engineering.
3. The candidate must have a minimum level of academic training: MS in a recognized biomedical engineering program or an M.D.
4. The candidate must have a minimum level of experience, including a period of residency of 1 year plus 2 years in the field of health care.

Consideration will be given to special cases, such as biomedical engineers from other countries who meet requirements (1) and (2) and have equivalent qualifications to those proposed in paragraphs (3) and (4).

It is recommended that certification be portable between provinces to the same extent that the engineer is portable.

Procedures for Certification

Preferred Scheme (Indirect Method). CMBES has considered forming a peer group (certification board) that would be the reviewing body on behalf of the provincial engineering associations. Certification procedures considered include:

1. Application to Provincial Association of Professional Engineers by prospective applicant
2. Applications collected by associations and forwarded to CMBES certification board for assessment
3. Provincial association awards certification to successful applicants on recommendations of the certification board.

Alternate Scheme (Direct Method). If the provincial associations do not wish to award certification, then the CMBES peer group (certification board) would become the certifying body, and the professional associations would be bypassed.

Hospital Residency Programs

CMBES has considered making a submission to several granting agencies to finance completely two to three in-hospital training programs for medical engineers in Canada. The program could provide broad training and therefore may require a tie-in with provincial health care rather than just one hospital. The program must be administered by a university having a biomedical engineering program. The proposed grants to the trainees should be substantial to cover sufficiently living costs plus travel and books. All additional expenses incurred by the hospital and university for equipment, training, and supervision should be underwritten as well. These grants may be interim, so there must be provision for long-term university hospital take-over of aid program.

Medical Equipment Technician/Technologists

CMBES has considered plans to take steps to examine the need for certification of technicians and technologists employed in medical equipment technology (maintenance, design, and research).

15

PROFESSIONAL REGISTRATION*

A. Zara

Philosophy of Registration

All professions require registration or licensing to practice before the public, and this includes the professions of law, medicine, dentistry, architecture, accounting, and engineering. Professional registration is deemed essential to protect the public safety and the public welfare against the incompetent and the charlatan.

Registration for the engineering profession commenced in 1907 in the state of Wyoming. Today, registration to practice professional engineering is required in all 50 states, the District of Columbia, and in the territories of Puerto Rico and the Canal Zone. Mexico and provinces and territories in Canada also have registration requirements.

In the early history of engineering registration, many engineers voiced violent opposition to registration as a tax on their practice in the field of their competence. Those who are competent have raised no serious objection to having their competency certified because they are ridding themselves at the same time of competition by the noncompetent.

A professional is judged by the qualifications of all who use its name, by the failures of the incompetents and the conduct of the unworthy, unless a clear dividing line is established in the public recognition between the lawful practitioners of the profession and those who are not admitted to practice. A profession should be empowered to disown those who hold themselves out as belonging to it without proper qualifications or character and to bar the unfit and the unprincipled who seek to practice in its name. The public expects a trusted profession to maintain high

*The editors wish to thank M. F. Lunch and P. E. Ellis of the National Society of Professional Engineers for their input to this chapter.

standards of qualification and to clear its ranks of those who do not meet those standards and whose pretensions and activities would degrade its good name.

Without registration laws, there is no way to (*a*) prevent the practice of engineering by the nonengineer; (*b*) stop the misappropriation and abuse of the designation "engineer"; (*c*) oust from the profession those who prove incompetent and unworthy; and (*d*) preserve to the qualified engineer his rights of practice against restriction, encroachment, and unqualified competition.

The work of no other profession more truly concerns the safety of life, health, and property than does engineering. Protection of the public in its practice provides legislative justification and establishes constitutionality of registration legislation. Protection of the profession, its standards, and its standing is an associated benefit. But the two benefits are inseparable.

Registration places the force and sanction of the law behind the desire of the profession to maintain a clearly recognizable line of demarcation between the efforts and aspirations of the profession to maintain high standards of qualification and ethical practice.

Legal Basis for Registration

Legal registration of members of the engineering profession is an exercise of the police powers inherent in every state for protection of the public health and public safety. Such registration gives assurance that only those persons who meet fixed educational and experience requirements may practice engineering.

Practically every design, operation, and process undertaken by the engineer has public implications. Engineering, therefore, comes under the police powers of the state.

Regulation is achieved in two ways, either by protecting the use of the title or by regulating the actual practice of the profession. Both methods have been declared constitutional by the courts.

Uniformity is difficult to obtain because each state is rightfully an independent commonwealth and has a right to establish its own police-power regulations. To obtain a measure of uniformity, however, engineering practitioners have developed a "model law" that has been used as a guide for many years. That law has been revised and brought up to date repeatedly since first drafted, the most recent edition having been made in 1972 by the National Council of Engineering Examiners, an organization composed of all the state registration boards.

However, even if complete uniformity of laws could be obtained, differences in interpretation and administrative procedure that exist among the state boards charged with their administration would probably bar likeness in operation of engineering registration from one state to the next. Uniformity, which will permit wider reciprocity, is a goal toward which engineering organizations and the members of the registration boards through their national organization are toiling.

So far as the two methods of regulation are concerned, each has its peculiar advantages and disadvantages. For example, in protecting the title, no difficult definition of engineering is needed, yet large discretion must be exercised by registration boards in dealing with nationally accepted groups that have commonly used the title, that is, locomotive enginemen who are almost universally called engineers. To regulate the practice of engineering, similarly, the law must provide a definition of engineering that will distinguish its activities from all others. Upon this snag, some state laws encountered constitutional difficulty during the earlier years of registration. The NSPE model-law definition, which has been upheld in many states, provides:

> The term, "Practice of Engineering," within the intent of this Act, shall mean any service or creative work, the adequate performance of which requires engineering education, training, and experience, in the application of special knowledge of the mathematical, physical, and engineering sciences to such services or creative work as consultation, investigation, evaluation, planning, and design of engineering works and systems, planning the use of land and water, teaching of advanced engineering subjects, engineering surveys, and the inspection of construction for the purpose of assuring compliance with drawings and specifications; any of which embraces such services or work, either public or private, in connection with any utilities, structures, buildings, machines, equipment, processes, work systems, projects, and industrial or consumer products or equipment of a mechanical, electrical, hydraulic, pneumatic or thermal nature, insofar as they involve safeguarding life, health or property, and including such other professional services as may be necessary to the planning, progress and completion of any engineering services.
>
> A person shall be construed to practice or offer to practice engineering, within the meaning and intent of this Act, who practices any branch of the profession of engineering; or who, by verbal claim, sign, advertisement, letter-head, card, or in any other way represents himself to be a Professional Engineer, or through the use of some other title implies that he is a Professional Engineer or that he is registered under this Act; or who holds himself out as able to perform, or who does perform any engineering service or work or any other service designated by the practitioner which is recognized as engineering.

A number of corporations in this country are following a policy of not permitting engineering employees to be designated by the title, *engineer* unless they have a professional license. For example, Allis Chalmers Manufacturing Company restricts certain sales employees in a statement by its general manager of sales and served, as follows:

> I am sure that many of us feel that it would be desirable, and under certain circumstances, a distinct advantage to use the title "Engineer" on calling cards, in correspondence, and sometimes verbally during our negotiations with customers.
>
> All states have laws requiring the registration of those involved in engineering, particularly as it might affect the health, safety and welfare of people. The use of the title "Engineer" bears certain restrictions.
>
> Because of this, it is the policy of the company not to use the title field or sales engineer or any other combination of title wording involving the word "Engineer" unless the individual is registered in accordance with state laws.

Here is another from the director of research and development of Bay State Abrasive Products Company, the third largest abrasives manufacturing concern in the world.

> The term ''Engineer'' should be omitted from all titles of Bay State employees unless such person is registered as a professional engineer in the Commonwealth of Massachusetts;
>
> The use of this title may be continued provided such person is now so registered or has made application for registration. If such applicant is turned down,the term ''Engineer'' must be dropped from his title and one of the following terms used;
>
> In the Research and Development Department and in the Quality Control Department, the term ''Chemist'' or ''Ceramist'' shall replace the term ''Engineer'';
>
> In the Industrial Engineering Department the term ''Analyst'' shall replace the term ''Engineer'';
>
> In Plant Engineering Departments the term ''Machine Designer'' shall be used; The use of the title ''Sales Engineering Department'' shall be continued provided the Manager of this department is or becomes a registered professional engineer; and the term ''Engineer'' shall be changed to ''Abrasive Specialist'' for outside personnel of the Sales Engineering Department and any non-registered inside men shall be known as ''Technical Service Men'' unless they become registered.

There are many more, but the pattern is the same.

Engineering management has shown an expanding recognition and concern for the benefits to the company and the individual engineer in ways other than title alone. Western Electric Company has informed its engineering staff that registration ''enhances recognition of our engineering organization by the public.'' The Mellon–Stuart Company, Pittsburgh, Pennsylvania, gives a salary increase to its engineer employees who become registered.

The British Columbia Power Commission now requires registration as a condition of employment for employees involved in the practice of engineering, and as a condition for obtaining or retaining the job title 'Engineer' within the organization. Employees engaged in professional engineering have 24 months to apply for registration. Failure to comply may constitute grounds for termination of service. Those unable to secure registration will lose the job title ''Engineer'' and will be reclassified by title and pay range, which may be lower than the engineering position formerly held. The reclassified positions ''shall not be perpetuated beyond the tenure of the incumbent concerned.''

DuPont's engineering department encourages registration, particularly in the state in which the engineer is working, in this policy statement: ''The attainment of professional registration is considered a mark of progress and carries with it recognition that the individual has reached a professional level.''

Underwriters' Laboratories, which issues the ''UL'' tag that appears on electrical appliances, has moved into vigorous support of engineering professionalism through registration. Approximately one-third of the present engineering staff have obtained registration, and a substantial number of staff engineers are preparing for the examinations. The UL statement follows (in part):

> Inasmuch as our organization is primarily an engineering organization, it is incumbent on our engineering staff to advance both their professional knowledge and their professional status in every proper manner, and one of the most important steps in this direction is qualifying under existing laws as a Professional Engineer.
>
> Professional Engineer registration is covered by law in every state, and it is becoming more and more necessary to have such recognition in order to qualify as a professional man. In addition, all of us have an obligation to support efforts to clarify the status of engineers for the protection that affords the public.

The US Bureau of Public Roads has requested its registered professional engineers to display their professional license. ''In this way, visitors to our offices can be made aware of the professional stature of the staff,'' an interoffice memorandum advised the engineers. The bureau encourages its engineers to become registered ''and to display with pride the certificates which they receive for this accomplishment.''

Most of the founder engineering societies have been weighing the merits of engineering registration as a requirement for top membership grade. ASCE adopted such a requirement in 1958.

With the growth of unions, many employed engineers have found themselves forced to join bargaining groups primarily intended to embrace technicians. Under the Taft-Hartley Act, professional people have the right to a separate vote on union representation but must first prove their professional status. Registration is one of the most convincing proofs that can be offered. In firms in which unionization of engineers is a problem or a matter of concern to management, registration can be a clear signal, by the engineer, as to which side he is on—management or labor—and what he hopes to be—professional or technician. No other single step can the engineer take to declare his position so firmly as the one to register.

PART IV

INSURANCE, LIABILITY, AND LEGISLATION

16
INSURANCE AND MALPRACTICE

K. L. Kayser

In the past, the only parties involved in medical malpractice suits were patients versus doctors and hospitals. One of the reasons for this was that some individuals owned very little; consequently there was no point in suing. However, in the United States, the wages of hospital personnel have risen in recent years more rapidly than the wages of the United States population in general. Thus, this has made all hospital and health-care employees a much more appealing target for lawsuits, together with the hospital and doctor. At the present time, it is a common practice to sue everyone conceivably connected with the alleged injury.

Generally speaking, and without resorting to technical legal language, a lawsuit is initiated if a person believes that he has suffered an injustice or a civil wrong. He may then seek compensation through legal proceedings. Because the legal process is quite difficult and complicated, lawyers are engaged by people to aid them in utilizing the legal process. Thus, in practice, persons usually seek legal action through their attorneys, and attorneys also provide the defense.

A lawsuit is initiated by filing a complaint in a court. The person who seeks the damages is the plaintiff. The person on whom action is being taken is the defendant. The complaint is a carefully drawn legal document and contains the conditions that the plaintiff must prove in order to win his lawsuit. Generally, the court will summon the named defendants by issuing a summons. At this point, a person becomes a defendant and must defend himself against the plaintiff.

In most cases, the primary basis for complaint against a medical practitioner is negligence. Proven negligence in the legal sense involves the following three elements.

Standard of Conduct. A standard of conduct for the type of activity the defendant was engaged in must be established.

Damages. It must be shown that the plaintiff suffered an actual loss of something.

Relationship. It must be shown that the damages resulted from deviation from the standard of conduct by the defendant.

Under the general principle that a man is presumed innocent until proven guilty, the burden of proof rests with the plaintiff. However, in a hospital situation, in which a patient has little if any control over his treatment and may even be totally unconscious, the law recognizes that the burden of proof is unreasonably difficult for a plaintiff and can shift it to the defendant. In other words, negligence may be presumed until proven otherwise.

This shift of burden may make the defense of a medical malpractice suit difficult and expensive. Specialized investigation, expert witnesses, and highly specialized and expert legal counsel are required. In addition, a large expenditure of time by the defendant himself may be required. Rules of evidence may shift to favor the plaintiff. This, coupled with the emotional appeal of a severely injured plaintiff, can paint a dismal picture for the defendant.

What is the role of an insurance company in such a lawsuit? Insurance contracts are detailed documents in which the insurance company, in general, agrees to *defend* lawsuits and pay judgments against a *named insured.* The contract will state the limitations of these services and a premium charged. An insurance company is much better equipped to defend a lawsuit than an individual. They either employ or know where they can hire the proper legal counsel and investigational help. They know which expert witnesses will testify to their advantage. They can, in general, defend themselves more competently and inexpensively than an individual. It is also obvious that an insurance company can pay lawsuits more easily than a defendant.

Insurance companies also have ample liquidity. They can bargain very skillfully, with cash readily available, and thus solicit a plaintiff to settle for a smaller cash settlement now rather than hold out for the possibility of a larger sum at a later date.

A key phrase in insurance contracts is ''named insured.'' There are at least two possibilities for inclusion by this term. ''Named insured'' may have his name printed on the policy, which leaves little doubt as to who is insured. Second, the named insured can be identified in some other way; employee, agent, servant, etc. Here, whether or not a person is the named insured may be in doubt, and the matter may have to be settled in a separate court case.

There seems to be widespread misunderstanding about the liability of a superior (doctor, hospital) and an agent (employee). Whereas it may be true that the superior is liable and responsible for the acts of his agents, he is not solely responsible. The agents are responsible in their own right unless they can prove otherwise. A person always lives with his own negligence. A superior lives with his own negligence and the negligence of his agents. That a superior is responsible for the acts of his agent in no way absolves the agent. The superior's insurance policy may list an agent as a named insured, or it may not, as outlined previously. In general, the insurance policy covers judgments against the superior for acts of the superior's agents. *This clause offers no protection whatsoever for the agent.*

Assume that an agent is being sued and that both the doctor's insurance and the hospital's insurance companies deny him defense. The agent would then have to hire his own lawyer and prove in court that he indeed was acting as an agent of the doctor. In this endeavor, the agent may find himself in a position of opposing his superior's insurance company in establishing this fact. When the case is closed, the agent may have to pay his own legal expenses and any judgments against himself. In addition, the superior's insurance company can sue the agent (this is called subrogation) for judgments that it paid on behalf of the superior for negligent actions of the agent. Also, the insurance company can sue the agent for legal expenses incurred in defending its insured. In defending the lawsuit, an insurance company may find that it is to their advantage to place as much of the negligence as possible on an agent and then try to show that the agent was responsible for these actions in his own right. This places the agent in the position of having not only to oppose the plaintiff but also the other defendants.

Some insurance policies have minor employees, such as agents, as the named insured; other policies do not. The only way that a person can ascertain this with any degree of assurance is to read the actual wording of the policy. Policies that will "defend and pay in behalf of employees" do offer protection; policies that will "pay in behalf of the superior for acts of the superior's employees" offer no protection to the employee.

There are several other aspects of insurance that should be pointed out. Double insurance often affords less protection because both companies may deny responsibility; therefore, if you work for a hospital and are covered by the hospital's insurance policy and then take out your own insurance policy with a different company, both companies can deny responsibility. Therefore, it is important to be completely candid in applying for your insurance and to avoid the occurrence of double coverage. If you do any amount of work that is not done as an employee of a hospital, it may be desirable to obtain your own insurance policy to cover these activities. In this case, it would be desirable to have the second policy with the same insurance company covering the hospital. In general, it is always best to have one insurance company covering everyone involved. In this way, it is much easier to present a common front and unify opposition to the plaintiff.

It is extremely important to be properly insured. Professional people owe their clientele this type of financial responsibility. It is quite possible to keep the major portion of one's assets in trusts, etc., and thus out of the hands of people who hold judgments. It is also possible to declare bankruptcy and escape most if not all of the payment of a judgment. These techniques, however, jeopardize a person's relationship with his coworkers and can cause irreparable damage to a professional's reputation.

17

THE CLINICAL ENGINEER AND INSURANCE

A. E. Hertzler Knox

Fire, explosions, a car accident, workmen's compensation, hospitalization, and life are common denominators for insurance. All are fairly predictable as to costs over the past decade, with any increases consistent with general economic trends.

One type of insurance, however, has broken out of this pattern and is showing a sharp increase in both cost and frequency of loss. This is liability insurance for hospitals—liability for damage to a patient or a person resulting from some action under the control of the hospital. This insurance is often referred to as "malpractice." Claims may arise from a slip on a wet floor to intricate professional errors involving patients, procedures, or pills. During the past decade, patients injured through a hospital's or institution's negligence have been awarded ever-increasing payments for their injuries until today \$300,000 and \$500,000 awards are no longer a rarity.

Basic Concept of Insurance

Insurance is merely the sharing of the cost of an expected risk common to many people that can be expected to occur within a given period of time. For example, if 100 people can predict that five of them will die within 1 year, and they decide each dead person will need \$500 for burial, one simply multiplies five deaths times \$500, and the amount needed is \$2500 annually. Thus, for any one of the 100 persons, an annual payment of \$25 will ensure his receiving a \$500 burial payment. In today's world, one must add administrative costs for bookkeeping, collections, etc., so that the added cost will be shared by all 100 members, making the annual payment x dollars more than \$25, depending on the efficiency of the administrator (or in today's parlance—insurance company).

Hospital Application

If a group of five hospitals has been having liability losses of $50,000 annually for the past 5 years, one can anticipate paying out $250,000 over the next 5 years if all factors were to remain constant. From the previous example, it is obvious that to insure any possible loss would require each hospital to pay $10,000 annually for 5 years or $50,000 for the total period, plus administrative costs and profit. Herein lies the gamble in insurance; if a hospital has no losses for 5 years, it is out of pocket $50,000. However, a single loss in any one year of $75,000 would place it far ahead of the game.

However, there are two basic problems in this simplistic approach. Either more frequent or more expensive losses might occur, or the reverse may be true. How does the insurance industry approach these almost inevitable variations? Initially, the premium must be based on past experience and trends indicating changes that can be anticipated. A marked increase in losses over the predicted figure can only result in an increased premium if the insurance company is to remain solvent, or the hospital's insurance must be canceled.

What happens if the hospital's losses are decreased markedly? The policy can be written so that retrospective ratings will return to the hospital any excessive premiums over the losses anticipated. This decreases the hospital's insurance expense and prevents unconscionable profits accruing to the insurance company. However, effective documented loss control programs are a prerequisite here.

One insurance company, the Hartford Insurance Group, for example, has made a commitment to assist its insured hospitals in decreasing the number of injuries from all causes through established and newly evolving methods of loss control. In 1969, the proliferation of medical devices of electronic derivation was first making its impact felt. However, in retrospect, the trend toward increased financial losses due to liability had begun to shoot upward early in the 1960s.

Since 1969, Hartford has markedly expanded its loss-control staff of engineers, hygienists, and consultants and now has a division of hospital safety headed by a qualified bioengineer. As a result of this pool of talent, Hartford has been able to carefully examine critical cases of liability exposure, ranging from $50 to $500,000. In the majority of these cases, when biomedical equipment was involved, it was determined that the presence of a functioning clinical engineer in each hospital involved would have prevented the accidents leading to these suits for malpractice liability claims.

Although the current "in" thing is electrical safety, how many individuals have heard seemingly endless pitches on isolation grounds and milliamp leakage currents? We have many areas and devices in hospitals in which the danger is not necessarily electrical. For example, consider a well-known respirator unit normally used on an intermittent basis. Within the past year, Hartford had a claim resulting from the failure of a rubber-belt drive on this unit when it was put into continuous operation for many consecutive hours. Because of the belt failure, the patient died from lack of oxygen. Lesson: equipment control program, proper and frequent maintenance, and dissemination of knowledge that those particular belts were known to fail under continuous usage.

Another example recently took place in a new, modern ICU with all the latest advances in electrical safety. A portable X-ray unit was moved into position next to one of the four beds. One of Hartford's loss-control men made contact with the bed and the X-ray unit in a manner typical of an everyday nurse or technician. As a result, he received enough current to knock him across the room. Duplication of this contact situation, interposing electrical measurement devices instead of relying on the electrical stimulation of human muscles, revealed that the X-ray unit and all four of the new ICU beds were literally death traps. The recommendations, needless to say, involved correction of this problem before Hartford could approve the use of this "modern" ICU.

The following are some suggestions that will benefit hospitals, its patients, employees, and others involved.

First, the need for proper education and training: education of a hospital administration in the far-reaching responsibilities of their job, and the critical need for a hospital to have a clinical engineer if accidents are to be brought under control; training not only of administrators and doctors but also of hospital staff (through courses offered by universities, etc.) to properly use medical devices and promptly report their malfunction. If doctors and hospital staff personnel could be indoctrinated with the need to check the latest maintenance data sheet in the same way they look at the label of a vial of medication before they use it, many problems could be prevented.

Second, establishment of an equipment control program. There are many good articles on how to organize an equipment control program. Basically, such a program depends on the following.

1. Procurement of equipment by the purchasing agent only after approval by the clinical engineer
2. Specifications of equipment that satisfy the physician's expectations for its use subject to safety, availability, or possibility of modification to meet that use
3. Inspection of equipment on receipt for malfunctions, standards, and safety
4. Instruction in usage of all equipment
5. Maintenance programs that are realistic, effective, and ongoing
6. Records systems for each piece of equipment

Elements of an Equipment-Control Program

Procurement and Specifications

In the October 19, 1972, New England Journal of Medicine, an editorial calling attention to the results of the AAMI-FDA National Conference on Medical Device Standards commented:

> The physician has been carried into deep waters where his lack of expertise in evaluating sophisticated medical instrumentation is often evident. In the absence of recognized specifications, performance criteria, test methods, and other standards, the purchasing agent is left with little but the physician's personal opinion and a host of manufacturers' claims on which to base a sound economic choice. Medical institutions, guided for so long by senior physicians and administrators untouched by these advances in engineering and technology, are too often lacking in personnel skilled in selecting or maintaining electronic, mechanical, or other sophisticated medical equipment.

This editorial should be a must in a basic learning kit because it stresses the importance of the clinical engineer's place in today's medical care.

Seven Basic Tips for Buying Medical Equipment

1. *Do not necessarily buy the cheapest.* (It may be the most expensive to operate.) Consider what it will cost to purchase the item, operate it, and maintain or repair it. It may be difficult to estimate operating costs. It should include batteries if they are used; electrodes; cables; and other expendables. Assign a cost to downtime for repair, as well as to actual direct repair cost, if possible.

2. *Approach the first production unit with caution.* Someone has to buy the first unit, but it does not have to be you. There may be a possible lack of field experience that may actually make the unit less desirable. Some equipment has worked well in the prototype stages, but when the transition to full-scale production is made, it performs with less than desirable results. In some cases, it has taken 6 to 12 months to remedy the situation.

3. *Seek the opinion of others.* Doctors frequently seek opinions from their colleagues in medical situations. Do the same with the equipment you purchase. Start out by knowing what your specific requirements are as they exist for your hospital. Establish a specification. Then ask for the opinion of other hospitals or doctors who are using this same equipment. Find out what their operating experience has been. Has the equipment lived up to its expectations? Has the company lived up to its promises? Go and visit an institution in which there is a similar piece of equipment and see what it looks like and how it functions for yourself. Some equipment looks more used in months than others do in years. You may be surprised that those fancy alarms may be good during a demonstration but for practical purposes may become a frustration to the nursing staff because they are influenced too frequently by artifacts. If possible, ask for a 2-week trial period so you can get your own practical experience. You may also want to consider having the equipment evaluated by an outside concern. There are several reliable firms for this type of evaluative service.

4. *Check equipment on delivery.* It is reported that upward of 40–50% of the equipment delivered is defective in some way. Be sure it is repaired before you use it. It may take months to get it repaired if you have paid for it; however, if the salesman has not received his commission, you can be sure you will get it fixed much faster.

5. *Require a performance and safety check as a condition for sale.* Do not establish that it is unsafe after the equipment is installed and about to or already being used. Be sure it will meet your safety requirements before you purchase it. Whether it is a big item or a small item, have the manufacturer rectify any safety problems before it is delivered. When it arrives, it should be checked for performance against the manufacturer's stated specifications and your safety requirements. This should be done at the hospital or through a third-party, impartial service.

6. *Service training.* One of the biggest problems in getting the proper expected use from the equipment is adequate training of the people using the equipment. It is reported that 80–90% of equipment problems are "cockpit problems," that is, they are problems of operator ignorance or error. This is particularly important where the equipment must be operated by a variety of personnel. This training should cover all shifts and should encompass several days' time to be able reasonably to cover all of the personnel working full time and part time in the hospital. A good idea is to be sure to provide refresher training instruction after the equipment has been used for a short while. At this time, the people using the equipment will understand the various aspects of its operation much better. Training must also include maintenance people. Many times, problems can be resolved quickly by a maintenance man if he has been given some degree of training. Insist on a duplicate set of operating and maintenance manuals.

7. *If you cannot maintain it, do not buy it.* Remember, equipment will not operate forever without a certain amount of care. A regularly scheduled preventive maintenance program should be contemplated before equipment is purchased and implemented when it is received.

Condition of Sale (Suggested)

It is understood that the electrical equipment in the purchase order must meet certain standards set forth by ____________________________ Hospital. No payment shall be made to the manufacturer or his authorized representative unless the following standards are met:

1. The equipment shall pass either of the following electrical leakage tests:

a. ____________________________ 500 μA leakage from the equipment case, controls, and electrodes to ground (AAMI Type B)

b. ____________________________ 10 μA leakage from the equipment case, controls, and electrodes to ground and 50 μA leakage from the equipment case, controls to ground (AAMI Type A for electrical patient areas)

2. The equipment shall pass the tests in Step 1, operating off a standard 115-V, 60-Hz power line with the equipment in the following modes: grounded, ungrounded, and ungrounded with reverse polarity.

3. The equipment shall be supplied with a standard NMEA or UL-approved three-wire power-line cord.

4. The equipment shall pass all of the specification performance tests as advertised by the manufacturer of the equipment. All tests will be performed at __________________________ Hospital by its biomedical engineer or name of third-party evaluator.

5. The equipment, after passing Steps 1 through 4, will then be placed in operation for a 30-day evaluation. If at the end of the 30-day period the equipment does not perform to the satisfaction of the hospital staff, the equipment will be removed from the hospital at the equipment manufacturer's expense, and no charge whatsoever shall be made to ________________________ Hospital.

6. Upon being placed in operation, ________________________ hours of in-service instruction to the hospital staff will be provided. Two complete sets of operating instructions, schematics, and maintenance manuals for each separate identifiable item of equipment shall be provided.

Inspection of equipment on receipt

Manufacturers have increasingly been the target of product liability suits, their counterpart to the medical-hospital professional liability (malpractice) suits.

A senior vice-president of the Hartford Group, speaking at a national convention of insurers, commented on the rapid rise in lawsuits based on product liability from 50,000 in 1960 to 500,000 in 1970, with an equally dramatic increase in financial awards for personal injuries and deaths resulting from faulty products.

Figures from the literature of medical devices seems to indicate that as high as 40–50% of medical devices may be defective in some way on delivery. Hartford recommends that a performance and safety check be made a condition of sale.

In the editorial in the *New England Journal of Medicine* quoted previously, the majority of manufacturers of medical devices are complimented (and justly so) for their efforts to promote standards, educate users, and furnish maintenance and training information for their products. Their cooperation has been crucial in achieving the present status of medical-device development and standardization. The clinical engineers working closely with the physicians on specification requirements, evaluation, and record keeping will hasten production of the safest and most effective medical devices.

Instruction in Usage

Some people call this "service training." It applies to anyone who will use any medical device in a medical institution or setting. Dr. Joel Nobel of the Emergency Care Research Institute, Philadelphia, Pennsylvania, has found that approximately 50% of the problems with medical devices are caused by operator error.

Advice in the area of medical devices includes a recommendation that individuals should acquaint themselves with health-device publications. Programs for BMETs are a source of assistants or staff for the clinical engineer. Numerous companies are now offering electrical-safety and equipment-inspection contracts.

Such companies will more than pay for the annual subscription cost if your institution is planning on contracting for such services.

Maintenance Programs and Records

These two items cannot really be separated since each is meaningless without the other. However, aside from the obvious need for maintenance and record keeping, there are several areas of advantageous fallout from such formal procedures.

The cost: benefit ratio is a well-understood term today. If less downtime can be shown on one type of medical device than on another, then the recommendations on purchasing are more respected and meaningful. If one piece of crucial equipment is known to require maintenance after seven times of use, it may save a life to back up your equipment with a spare. Replacement needs can be documented when downtime and costs of repair begin to mount.

Improper use of medical devices can be pinpointed and proper training instituted when records show that use by a particular department routinely results in the need for maintenance.

An important aid for record keeping has been the use of the International Classification of Diseases, Adapted (ICDA-8). This is a coding system for all types of diseases and injuries or accidents in use in most medical-records libraries of hospitals across the country. This system also has various types of accidents coded as to method of causation. For those who are interested and have a computer orientation, it is suggested that ICDA is further considered for a ready-made entry into the development of a meaningful data base, which is currently lacking in the field of medical care.

This lack of hard data makes it impossible to estimate the actual cost of accidents occurring annually in the medical-care system. Medical care is now the third-ranking industry in the United States dollarwise. It is costing the American people approximately $75 billion annually.

Much of this cost cannot be pared because of the high percentage of employees per patient required in our present system. However, the insurance costs of professional liability cases can be markedly affected by an intelligent clinical engineer making the medical-care system a safer and more efficient environment for the patient, the doctor, and the hospital employee. To further the importance of a clinical engineer's position, the Joint Committee on Accreditation of Hospitals is now advising the initiation of such a position or a contract service. The Hartford Insurance Group is making available to its insured hospitals advice, reprints, inspections, and assistance in the entire area of hospital safety. It is suggested that the loss control department of a hospital's insurance carrier be consulted for assistance in selling various programs to administrators, developing program and staff, or arranging support for a full-scale safety survey of an institution's medical devices. Only in this way can the serious increase in insurance costs be reduced. What is perhaps even more important is that clinical engineers hold the key to saving an untold number of lives.

18

HOW MEDICAL-DEVICE LEGISLATION AFFECTS HEALTH-CARE PROFESSIONALS

M. J. Miller

Manufacturers of medical devices have long recognized that medical-device legislation, which after several years of consideration became law (PL 94-295) on May 28, 1976, in the United States will have a significant effect on the design, manufacture, and distribution of medical equipment. Less obvious but equally significant are the new responsibilities, potential limitations, and benefits of the new law to physicians and health-care personnel.

Responsibilities

1. Professional societies and professionals have a responsibility to help select the most qualified experts to serve on device classification and scientific panels, which will help the FDA make technical and scientific judgments.
2. Professionals and their societies have a responsibility to review and question scientific decisions by the advisory panels and the agency.
3. The professions must assume more responsibility for standards development and review.
4. Health-care professionals must realize that medical devices purchased or used that violate provisions of the new law may create presumptions of negligence in malpractice suits involving medical devices.

Limitations

1. Certain "special order" devices for individual patients can now only be made available by companies on a limited basis.

2. The use of new or improved devices of an investigational nature are subject to FDA application and approval and new informed-patient-consent requirements.

3. HEW, under stated circumstances, must order physicians and other ''health professionals'' who prescribe or use a ''defective'' device to notify patients of risks presented by the device and of any action that should be taken to reduce or eliminate risks. Query: What if the physician disagrees with the Agency that an individual patient should be informed? There may be serious legal and moral considerations.

4. The secretary may limit the use of ''restricted devices'' to certain health-care professionals to assure the safe and effective use of devices. (The extent of this authority is unclear.)

5. The secretary has the authority to require a manufacturer, distributor, or importer of a device to disclose the identity of a patient when required for the ''medical welfare of an individual, to determine the safety and effectiveness of a device, or to verify . . . information submitted'' under the law.

Benefits

1. The regulatory controls provided by the law will undoubtedly require manufacturers to be more exact in the design and manufacture of their products.

2. Unsafe and ineffective devices may be quickly removed from the marketplace.

3. Health-care professionals will receive much more information from the FDA and companies on use, maintenance, installation, and hazards of devices.

4. Manufacturers may have to assume more financial responsibility for repair, replacement, or refund of defective devices, which may reduce the financial burden on health-care professionals and facilities. (This area of authority is almost unprecedented in its potential impact on manufacturers, users, and health-care facilities.)

The Congress's intent, obviously, is that the positive implications by far outweigh the negative implications. The effect of the law on health-care professionals will be determined, to a great extent, by how well they understand the law and how they assume new responsibilities created by the law.

Device Law Summary

Definition

A ''device'' is defined as an instrument, apparatus, implement, machine, contrivance, implant, *in vitro* reagent or other similar related article, including any component, part, or accessory, which does not achieve any of its principal intended purposes through *chemical action* within or on the body of man or other animals and which is not dependent on being *metabolized* for the achievement of its principal intended purpose. The primary differentiation between a device and a drug and other products is the words "chemical action" and "metabolized."

Medical Device Classification

The law contemplates that all medical devices will ultimately be placed into three regulatory categories that will determine the type and extent of regulation applied to any medical device. All medical devices will be classified by expert panels (made up of medical, technical, consumer, and industry experts) into Class I, General Controls; Class II, Performance Standards; and Class III, Premarket Approval.

Classification panels may assign a device to any or all regulatory categories. In addition, a single medical device may be classified into different regulatory categories depending on the different uses to which a medical device may be put that may require different regulatory considerations.

Classification will be determined by the available evidence on safety and effectiveness. Criteria for determining safety and effectiveness are set forth in the law and require that consideration be given to (*a*) the persons for whose use the device is represented or intended; (*b*) the conditions of use prescribed, recommended, or suggested in the labeling; and (*c*) weighing of any probable benefit to health from the use of the device against any probable risk of illness or injury from such use.

Effectiveness will be determined by two types of evidence. The first is on the basis of "well-controlled investigations" as described in regulations of the FDA. The second is "valid scientific evidence" acceptable to the secretary under prescribed criteria.

Determinations of safety and effectiveness are relevant for purposes of classification, establishing performance standards, review of premarket approval applications, and for determining effectiveness whenever it is required in the amendments.

Criteria for Classification

General Controls. A device shall be assigned to general controls by a classification panel if general controls will provide a reasonable assurance of safety and effectiveness, or if there is inadequate information on safety and effectiveness, provided that the device is not represented for a use in sustaining or supporting human life or for a use that is of substantial importance in preventing impairment of human life and does not present a potential unreasonable risk of illness or injury.

Performance Standards. A classification finding must be made that general controls are insufficient to provide a reasonable assurance of safety and effectiveness, that standards would be sufficient, and that there is sufficient information available about the device to establish a standard.

Premarket Approval. This classification assignment requires a decision that there is not enough known to determine if general controls would provide a reasonable assurance of safe and effective performance, and not enough is known to establish a performance standard. A device will be assigned to Class III if (*a*) it is intended for use in supporting or sustaining human life or if of substantial importance in preventing impairment of human health; or (*b*) it presents a potential unreasonable risk of illness or injury.

Classification Procedures

Device classifications will be based on the recommendations of the classification panels established under the law. The classification panels are required to make classification recommendations to the FDA within 1 year of the date the funds are appropriated to implement the new law for devices on the market the day the law is passed.

"New" devices or devices placed on the market after enactment date that are not of the same type and are not substantially equivalent to those on the market on enactment day will automatically be placed in premarket approval and cannot be commercially marketed until either an application is approved or the device is reclassified into standards or general controls.

There are two further categorizations of premarket clearance devices that must be understood for purposes of classification and the application of transitional provisions. For definitional purposes, these premarket approval devices can be categorized as "old" and "me too" devices. "Old" devices can be described as those devices on the market on enactment day. "Me too" devices can be described as devices marketed after enactment day that are of the same type and are substantially equivalent to devices on the market on enactment day.

Devices first marketed after enactment day but that are of the same type and substantially equivalent to devices on the market on enactment day (i.e., "me too" devices) for classification purposes are treated the same as devices on the market on enactment day (i.e., old devices).

It is also useful to define as "critical" devices those devices that are implants of life-supporting and life-sustaining devices.

Critical devices will be classified into premarket approval unless FDA determines that premarket clearance is *not* necessary to provide reasonable assurance that there is safety and effectiveness and provides appropriate documentation supporting this decision.

After the FDA has received its recommendations from the classification panels, required after the 1-year period, the FDA will publish *proposed* recommendations for classification of all medical devices. After public comment, regulations will be published that will assign each device or class of device to one or more classifications. Proposed classification does not require any action by the manufacturer. After reviewing comments, the secretary shall publish a final classification.

Acting on the recommendation of the classification panel or on his own action, the secretary may exempt in whole or in part devices classified in general controls from registration and listing, records and reports, and good manufacturing practices requirements.

The secretary may, on his own initiative or on petition of an interested person, by regulation change a device's classification and revoke, because of the change of classification, any regulation or requirement in effect under Section 514 or 515 with respect to such device.

Classification recommendations from panels shall include (*a*) a summary of the reasons for the recommendation; (*b*) a summary of the data on which the recommendation is based; (*c*) an identification of the risk to health (if any) presented by the device with respect to which the recommendation is made; and (*d*) to the extent practicable include a recommendation for the assignment of a priority for the application of the premarket approval and standards sections of the law.

A regulation changing the classification of a device from Class III to Class II may provide that such classification not take effect until the effective date of a performance standard.

"New devices," which are automatically classified into Class III, shall remain in Class III until the effective date of an order of the secretary classifying the device into Class I or Class II. A manufacturer or importer of a device automatically classified in Class III because it is a "new" device may petition the secretary for the issuance of an order classifying the device into Class I or Class II after referring the petition to an appropriate classification panel.

Types of General Controls

Adulteration. The amendments supplement existing adulteration provisions of existing law and deem a device to be adulterated if it does not comply with an established performance standard to which it is subject, if it does not comply with premarket approval or product development protocol provisions, if it is a banned device, if it is in violation of good manufacturing practices, or if it fails to comply with an investigational use exemption.

Misbranding. The law requires the use of established device names on product labels and type size at least half as large as the proprietary name used. FDA has the authority to set the official name of a device, which would become its established name. Misbranded devices are devices produced in unregistered facilities, those devices not listed with the FDA, devices not in compliance with a uniform system of identification, and restricted devices not meeting labeling requirements. Misbranded devices would also include devices that fail to conform with the applicable labeling requirements of a standard. A device would also be misbranded when it fails to comply with the notification and other related remedies or when there is a failure or refusal to comply with the records and reports regulations established by the FDA.

Prohibited Acts. The amendments revise existing law to clearly state prohibited acts, which result from violations of provisions of the bill pertaining to classification, standards, premarket approval and product development protocols, banned devices, notification and other remedies, and provisions pertaining to custom devices, trade secrets, restricted devices, good manufacturing practices, investigational use devices, and other requirements of the bill.

Registration and Listing and Advance Notification. Manufacturers and processors of devices are required to register their facilities initially and annually thereafter with the FDA; initially list all devices with a 6-month update on new products in June and December; and to notify the FDA 90 days prior to the introduction or delivery of a device for commercial distribution. It is unclear whether or not advance notification is required for substantially new devices only. Advance notification requires that the manufacturer make a determination of the device's classification or the absence thereof with an explanation of determination and actions taken by the manufacturer to comply with a performance standard or premarket approval if applicable to the device.

Banned Devices. The FDA has the authority to ban a device from the market when it is established that the continuing availability of the device presents either substantial deception to the public or an unreasonable or substantial illness or injury. The secretary has the authority to ban a device upon a proposed regulation if the deception or risk of illness or injury presents an unreasonable, direct, and substantial danger to the health of individuals. In this case, the product will be removed from the market on the date of the publication of the proposed regulation. After opportunity for an informal hearing, the proposed regulation will either be affirmed, modified, or revoked. At that time only would appeal to the courts be permitted.

The law provides both procedural and substantive checks on the use of this remedy because of the extreme authority provided the secretary.

The FDA must make a positive determination that additional labeling or changes in labeling would not be adequate to correct or eliminate the deception or risk. If labeling would rectify the problem, the manufacturer must be given the opportunity to comply with the agency directives on labeling.

Notification. When the secretary finds that a device presents an unreasonable risk of substantial harm to the public health, and notification is necessary to eliminate the risk or harm, and no more practicable means is available to eliminate such risk, he may issue an order to assure that adequate notification is provided, by the persons and means best suited under the circumstances involved, to all health professionals who prescribe or use the device and to any other persons, including manufacturers, importers, distributors, retailers, and device users. Patients are to be notified of the risk unless the secretary determines that notice would present a greater danger to patients' health than no notification.

The secretary may require that physicians and other health professionals provide for the notification of the individuals treated with the device of the risk presented by the device and of any action that may be taken by or on behalf of such individuals to eliminate or reduce such risk.

Repair, Replacement, or Refund. Manufacturers, importers, and distributors or any combination of them may be required to repair a device, replace a nonconforming device, or refund the purchase price whenever the secretary determines that the device presents an unreasonable risk of substantial harm to the public health; the device was not properly designed and manufactured according to the state of the art when produced; the unreasonable risk was not caused by a third party's failure to exercise due care in the installation, maintenance, repair, or use of the device; and a notification order would not be adequate to eliminate the unreasonable risk.

Manufacturers would submit plans for repair, replacement, or refund to the secretary for approval, and if unsatisfactory, the FDA may revise or develop an appropriate plan.

Records and Reports. The FDA is provided the authority to prescribe regulations for records and reports by manufacturers, importers, and distributors. Records and reports will be limited to necessary procedures and submissions that are not unduly burdensome, and required records and reports must be fully explained as to their purpose. Patient identity will generally be protected. Records and reports for Class I devices may not require maintenance or submission of information not in the possession of the manufacturer, importer, or distributor.

Good Manufacturing Practices (GMPs). The FDA is authorized to develop GMP regulations, in consultation with an advisory committee of nine persons, to which manufacturers must adhere.

Manufacturers may obtain exemptions or variances from GMP requirements on petition and on demonstration that compliance with a requirement is not necessary, or if a variance is sought, that a suggested alternative approach is adequate.

Related to the GMP authority is an authority that permits the FDA to establish categories of products for the purpose of defining the degree of distribution traceability needed to protect the public health. No regulation promulgated under the act may require traceability for a type or class of device unless it is necessary to assure the protection of the public health.

Custom Devices. The custom-device exemption permits a physician or other health-care professional, designated by regulation, to order a device that deviates from an applicable performance standard or approved premarket review or product development protocol application. To qualify for the custom exemption (*a*) the device may not be generally available in finished form for purchase or offered for commercial distribution; and (*b*) the device must be intended and made in a specific form for an individual patient named in an individual practitioner's order, or the device must be intended to meet the special needs of the practitioner in the course of his professional practice. Custom devices may not be generally available to or used by other practitioners.

Restricted Devices. The FDA has the authority, by regulation, to restrict the sale, distribution, or use of certain devices. Devices that require the written or oral authorization of a practitioner licensed by law to administer or use the device and/or are subject to such other conditions as the FDA may prescribe are considered as restricted devices. Restrictions on sale, distribution, or use are necessary when the FDA finds that a device has a potential for harmful effect or because the collateral measures for use are such that there cannot be reasonable assurance of safety or effectiveness. No restriction may limit the use of a device to persons with specific training or experience unless the limitation is required for safe and effective use. In addition, restrictions may not exclude a physician from using a device solely because he is not board eligible or board certified in a medical specialty.

Administrative Restraint. The FDA is authorized to detain temporarily a device suspected to be adulterated or misbranded for a period not to exceed 20 days unless the FDA determines that a period of up to 30 days is needed for a seizure or injunctive action. Detention must be approved by a higher FDA official. Detention orders may be immediately appealed to the FDA. Within 5 days the FDA must, after opportunity for an informal hearing, either confirm or revoke the order under appeal.

Performance Standards

The law does not specifically define a performance standard. However, the effect of and what shall be included in a performance standard is partially described in the following provisions:

First, a performance standard shall include provisions to provide reasonable assurance of a device's safe and effective performance.

Safety and Effectiveness

The phrase "safety and effectiveness" and qualifying rules will be used to judge standards and whether or not they serve the intended regulatory purpose.

The safety and effectiveness of a device are to be determined (*a*) with respect to the persons for whose use the device is represented or intended; (*b*) with respect to the conditions of use prescribed, recommended, or suggested in the device labeling; and (*c*) weighing any probable risk of illness or injury from such use.

The House Committee Report states that the criteria for safety and effectiveness are intended by the committee to include reliability of a device.

In some instances, the safety and effectiveness of a device intended for use only by health professionals will not be evaluated in terms of suitability for use by lay individuals. This is the case in which the persons for whom the use of the device is represented or intended may be primarily health professionals.

As noted, the requirements of safety and effectiveness are to be determined on the basis of conditions of use prescribed, recommended, or suggested in labeling. This is not intended to preclude the secretary from considering the actual uses to which a device is put or those uses promoted through advertising. Thus, the law, according to the House report, may broaden the secretary's authority to assure that every device is appropriately labeled. This labeling authority could include labeling intended for patients, health professionals, or both.

The phrase "conditions of use" is intended to include consideration of the environment in which a device is to be used.

The key concept that the safety and effectiveness of a device are to be determined "weighing any probable benefit to health from the use of the device against any probable risk of injury or illness from such use" makes it clear that the legislation recognizes that products having the power to be useful in the healing arts also have the potential to do harm and that the determination of safety and effectiveness is to balance carefully these considerations.

As a general rule, device *effectiveness* is to be determined on the basis of well-controlled investigations by qualified experts, including clinical investigations when appropriate, from which it can be concluded by qualified experts that the device will have the effect it purports or is represented to have. This requirement is derived from existing provisions of the act relating to drugs.

The legislation does provide, however, that the secretary may authorize that the effectiveness of the device be determined on the basis of valid scientific evidence other than the well-controlled studies required by the general rule.

Other Standards Requirements

The second category of standards requirements provides that a performance standard established under the law shall, where necessary to provide reasonable assurance of its safe and effective performance include:

1. *Provisions respecting the construction, components, ingredients, and properties of the device and its compatibility with power systems and connections for such systems.* This provision obviously permits the FDA to develop standards, where necessary, that will dictate the design characteristics of certain medical devices and to develop "standardization" or system compatibility standards.

2. *Provisions for the testing (on a sample basis or, if necessary, on an individual basis) of the device or, if it is determined that no other more practicable*

means are available to the secretary to assure the conformity of the device to the standard, provisions for the testing (on a sample basis or, if necessary, on an individual basis) by the secretary or by another person under the direction of the secretary. This permits the FDA or an agent of the FDA to individually or lot sample or test each device to assure the conformity of the device to a standard. The burden for testing may also be placed solely on the manufacturer.

3. *Provisions for the measurement of the performance characteristics of the device*. According to the House Committee Report, this refers to testing procedures or methods that are the means by which conformance to standards are to be evaluated. This may also include quality-control procedures, means by which users may ascertain device performance, and methods for use by the secretary in judging compliance with the standard.

4. *Provisions requiring that before the device is introduced or delivered for introduction into interstate commerce, for commercial distribution, the results of each or of certain of the tests of the device required to be made under the law show that the device is in conformity with the portions of the standard for which the rest or tests were required*. Here the burden will be on the manufacturer.

5. *A provision requiring that the sale and distribution of the device be restricted but only to the extent that the sale and distribution of the device may be restricted under other provisions pertaining to restrictions on device use*.

6. *A third category of requirements provides that standards shall, where appropriate, require the use and prescribe the form and content of the labeling for the proper installation, maintenance, operation, and use of the device*. The committee report indicates that the provisions of the standard requiring labeling for the proper installation, maintenance, operation, and use of the device may, where appropriate, include instructions or warnings, information as to storage and transportation, expiration dates, results to be expected from the device, ranges of accuracy of diagnosis, instructions as to the proper care of the device, and equipment to be used with the device. Where necessary, labeling may also specify that the device is to be only considered safe or effective when used by or in the treatment of a patient who has been tested under certain diagnostic procedures by an appropriately skilled person and found to have an illness or condition for which the device is indicated.

It is important to note that the manufacturer will be subjected to two forms of labeling authority. First, a general labeling authority under the "general controls" provisions of the law; and second, a labeling authority set forth in standards. Presumably, the labeling requirements under standards will be very specific concerning the areas mentioned above. For example, during the development of a standard, the FDA may determine that an appropriate way to regulate an essential characteristic of a device is to assure safety and effectiveness by labeling rather than by a performance standard.

The House committee expects that a demonstration that a device is in conformance with portions of the standard for which tests are required would ordinarily be implemented through procedures whereby manufacturers either certify to the purchasers that the device conforms to an applicable performance standard or periodically make such a certification to the secretary.

The committee indicates that the provisions authorizing testing permit both clinical testing and testing relevant to technical characteristics of the device. The report also makes it clear that in certain instances the secretary will require third-party testing of individual devices.

In summary, the FDA has few limitations on what it might construe to be a medical-device standard. As a matter of fact, the conference report eliminated a provision in the law that stated that a performance standard established under the law may not include any provision not required or authorized by the subsections outlined above.

If a device is classified in Class II, it will be required to conform to an applicable performance standard only after promulgation of a regulation establishing the standard and only upon such date as the secretary makes the standard applicable to the Class II device, which can generally be no earlier than 1 year after the promulgation of the regulation establishing a standard. If the secretary reclassifies a Class III device into Class II, he may provide that the reclassification not take effect until the effective date of the performance standard for such a device. General controls will also continue to apply to a Class II device unless specifically superseded by a provision of the standard.

The outline of an FDA medical-device standard may be similar in approach to the outline presented in the AAMI *Draft Standard Guidelines*. This guideline at least provides a frame of reference.

Establishing and Promulgating Standards

The following is a sequential walk through the process or procedures envisioned by the law by which manufacturers and investigators are affected by the standards provisions.

First, as has been described earlier, the manufacturer or investigator will have his device classified or reclassified by a classification panel and the secretary.

Second, the secretary will initiate a proceeding for the development of a performance standard by a publication in the Federal Register of a notice of an opportunity to submit to the secretary a request (within 15 days of the date of the publication of the notice) for a change in the classification of the device based on new information relevant to its classification. In other words, the first step in any proceeding for a federal medical-device standard is providing an opportunity for reclassification of the medical device into another category of regulation (i.e., Class I or Class II).

Third, if the secretary receives a request for a change in classification, he shall within 60 days of the publication of such notice and after consulting an appropriate panel either deny the request for change of classification or give notice of his intent to initiate such a change.

Fourth, if no reclassification occurs, the secretary then publishes in the Federal

Register a notice inviting any person, including any federal agency, to submit to the secretary within 60 days (*a*) an existing standard; or (*b*) an offer, within 60 days after the date of the publication notice, to develop such a proposed standard. This notice shall specify the following: (*a*) a period within which the standard is to be developed; (*b*) a description or other designation of the device; (*c*) a statement of the nature of the risk or risks associated with the use of the device and intended to be controlled by a performance standard; (*d*) a summary of the data on which the secretary has found a need for initiation of the proceeding to develop a performance standard; and (*e*) identification of any existing performance standard known to the secretary that may be relevant to the proceedings.

Both the statement of risk and summary of data should include pertinent portions of classification panel recommendations with respect to the device.

Fifth, at this point in time, the secretary can either accept an existing medical-device standard developed by a government agency, including the FDA, or accept a voluntary medical-device standard or an offer or offers to develop a standard from a government agency or private entity. The committee report states:

> The committee also understands that several "voluntary" medical device standards have been developed or are in the process of being developed by various standards-setting organizations. If the Secretary determines that a standards-setting organization has appropriate qualifications and that a voluntary standard has been subjected to appropriate scientific consideration, it may be accepted, in whole or in part, as a proposed performance standard.

Sixth, if the secretary determines that a performance standard cannot be developed by a federal agency or that a performance standard has not been issued, has not been adopted, or is not being developed by any federal agency or by any other qualified entity and does not receive a performance standard in existence, he may accept an offer to develop a standard from an appropriate private or public contractor.

The law permits and encourages the FDA to rely heavily on federal agencies in performing its function under the standards section of the bill. The FDA may rely on a qualified government agency to develop a standard rather than accepting an offer from a private entity.

The law implies or encourages the secretary to approach standards with the following priorities:

1. Obtain an existing standard from a qualified government agency or, if there is no other existing standard, have a government agency develop a standard
2. Adopt an appropriate "voluntary" medical-device standard that has been developed by a standards-setting organization
3. Contract with a qualified organization for the development of a performance standard

In the last category, the secretary may accept an offer or offers to develop a performance standard if he determines that the offerer is technically competent and qualified under certain criteria.

The qualifications of an offerer are that the offerer be qualified to develop a standard and is technically competent to undertake and complete the development of an appropriate performance standard within the period specified in the notice. In determining the qualifications of an offerer to develop a standard, the Secretary shall examine the offerer's financial stability, expertise, experience, and any potential conflicts of interest, including a financial interest in the device for which that standard is to be developed.

A key phrase in the law is a "business entity" offerer. If the offerer is a business entity, it must comply with the following provision:

> The Secretary shall by regulation require that an offeror of an offer to develop a proposed performance standard submit (and if the offeror is a business entity, require that appropriate directors, officers, and employees of, and consultants to, the business entity submit) to the Secretary such information concerning the offeror as the Secretary determines is relevant with respect to the offeror's qualifications to develop a proposed performance standard for a device, including information respecting the offeror's financial stability, expertise, and experience, and any potential conflicts of interest, including financial interest in the device for which the proposed standard is to be developed, current industrial or commercial affiliates of the offeror, current sources of financial support for research, and relevant business entities in which the offeror has a financial interest.

The secretary may contribute to the offeror's cost in developing a medical-device standard if the secretary determines that such contribution is likely to result in a more satisfactory standard than would be developed without such contribution.

Standards developed by offerers are subject to regulations providing that

1. Performance standards be supported by such test data or other documentation or materials as the secretary may reasonably require
2. Notice be given to interested persons of the opportunity to participate in the development of such performance standards and require the provision of such opportunity
3. Records be maintained to disclose the course of the development of standards, comments and other information submitted by any person, and such other matters that may be relevant to the evaluation of standards

As noted earlier, in the event that no person or organization submits a standard, the secretary does not accept an offer to develop a standard, or where the secretary has accepted an offer but determines that the offeror is unwilling or unable to develop the standard or the performance standard is unsatisfactory, the secretary may proceed to develop a performance standard.

When the secretary does develop a performance standard, certain due-process requirements apply, such as: Notice must be given to persons of the opportunity to participate in the development of such a performance standard, and such opportunity must be provided; the maintenance of appropriate records; and other requirements pertaining to notice and opportunity for participation.

After the development or acceptance of a standard, the secretary initiates proceedings that lead to the promulgation of a mandatory standard. First, however, the secretary must propose the standard with the notice of proposed rule making with an opportunity for comment. The notice of proposed standard must set forth proposed findings with respect to the degree of risk or illness or injury designed to be eliminated or reduced by the proposed standard.

The secretary also has the authority to terminate the standards proceedings with reason, but a notice of termination must be accompanied by a notice of a proceeding for a reclassification of a device into either Class I or Class III, or both.

After the expiration of the period for comment on a proposed performance standard and after consideration of such comments and any report from an advisory committee, the Secretary promulgates in the Federal Register a regulation establishing a performance standard, or, once again, he may publish a notice terminating the proceeding, with reasons, with the notice of an intent to reclassify the medical device into Class I and/or III.

During the rule-making proceedings leading to a medical-device standard, the secretary, on his own or upon the request of an interested person, unless the secretary finds the request to be without good cause, may refer a proposed regulation for the establishment, amendment, or revocation of a performance standard to an advisory committee of experts for report and recommendation with respect to any matter involved with the proposed regulation that requires the exercise of scientific judgment. The committee must respond within 60 days with reports and recommendations. The advisory panels may not be classification panels, but individual members can serve on both types of panels.

A regulation establishing a performance standard shall set forth the dates on which the standard shall take effect. No standard may take effect before 1 year after the date of its publication unless the secretary determines that an earlier effective date is necessary for certain devices for the protection of public health and safety. For example, a standard that has been established for a device that has been reclassified from Class III to Class II may have an earlier effective date. The bill indicates that such an effective date shall be established so as to minimize, consistent with the public health and safety, economic loss or disruption or dislocation of domestic and international trade.

The committee report indicates that "stockpiling" of nonconforming devices is discouraged since standards will apply to all devices in commercial channels on their effective dates.

A proposed amendment to a performance standard may be made effective on its publication if the secretary determines, after an opportunity for an informal hearing, that such action would be in the public interest. This will permit innovative devices, prior to an amended standard, to be marketed and will not prohibit the marketing of nonconforming devices during the proposal stage. The committee report indicates that the expedited approach is intended to stimulate desirable changes in "standardized" products without penalizing manufacturers of products on the market that conform to existing standards.

Premarket Clearance Standards

The premarketing clearance authority provided HEW under the bill permits a manufacturer to deviate from an FDA standard if, in an application for premarket clearance, the manufacturer presents adequate information to justify any deviation from such standard. Otherwise, a manufacturer of a Class III device must show that he meets the provisions of a medical-device standard in his premarket clearance application. It should be noted that failure to conform with a standard will enable the secretary to withdraw an approval of a premarket clearance application. In addition, a product development protocol, for purposes of an approved completed protocol application, requires that applicable standards be conformed to or noncomformance justified.

Priorities for Standards

The law states that in making their classification recommendations the panels shall also establish a priority for standards promulgation by the secretary.

Judicial Review

The medical-device law provides that the following decisions pertaining to standards may be reviewed by the courts:

1. A final classification or reclassification changing the classification of a device
2. The promulgation of a regulation establishing, amending, or revoking a performance standard for a device

Premarket Approval

Despite formal classification of a device into Class III or premarket approval, the law provides that "old" and "me too" devices are not required to have an approved application for premarket approval until the FDA promulgates a regulation requiring an application. This regulation is in addition to the regulation classifying the device.

Although the law imposes no deadline on the FDA for regulations requiring applications, the law provides that the earliest date that old and "me too" devices can be required to have an application for premarket approval is 30 months after the publication of the regulation that classified the device. In addition, the regulation must provide at least 90 days after the promulgation of the regulation for the submission of the application.

As noted earlier, "new" devices are automatically placed into premarket clearance until reclassified.

The FDA will publish the proposed regulation requiring premarket approval in the Federal Register, which must contain the findings on the degree of risk sought to be eliminated or reduced and must provide an opportunity (within 15 days) to request a change of classification based on new information about the device. If a reclassification petition is filed, the FDA must consult with the appropriate classification panel and within 60 days either deny the petition or begin an action to reclassify the device. If there is no petition to reclassify, the FDA will proceed to publish a final regulation for premarket approval or publish a notice of termination and reclassify under statutory requirements.

A premarket approval application will provide the FDA with reports of investigations on the safety and effectiveness of the device; a statement of its components and principles; a description of the methods, facilities, and controls used for its manufacture; a reference to any performance standard that would be applicable to the device if it were a Class II device; a sample of the device, where practicable, and, if submission of a sample is not practicable, the location of a sample; specimens of labeling; and such other information that the FDA, with the concurrence of appropriate reclassification panels, may require. After the application has been referred to the appropriate classification panel for study and submission of a report respecting approval of the application, the FDA is to approve or disapprove the application within 180 days of its receipt unless a greater period of time is agreed on by the FDA and the applicant. No agreement to extend review time may be made for a Class III device on the market on the day the amendments were passed unless the FDA finds that continued availability of the device is necessary for the protection of the public health.

An application may be denied if it fails to show reasonable safety or effectiveness of the device, conformance with good manufacturing practices, appropriate labeling for the device, or lack of conformance to an applicable standard that is a requirement for approval.

Any application may require restrictions on the sale or distribution of the device.

Product Development Protocol

The product development protocol and the notice of PDP completion is an alternative to the premarket approval application process.

The House committee report ". . . recognizes that many devices are subject to frequent modification during development. For this reason it has designed a provision . . . whereby the investigation of a device and the development of information necessary for its approval are merged into one regulatory mechanism." However, the language of this section does not restrict it to modification of existing devices.

The PDP approach for a device is dependent on the FDA's decision that the approach is appropriate in lieu of an application for premarket approval. The FDA cannot, however, require the PDP procedure.

Assuming that FDA approves the PDP process, the manufacturer must obtain approval of a protocol that describes the device to be developed, describes any preclinical or clinical trials to be conducted on the device, including results to be expected, and any other relevant information. The protocol must be approved or disapproved within 120 days of receipt.

The product development protocol approach includes the investigational process, whereas the premarket approval application process more clearly delineates (or separates) the investigational-use exemption and the application process. There are at least four apparent differences between the investigational-use exemption provided in the bill and the PDP investigation procedure found in the premarket approval section of the law. These are as follows:

1. The clinical testing protocol is to be decided by a local institutional review committee under the investigational exemption and by a classification or advisory panel when the PDP is utilized.
2. Once the investigational device process is completed, the manufacturer must still complete the premarket application process, whereas under the PDP, there is a second stage in the statute that leads right into the premarket-approval process.
3. Investigation can begin more quickly under the investigational device exemption. Investigation can begin after 30 days after an investigation application is filed unless the FDA forbids further investigation, whereas under the PDP, the FDA simply refers the protocol to the classification or advisory panel for review.
4. Progress reports and a complete record on completion of the PDP are required but not under the investigational use exemption.

After the protocol has been accepted, the manufacturer must submit a notice of completion of the PDP. Such a notice will include a determination that there is no reason bearing on safety and effectiveness why the notice should not be approved; data on which such determination is based; and the results of any preclinical or clinical trials required by the protocol. Within 90 days after the notice of completion is submitted, the FDA is required to either issue an order declaring it completed, or, after affording an opportunity for an informal hearing, issue an order declaring it not completed.

The FDA may declare a PDP not completed if it finds a failure to comply with the requirements of the protocol; that the results of the trials differ substantially from those required by the protocol; or that there is a lack of showing of safety and effectiveness of the device.

A completed and approved PDP approval has the same effect as an order approving an application for premarket approval.

The law sets forth such conditions under which applications and PDP completions may be revoked.

Exemption for Investigational Use of Devices

An exemption for the investigational use of a device must be obtained if the investigation would result in violation of provisions of the act pertaining to misbranding, registration and listing, performance standards, premarket approval, banned devices, records and reports, listing and certification of color additives, restricted devices, or good manufacturing practices. Almost all, if not all, "new" devices will require an exemption regardless of how they are classified.

It is important to note that the classification of a device into Class I, II, or III has no effect on whether or not the device must obtain an investigational exemption. Earlier versions of Congressional bills required an investigational exemption only for premarket approval devices. This was changed in the final law.

Within 120 days after enactment, the FDA will, by regulation, establish procedures and conditions under which investigational exemptions will be granted. The investigator will submit an application to the FDA and will maintain records and make reports to the FDA as necessary to assure compliance with the conditions for exemption to allow for agency review of the progress of the investigation. The procedures and conditions may vary depending on the scope and duration of clinical testing to be conducted, the number of human subjects involved, the changes contemplated in the device during investigation, and whether the device is being tested for ultimate commercial distribution.

When human testing is involved, the investigator must develop a plan for proposed clinical testing that must be submitted to a local institutional review committee or, if none exists or is inadequate, to the FDA for approval. If other investigators are involved, the primary investigator must obtain a signed agreement from other investigators that the testing will be under the principal investigator's supervision and that informed consent will be obtained from each human subject or his representative. These agreements will be submitted to the FDA.

Informed consent must be obtained from each human subject or his representative. Although the details of informed consent are not in the new law, legislative history instructs the FDA to develop regulations to cover all elements of informed consent as set forth in the Senate bill. This regulation must ultimately conform to the recommendations of the National Commission on the Protection of Human Subjects of Biomedical and Behavioral Research when they are adopted.

Applications for an investigational-use exemption are deemed to be approved on the thirtieth day after their submission unless specifically disapproved by FDA and notice of disapproval is provided to the applicant.

Protection of Trade Secrets

First, Section 301(j) of the Federal Food, Drug, and Cosmetic Act prohibits the using by any persons to his advantage or the revealing of any information acquired under relevant sections of the amendments concerning any method or process that as a trade secret is entitled to protection. Second, the general federal confidentiality statute prohibits officers and employees of the United States from divulging information that concerns or relates to trade secrets. Third, the Freedom of Information Act contains a provision that exempts "trade secrets and financial information that is privileged or confidential" from the requirement of mandatory public disclosure.

As a general rule, safety and effectiveness data for premarket approval devices filed within the trade-secret exemption and regulations would preclude the disclosure of such data unless the applicant has previously made the information public; the device has been disapproved or withdrawn from the market; or the device has reached the stage at which it may be marketed without submission of such data to the agency for approval.

Since the secretary will not be able to determine the confidentiality of safety and effectiveness data submitted for devices until he makes a final decision on classification, safety and effectiveness data and information submitted to a panel, except for material that has been previously disclosed to the public, shall be considered confidential until a decision on final classification is reached.

There is considerably less protection for information submitted to the Secretary for Class I and Class II devices.

Trade-secret information may not be used by the secretary as the basis for reclassification of a device from Class III to Class II or as the basis for the establishment or amendment of a performance standard for a device reclassified from Class III to Class II.

The law authorizes the secretary to release information exempt from disclosure to a person not in his employment if such a person requires the information in connection with an activity undertaken by contract with the secretary if, as a condition of a release of such trade secrets or other confidential information to contractors, the secretary shall require that the person receiving a tape prescribe security precautions.

The law has a new provision that would require the secretary to promulgate regulations under which a detailed summary of information on the safety and effectiveness of a device, which was the basis for major decisions made by him with respect to a device, be released to the public. Such summaries are required to include information respecting any adverse effects of the device on health. By regulation, the FDA is required to develop a content of summaries for each of the following actions:

1. Issuance of an order approving, denying approval of, or withdrawing approval of an application for premarket approval or on advisory committee recommendations thereon
2. On issuance of an order revoking an approved premarket development protocol, declaration of approval or nonapproval of a protocol, revoking the approval of a protocol, revoking the approval of a protocol previously declared completed, or on advisory committee recommendations thereon
3. On issuance of an order approving an investigational-use exemption for a previously banned device or an order disapproving or withdrawing approval of such exemption

As a general rule, the release of summary information for a particular device will not be made until the FDA makes a final determination that the device cannot be approved and all legal appeals have been exhausted. In addition, no summary, after release, may be used to establish the safety or effectiveness of another device for purposes of the act.

Inspections

The new law grants the FDA authority to inspect certain records, which supplements the FDA's existing authority to inspect the establishments of device manufacturers, including equipment, materials, containers, and labeling.

A distinction is made, relative to the FDA's inspection authority, between restricted devices and other devices.

All records required to be maintained under the records and reports section or the section pertaining to investigational exemptions for devices may be reviewed during an FDA inspection. The inspector is authorized to verify the contents of records and make copies of the records.

Where restricted devices are involved, inspectors are authorized to inspect records, files, papers, processes, controls, and facilities to determine if such devices are adulterated or misbranded.

State and Local Requirements

As a general rule, no state or political subdivision may establish or continue in effect any requirement, under the new law, that is different from or an addition to requirements under the federal law related to the safety or effectiveness of the device or other matters concerning the devices addressed in the federal law. There are two important exemptions. The state or locality may petition for an exemption where the requirement would be more stringent than a requirement under federal law or the requirement is necessary because of compelling local conditions.

Exported Devices

Devices that do not conform to existing law and the new law may be exported if (*a*) they conform to the specifications of a foreign purchaser; (*b*) they are not in conflict with the laws of the country of destination; (*c*) they are labeled on the shipping package for export; and (*d*) they are not sold or offered for sale in domestic commerce. In addition, the new law applies these conditions with additional conditions for export of devices that do not comply with an applicable performance standard or a requirement relating to premarket approval. Such nonconforming devices may be exported if the FDA determines that exportation is not contrary to public health and safety and has the approval of the country of destination.

There are specific provisions with important but limited applicability that are not covered by this summary, including transitional provisions for new drugs that are now devices; color additives; presumption of interstate commerce; small manufacturer assistance; and judicial review of agency action.

The legislative history for this law includes House Report 94-853; Senate Report 94-93; and Conference Report 94-1090. All of these documents may be ordered from either the House or Senate Document Room, U.S. Capitol, Washington, D.C. Public Law 94-295 may be obtained from the Superintendent of Documents, Washington, D.C. 20402.

PART V

MANAGEMENT AND HOSPITAL-ADMINISTRATION PREMISES

19

TECHNOLOGY IN MANAGEMENT OF MEDICAL CARE

J. H. Busser, G. Arbona, M. Arnold, R. F. Bridgman, A. Brodziak, W. Hobson, D. Jurela, J. Van Der Maas, I. Margan, J. W. Owen, L. Petrovic, M. Prywes, A. Remond, G. Thomas, R. Tomovic, M. J. Van Trommel, D. Salinas, and G. Zarkovic

Management is the art and sometimes the science of deciding between alternatives and manipulating the appropriate tools to accomplish the task. Clearly, if managers are to arrive at the best possible decisions, they must know and fully comprehend the numerous alternatives. One of these alternatives is the application of various forms of technology to solve modern management problems—health-care-management problems being no exception.

The goal of management in the health services is to provide the best possible health care efficiently and effectively, thus satisfying the needs of the consumer (patient) and the professional standards of the provider (the health-care worker).

The term "health care," as it is used here, includes any type of care provided by physicians, nurses, dentists, allied health professionals, and others and does not distinguish between preventive, diagnostic, therapeutic, and rehabilitative services or between physical, emotional, and social components of health and disease.

In this context, then, health-care management relates to the functions of planning, organizing, implementing, controlling, and evaluating the delivery of health services. Primary emphasis is placed on those problems and technologies associated with *primary care* and, in particular, the first level of contact—*primary contact* between the individual in need and the provider of the needed care. A health-care system is composed of individuals and groups of professional people who cooperate and pool their skills in order to improve the health of a given population. Usually, they are united in an organized grouping or institution.

It is the function of health-care management to optimize the structure and reap the greatest benefits from the investment of human, material, and financial resources. It is also important for management to be aware that goals shift from time to time in response to changing social conditions; so good management is flexible management, alert to changes and able to react to them. The organizational structure must be dynamic rather than static.

There is a vast store of knowledge in the field of management. For several decades, technology has been exploited as a planning and management aid for industry, the military, and in some sections of government, yet these techniques are not well known in the health-care management field and are not often used. It is strongly recommended that an investment in time and money for education and training of managers of health-care systems be made in order that they may benefit from this accumulated knowledge.

The Problem

There are enormous variations in the use of primary health-care services, with the average number of visits to health-care providers per person per year varying from zero to 15. Many people do not use health-care services when they should because they are unaware of the service, because the service is relatively inaccessible, because of language difficulties, or because of the expense involved. At the other end of the scale are those who go to health centers for help with problems other than health. Many in this group are faced with social and psychological problems that health-care personnel at these centers are not prepared to handle, while others use the service to obtain illness certificates to justify absences from work or school.

In some instances, the health-care system is regulated in a way that makes it necessary for a person to enter through the primary level; in others, the matter is left to personal choice. In both situations, technology can be of great assistance, particularly through the use of easily operated mechanisms for the transfer of information from and to the primary level.

Modern technology has not made a significant contribution to the organization and management of health-care-delivery systems. This is particularly important at the primary level of care. Its potential for gathering and processing information required for planning, administration, and education has not been exploited, nor has it been used to improve patient care. This situation exists not because techniques and technologies are lacking but because health-care managers are unaware of them or are unable to put them into practice. If technology is to serve well, it must be introduced and used by people who are committed to and responsible for its success. They must understand not only the technology but also the health-care system from the inside. Moreover, it must be recognized that the application of technology to health-care management will not result in cheaper service but in better-quality service for the same expenditure.

At the same time, it must be recognized that as individuals and societies we put a price on human life and suffering every day, albeit under different sets of rules that vary from individual to individual and from nation to nation. There are cultural variations in the style of management, just as there are variations in the perception of what is health. These differences in perception make it difficult to define a quality unit of measure that can be satisfactorily applied to a health-care system and that a system of technology can handle.

Part of the cause for the rapid advances in the cost of health care can be attributed to unavoidable factors, for example:

1. Technical progress and new life-saving medical procedures
2. Increased demand by low- and middle-income groups
3. Aging populations
4. Preventive medicine being applied to more of a given population
5. Increases in the number and skills of health care personnel

The rest of the problem of runaway costs is probably due to defective organization and management of health services that result in inefficiency. These include:

1. Lack of coordination of medical records between different health institutions (or even between different departments in the same institution) that results in duplication of diagnostic procedures
2. Poor geographical distribution of health-care institutions
3. Obsolete administrative practices
4. Competition between public and private sectors
5. Uneven qualifications of health-care personnel
6. High cost of hospital construction and equipment and under-utilization of the latter

The result of these deficiencies is a growth rate for health costs that exceeds the growth rate of the gross national product (GNP). In the 1950s, United States health costs were estimated to be about 4% of the GNP. Today, they are between 6 and 8% and in some regions are expected to reach 10% by the year 2000.

In the United States market economy, GNP is privately owned in the form of salaries, employee benefits, capital investments, company stocks, etc. About 50% of the GNP remains in private ownership. The government takes 25 to 30% of the GNP through taxes, and the remaining 25% is the "social budget." This, in turn, breaks down to 5% for medical care, 12% for sickness benefits and pensions, and 8% for family allowances.

Thus, health care is supported by funds collected from employees and employers and controlled by committees culled from the same two groups. Under these circumstances, public health care is allotted about 5% of the state budget or 0.0125% of the GNP. Since 0.7% is necessary to meet total expenditures, the public health authority in a market economy system is responsible for only a part of our health care, usually primary preventive services, public assistance for noninsured patients, and contributions to capital investment for health-care centers and hospitals.

When a market economy and industrial development have a high priority, the GNP increases 8 to 12% per year. Regrettably, this growth is not generally matched with a similar increase in the allocated budget for health. Much of the industrial investment goes into automation, which requires no large labor force that will contribute to the social budget, and health care itself is a labor-intensive industry.

Considerations

1. The health-care provider is a responsible individual and as such is accountable for what he does and how he does it.

2. An accounting and budgeting system is an essential component for the useful application of technology as an aid in the management process.

3. There are appropriate technologies available that can be profitably used to assist in the various functions of management, such as planning, organizing, implementing, administering, controlling, and evaluating the delivery of health-care services.

4. The introduction of technologies into health-care management must be undertaken by professionals from within the health-care system who are committed to the success of innovations.

5. Introduction of technology into health-care management will improve the quality of health care provided per unit of cost but will probably not reduce the overall cost of health care.

6. Management planning is a capital expenditure that is necessary for better health care, but it should not be expected to reduce health-care costs.

7. Technologies available today for use in the management of health-care-delivery systems include (*a*) mechanisms (hardware) for data collection at the primary contact level and for transmission and/or storage of the data for use at other levels in the health-care system; (*b*) techniques and methods for identifying populations at risk and assessing their probable needs for health care; (*c*) models for use in optimizing the ratio of cost to benefit under given sets of social and economic constraints; and (*d*) systems for collecting the data, which must be available before making decisions relative to (*c*).

8. At the present time, there is no ideal or universal method for health-care management and therefore no universally applicable technology to help in the process.

9. A vital component in the application of technologies to health-care management is the education of the manager. At the present time, this is best accomplished by users and nonusers of technology meeting to compare and learn from each other.

10. A body of knowledge exists that is relevant to the introduction of various levels of technology into various levels of management. What does not exist is an organized study of the transfer of these technologies into the health-care system. A great variety of management systems and technological aids to those systems are presently being tried and tested. None has been shown to be universally acceptable, particularly at the primary level of care, which for some reason has been the last level of care to be investigated. If available, such systems would also have great value in the teaching of medicine.

11. The universal computer-based management system is still in the future, but several small simple steps that could do a great deal to achieve better patient care and patient management are now possible. These simple steps are quite involved and will cost a great deal of money. To introduce uniformity will require costly changes in record-storage facilities (files, file cabinets) and the transcription of old records to new formats.

12. The institutionalization of health-care services must be recognized as a factor. This is happening. However, wherever and whenever institutionalization takes place, it is mandatory to include technology in its plan, for without it the institution cannot know what it is doing or how it is doing it.

13. In order to determine the appropriate territorial distribution of health-care centers, it is necessary first to identify the dynamic health needs of the population to be served. The answer is not a simple geographical distribution, particularly when modern transportation facilities are available.

14. There is an observable difference in the pattern of health-care use between populations. As the age of a given population increases, the health-care use expressed as an average number of visits per year increases for developed populations.

15. Medical staff presently take personal records and medical histories. With the rising level of education, it is increasingly possible for the patient, the patient's family, or paramedical staff to do this work, thus freeing the medical staff from clerical duties.

16. There is presently a lack of confidence in the effectiveness, completeness, and accuracy of examinations and laboratory tests carried out at various levels of the health-care system. This results in duplication of examinations, of forms to be filled out by patients and physicians, and of laboratory and other tests. This can be overcome by placing greater emphasis on the use of management technology and standardized record systems, for only in this way can the use of standard procedures be accepted.

17. While it is possible to standardize health-care services, it is not possible to predict a uniform outcome from such services because of the diversity among any given patient population. Further, because individuals are constantly evolving and changing, the response to health-care services will also shift, requiring a structure and management that responds in a dynamic way.

Recommendations

1. An urgent need exists for educating and training health-care managers in management technologies and the best techniques and methods for applying them. The health-care manager today is too little aware of the available options. In order to make decisions between the various possibilities, managers must be in possession of all the available knowledge.

2. It is strongly recommended that an investment in time and money for education and training of managers of health-care systems be made so that these systems may benefit from the accumulated management knowledge.

3. There is an urgent need to assign a higher priority to funds for planning purposes or to provide funds specifically for planning purposes. Funds for health care are universally small. Money used for planning is not available for use in providing health-care services. Present priorities assign money first to provide services, which usually leaves little or nothing for planning.

4. A need exists for permanent planning groups or committees for health-care management whose function is to investigate new techniques and technologies helpful in the planning and management of patient care; equipment purchase and maintenance; building design and construction; patient screening procedures; health-care-delivery systems and mechanisms; clinical management; use of computers and communication systems; work classifications and job descriptions; local and centralized patient record systems; and patient and physician identification.

5. Cooperative studies of many different systems of health-care services, including technology now in use, would be of significant value to management, as would further opportunities for experts in the use of modern technology and managers of health-care services to exchange information and experiences.

6. When planning for the application of technology to health-care management, it is essential that the people who are to use the technology be involved with its selection and implementation even if this requires their extensive education and training.

7. In order to reduce present duplication of patient records and record transcription and excessive use of physicians' time on such matters, it will be necessary to create central storage facilities for patient data with easily accessible output. However, such output must also be protected for confidentiality.

8. It will be necessary to develop simplified procedures involving modern technology designed to facilitate transfer of information from the primary contact level to other levels of the health-care system. It will also be necessary to institute uniform (standardized) quality-control procedures in taking patient data.

9. In order to overcome the present lack of physician confidence in data generated at other levels of the health-care system, it will be necessary to institute uniform (standardized) quality-control procedures in taking patient data.

10. The general practitioner or other generalist, such as the nurse-practitioner, can be the center of responsibility for the patient's destiny within the health-care system, assisted as needed by medical specialists of all kinds. This will require a restructuring of many organizational and institutional practices.

11. It will be desirable to restructure medical education institutions to place greater emphasis on primary medical care, for only in this way can the present trend of extreme specialization be reversed and an awareness of the needs of primary care become an essential part of medical education.

Health-care needs are the sum of (*a*) the level of medical care seen as desirable by the medical profession and as perceived by the patient; and (*b*) a delivery system that meets these needs to the mutual satisfaction of the recipient and the provider. Health care includes services provided by physicians, nurses, dentists, and allied health professionals, whether the service is preventive, diagnostic, therapeutic, or rehabilitative, or whether physical, emotional, or social factors are involved. The management of health care is a complex process that involves planning, organizing, implementing, administering, controlling, and evaluating health-care services so that the patient is rendered the best possible care at the least expense.

Problem Solving and Technology

The problem-solving process in health-care management is comprised of a series of steps. The number of steps and their order will depend on the complexity of the problem and the group involved, but in general, the following steps will be necessary, in the order shown:

1. List the goals of the health-care system for both the present and the future.

Before competent planning of health-care services can begin, the health-care needs of the target population must be clearly defined. The objectives of health services are threefold: to promote good health, to prevent disease, and to treat disease and disability beginning with primary care and ending with rehabilitation and resettlement in suitable employment.

The most significant organizational goals should be to foster systems of care that will provide each individual with a continuity of care. The distribution of health care is as important as the quality of the care distributed.

2. List the goals of the health-care management system.

Once the goals of the health-care system have been defined, it is possible to define the goals and objectives of a system for management that is designed to help achieve them.

Management involves planning, administration, and evaluation in order to function effectively. The goals and objectives must be clearly stated and the measurements and standards of performance clearly defined. A health-service organization has objectives and possible methods to achieve those objectives. But by whose standards? Clearly, the professional definitions of desirable health care may not coincide with that of an individual or of pressure groups in the community nor with that of the research worker. Each will be influenced by different factors, and these will determine whether the needs as they perceive them are fully met.

3. Determine the measurable criteria that can be used to evaluate success.

Prior experience has clearly demonstrated that health care quality (not economy) is the real measure of the success of health care and that it is virtually impossible to express this quality in units of money. This makes life difficult for the manager because the other elements with which he deals—time, space, people, material, education, and training—are usually evaluated and expressed in money units.

The manager is therefore faced with the need for equating elements in units that cannot readily be equated. One solution to this dilemma is to make arbitrary or intuitive equations. If this is done, it is mandatory to keep detailed records of these so that it will become obvious if the intuitive or arbitrary criteria are no longer applicable in a changing situation or perhaps that the initial assumptions need review.

Certain associations between socioeconomic factors and disease or risk of disease are well documented, and these are useful for identifying risk populations and projecting the potential need for services in a given population. The association of socioeconomic factors with the organization and management of medical care is less understood. We lack the data that would aid in estimating the potential consequences of changes in the health sector and shifts in economic development.

In order for decision makers to select a rational choice from among several alternatives, certain types of fundamental information are needed. These will require new methods of analysis and additional social policy research that will address the following problems:

(*i*) Although it is assumed that manpower, education, and economic development are interrelated, we do not know whether these can be generalized. For example, what effects do varying patterns of medical-care delivery have on a country's or an area's labor pool? What percentage of the labor pool should be employed in the medical-care system? How should this differ by stage of economic development? Is there an optimal ratio of use of manpower by different sectors of society (e.g., agriculture, health, industry) at varying levels of economic development? On what basis should "optimal" be judged—on economic growth as measured by GNP, on mortality rates, or on frequency of use of health-care facilities?

(*ii*) There is little adequate data on the capital investment in hospitals and other care facilities nor on whether real costs of providing medical care are rising or falling.

(*iii*) There is some evidence that as the level of education rises, so does the demand for medical care and for family-planning services. We can only speculate as to the reasons. If education alters the individual's perception and definition of illness and belief about causation and cure, then as the education level increases on a worldwide basis, will a corresponding demand for medical services be created? Should efforts be made to satisfy that demand, or should incentives and motivations be instituted to control them? Do we, in fact, have adequate scientific knowledge to consider motivation and incentive factors?

4. Describe what is being done now by management to meet the set goals.

A full description of what is being done by health-care management is required with as much detail as possible. Often, this initial analysis, when discussed with various people who are involved, will reveal further details otherwise unknown to the manager and points where simple remedies can improve management immediately, with or without technology.

5. List the resources available to management for use in meeting the goals.

Not until the health-care needs have been determined by the medical professional and/or the consumer can the resources necessary to satisfy them be evaluated.

Manpower resources are clearly one of the principal components, and accurate information on the available manpower and how it is used is essential to establish future manpower needs on a long-term basis and improve the effectiveness of short-term patterns of use. For this purpose, technology can maintain permanent inventories of available personnel as well as information about their skills useful in the health-care service. Moreover, economic use of available allied professional and auxiliary personnel is important, but none more so than those areas in which there is a shortage of trained professionals per capita.

There are cultural variations in the style of management as well as in the perception of what constitutes health and what constitutes illness.

The determination of health services involves two components: (*a*) the material input; and (*b*) the human input. The techniques used by commerce can be applied to the management of material resources, but the management of people is governed by the behavioral sciences. These are important differences when considering front-line care (domiciliary or primary) and second-line (hospital) care.

Planning must take into account all these resources, but its implementation may be different. There is no blueprint to which everyone can respond, but certain information and data are necessary and common to all.

Health care is a labor-intensive industry. Demographic, social, and environmental data are needed. These include but are not limited to:

(*i*) Periodic data, that is, sex, marital status, employment, education, mobility, ethnic groups, household facilities, crowding, transportation, etc.
(*ii*) Continuous data, that is, births, deaths, marriages, and migrations
(*iii*) Environmental data, that is, pollution levels, climate, population density, industrial structure, and housing standards

6. *List the constraints and boundary conditions on management in meeting the goals (social, geographic, medical, economic, technical).*

Other determinants of health services include political constraints, cultural and ethnic principles (e.g., care of the elderly), historical, economic (e.g., industrialization, GNP), epidemiological (e.g., distribution of disease), geographical (e.g., communication, roads, climate), and scientific and technological (e.g., computers, automation, and managerial science).

The economic constraints on the use of technology in the management of medical-care systems will vary, but where there are no competent accounting and budgeting systems it will be impossible to really manage. Poorly organized budgets (or no budgets at all) and uncertainties as to the extent of the appropriation for health care and when it will be received result in economic distress in many health-care systems and render the application of management techniques impossible. These and other economic constraints could be alleviated by a reassessment of the interaction between national and institutional goals and needs. Ways of implementing change have not been studied with precision if, indeed, they can be said to have been approached at all.

Many hospital administrators are compelled to purchase equipment from the lowest bidder—not necessarily the best—and this constraint often results in long and costly delays. Furthermore, hospitals located in cities usually have a greater need for emergency-care facilities, including special equipment to deal with special demands, yet this is often not considered in planning and budgeting for city-hospital services.

In addition to the constraints of economic, social, and technological factors, further constraints are imposed through duplication of services; fragmentation of effort; lack of continuity and communication; distrust and archaic professional attitudes; the size of the particular institution; the organization and interrelation of generalists and specialists; the influence of such factors as modern transportation, which gives mobility to both patient and physician; and the desirability of a particular distribution of benefits that can or may result from a particular distribution of effort, planning, and management at the primary and other levels of care.

7. *Identify points where technology could be applied to help achieve success.* Once the entire health-care process is analyzed, we can determine how technology can best be applied to increase its efficiency and effectiveness. Technology often exists, but it is not always true that everyone is familiar with its possibilities.

In general, the development of health-care systems on a regional rather than a local, isolated basis is desirable, and for this purpose new technology must be introduced. A central record center that would maintain information concerning the condition of a patient's health as well as his socioeconomic status would greatly aid health-care practitioners. For example, the introduction of a uniform "patient identification" folder similar to those used in various public service areas such as police record systems. These would include a separate sheet for each patient visit, bearing a uniform physician identification and description of the service rendered (with an abstract useful in record linkage to other levels of care) and places for other sheets bearing laboratory and other test results, hospital discharge information, and other appropriate records.

Planning will involve demographic information for which technology can be useful in satisfying the need for data collection, processing, and analyzing. Technology can maintain inventories, such as presently available services, including hospitals, health centers, convalescent homes, and other locations where health care is dispensed, as well as size, available equipment, outpatient and emergency services, financing, staffing, and provision for intensive and other special care.

The interpretation of data is important and should be done by doctors, engineers, statisticians, and social scientists working as a team and with the use of modern technology. Systems for quality control involving the entire health-care staff should be developed. This, in turn, would necessitate a standardization of diagnostic and treatment processes, medical audits, peer-review systems, and similar mechanisms. Technology can make this possible and do so at the least cost in professional personnel time.

In the operation of hospitals and other centers of medical care, modern techniques such as system and cost/benefit analyses must be further developed and applied to communities large and small, rural and urban. Many available techniques and technologies exist that can be exploited by management to improve the quality and efficiency of health care. For example:

(*i*) Recording diagnosis and treatment for each individual patient in a way that will ensure continuity of care
(*ii*) Maintaining and administering daily activities in the health service and monitoring the quality and quantity of the care provided. This is not only necessary to run the service efficiently but will also keep those who support the professional staff informed of progress and difficulties.
(*iii*) Surveillance of the general population to detect changes in the pattern of disease. This is particularly important in the case of infectious diseases.
(*iv*) Accumulate data needed as a base for clinical, epidemiological, and health-services research
(*v*) In some instances, health service personnel are required to respond to legal requirements, such as providing to appropriate authorities information about dangerous drugs
(*vi*) Cost/benefit and cost/effectiveness studies, including planned programming and budgeting systems
(*vii*) System analysis and flow charting
(*viii*) Program evaluation review techniques
(*ix*) Time and motion studies
(*x*) Job analysis and description with the objective of delegating certain duties to health-care personnel with less training, for example, medical assistants
(*xi*) The use of models, especially computer models, for hypothetical health service and epidemiological studies
(*xii*) Computerized records, including personnel, payroll, and accounting
(*xiii*) Automation in the laboratory
(*xiv*) Use of the computer as a diagnostic aid

The objectivity of technology when applied to the supervisory process can often eliminate or reduce the danger of damaging interpersonal relationships in instances in which collective action is required. For example, proper mechanisms not only improve patient care but also evaluate the quality of the care and the performance of individual professionals. Such problems as unnecessary surgery, over-and/or underuse of costly laboratory, X-ray, and similar procedures, and improper recording of clinical data can be identified. When these data are gathered in an impersonal way and presented to people whose sense of responsibility is usually well developed, there is generally no need for coercion to bring about corrective measures.

In many areas, particularly developing ones, the imbalance between the need and the available resources of manpower and money is a severe handicap to improving health care. While the application of technology can alleviate the manpower problem by developing a more effective allocation of skills, it must be remembered that modern technology is very expensive. Unless the cost/benefit ratio can be shown to be balanced in favor of benefits, developing areas should not be encouraged to make large capital investments for equipment and physical plants that may not be fully put to use. There is a pressing need to find ways to reduce the costs of modern technology so that it can benefit people in those areas in which financial resources are a major constraint.

In many cases, technology is easing the gathering, processing, and analyzing of health-care data in greater detail and in a shorter time than was possible before its advent. Such studies identify areas in which services are fragmented and duplicated.

To a large extent, however, modern technology has bypassed health care at the primary level, partly due to the high costs involved. In addition to reducing the high costs inherent in technological innovations, there is a need to adapt other modern technology now used in commerce and industry.

8. Devise several ways of meeting the goals with the available resources and within the boundary conditions.

There never seems to be one unique solution to any management problem, and management "style" already has been mentioned as one of the boundary conditions. This style may exert an undue restriction in planning for innovation. Resistance will often appear because of the difficulty in guaranteeing results, and there may be unwillingness to try anything because it cannot positively be shown how benefits will accrue. It therefore becomes necessary to present several alternatives so that the users of the system have (or think they have) a hand in deciding what is to be done and are thus motivated to see the proposed system succeed. While medical professionals (physicians, nurses, etc.) may readily admit that an appreciable part of their time may be wasted with an admittedly ineffective system, there is a resistance to change.

In order to avoid the pitfalls inherent in "grand master plans," it should be possible to plan for health-care needs on an individual area or regional basis and to make the planning flexible enough to respond to changing needs. Planning for health care means seeking ways to ensure that future health-care systems will be better than the present by restructuring the system to bring this about.

Competent planning in medical care, as elsewhere, requires the development of a visual picture of total plans. This should be as detailed as is necessary to identify essential activities. When details and specifics of a program are explicit, the inherent weaknesses become apparent, and any misunderstanding or misinterpretations can be rectified. The health-care plan, like any problem-solving process, must be logical and comprehended by the group involved. In addition, the plan should be one in which emotion and opinions are separated from fact and in which judgments are based on experience and sound information. If this criterion is met, it is reasonable to assume that a rational solution for problems will emerge.

Limited or poorly distributed health-care resources, coupled with a growing demand for service, have forced a reappraisal of health-care delivery. In developing areas, the planning emphasis is on the control of infectious diseases and the establishment of public health facilities. Effective planning for health-care services will vary, but in all cases it will be dependent on adequate data. These data may have built-in strengths and weaknesses, but they are essential because much that is technically feasible may not be a viable possibility when the available resources are considered.

Much of the emphasis in the past centered about planning hospitals for acute illnesses. This planning was, to a large extent, based on beds per 1000 population in the various specialties. Today, the bed ratios are based on current demand, which has been demonstrated to be an inadequate measure of need, ignoring as it does both the impact of outside medical service and socioeconomic conditions. There is often no effective planning organizational unit, and the layers of administrative authority may serve only to obstruct any serious attempt to establish one.

If it is demonstrated that technology can help with a given health-care-management problem and how its implementation can be achieved, it must be determined whether the costs of the technological innovation are justified by the benefits to be gained. Even more elusive is the capital that will pay for the change without any guarantee of immediate cash return or savings or even any guarantee of short-term improvement in patient care.

9. Make a preliminary decision, field trial(s), and evaluation(s) of possible system(s).

This step can be considerably enhanced by introducing program evaluation and review techniques (PERT), in which logical ordering of activities is stressed and helps to visualize a total plan. PERT has long served industry in controlling the time element of complex tasks and cost factors and in ensuring the best use of skilled and scarce manpower.

The best organization is one that considers the social and client perspective as well as the professional provider's perspective. Whatever the definition of health care, that organization is best that can recognize and adapt to shifts in population and opinions. The organization that serves best is also that which views health and illness in the context of the total ecology of disease in human communities.

Hospital administrators must ask themselves honestly whether they are ready to accept the technologist as a part of the managerial team or whether they will regard him as an intruder who must be tolerated temporarily. If the technologies of system analysis and data processing are to make a dynamic contribution to the health-care system, the practitioners must be permanently identified as active members of the managerial team and share in the decision making and responsibilities. Field trials on a small scale may be required in order to bring out unidentified problems, assess user acceptance and ways of improving it, and allow for use of feedback, modification, and improvement as a result of local knowledge.

10. Select the system to be used.

The evaluation criteria developed in the third step receive their most rigorous testing here, and their validity may determine the final success in choosing a useful system about which everyone feels assured.

11. Introduce and use the system (including training).

Introduction and use of any innovation must be preceded by thorough training of its users as well as by complete education in the benefits to be expected and the improvement in health-care quality that should result. Education for all members in the health-care industry needs to be basic, specialized, and continuing.

Candidates for top-level management need 2 to 3 years of interdisciplinary study. This requirement extends to health professionals who have managerial responsibilities. Refresher seminars in management techniques can be helpful not only to members of the health-care team but also to those in decision- and policy-making positions, such as hospital administrators and other department heads.

Improvement in any health-care-delivery system, no matter how obviously desirable it may be, requires the cooperation of groups of individuals who are the potential agents of change but whose vested interests may cause them to resist such change vigorously. Thus, along with proposed remedies, we need innovative approaches designed to overcome such opposition. Our options are often obscure and frequently must be invented rather than discovered.

12. Periodic evaluation (and possibly return to Step 1).

Periodic evaluation will help to reveal weaknesses in the final system as well as changes in the circumstances under which it operates. There must be feedback provided to the manager, and the paths for this feedback must be a part of the original plan. It is to be expected that periodic review and regular feedback will, from time to time, show the need for starting the entire planning procedure over again.

20

THE ADMINISTRATOR'S ROLE IN THE INTRODUCTION OF NEW TECHNOLOGY INTO THE COMMUNITY HOSPITAL

S. Jacobs, J. Bray, W. Seligman, D. Buchmueller, and A. Bennett

What is the administrator's role in the introduction of new technology into the hospital? Various types of technological advances must be discussed by hospital administrators in this regard.

Should the administrator actively try to keep abreast of new technology, or should he assume a passive role, wherein new technology is considered only when recommended by the staff?

Within the question lies a much more basic consideration, which administrators and their professional staff must understand. The basic concern is with the relationship between the administrator and his staff and vice versa. A mutual respect and an appreciation for the understanding of the overall needs of the institution must exist. If both parties realize they are each dealing with trained, competent, dedicated professionals, then a basis exists on which this subject can be discussed intelligently.

For example, if a pathologist comes to the administrator's office to discuss a mutual problem for the well-being of the institution, the probability of solving the problem is very good; however, a basic consideration is that the final decision will usually have to be made by the administrator. So what can the pathologist expect when he comes to the administrator's office with a request for new medical equipment? First, he should expect a receptive attitude; this is mandatory. Second, he should expect to deal with an intellect capable of understanding the request. Of course, the detailed knowledge of its implication in the laboratory rests with the pathologist, not the administrator. However, the pathologist must understand that the administrator has an understanding of the institution as a whole. In turn, the administrator must be able to understand what is proposed and how it will relate to the entire institution, community, and, most importantly, the patients. Conversely, what can the administrator expect when the pathologist enters? He should expect a receptive attitude combined with the intelligence to understand the concept that the new equipment will affect the entire institution.

Assume the pathologist requests a new device costing $750,000. The administrator expects that the pathologist has the intelligence and ability to understand what the new equipment signifies in terms of technical staff, tests per admission, costs for installation, implementation and operation, and finally, what it may do to overall costs per patient day. To do this, the professional must participate in budget and review sessions. We live in an age in which many people will look at a hospital as compared to other hospitals of like size and services and ask why do you want this? Why are you going to implement that? Why are your costs for laboratory services or costs per test higher than other hospitals?

It is obvious from the preceding that neither party can be the sole person charged with the responsibility for introducing innovative features into the hospital. In order to arrive at a meaningful answer, one must understand both sides of the question. One facet deals strictly with technical, scientific matters. The other is concerned with practicality, both in terms of expenditure resources and feasibility of implementation in the institution. Thus, when an innovative idea is suggested and accepted in a hospital, neither one party nor the other should take the overall credit for it. There are institutions in which the pathology department announces "the implementation of an SMA 12," or the administrator sends out an announcement stating that "he is proud to announce that the XYZ hospital now has such service." It should be a joint affair.

Similarly, in the pathology example, in view of the constraints that have been placed on hospitals and the ominous cloud that hangs over the administrators in terms of national health insurance, how can any party that contributes directly to the cost of providing medical care not help but share actively in the management of the institution? Should the burden of the cost of the expenditure or its justification be placed solely on the pathologist? If the pathologist has not concerned himself with this area, then he must have an open mind when the administrator agrees and the two discuss costs, staffing, etc. When the professional comes in, he should have considered these areas. If he has not, the administrator must bring these areas to his attention. Too often, only the medical aspect of the new life-saving device is pointed out by the professional.

It has been suggested that the final decision rests with the administrator. The question, then, is whether or not the administration has the responsibility to keep up-to-date actively with new technology. Should the administrator actively strive to keep abreast or ahead of his professional people by knowing what is available and what is not, or should he take a passive role and wait until the professional staff recommends new technology?

It is too simple to say yes or no. No administrator can live in a vacuum without being aware of new technological developments and expect only the pathologists, radiologists, etc., to bring innovative technology to his attention. It is imperative that all parties concerned have the necessary knowledge, background, and experience so that a meaningful decision can be reached. The pathologist is obviously the technical expert, but if the administrator lives in a vacuum, he cannot possibly understand the new development being explained to him. Therefore, all must have the proper background so that everyone concerned can effectively communicate with each other.

If a pathologist comes in and explains the details of an SMA 12, and the administrator has never even heard of it, he has failed to keep abreast of new developments. The administrator should at least know its function and that it could be used effectively in his hospital. Also, when the pathologist explains the details of the SMA 12, he must relate it in terms of patient usage and who on the medical staff is capable of utilizing this new device.

There are a number of ways of approaching the different technical problems involved in new medical instrumentation in order to achieve the same end. Should the administrator rely solely on the pathologist for information on instrumentation acquisition? It should usually be considered as a "joint venture" so as to arrive at a successful understanding. If another new device such as an XYZ is being considered, is it important to ask who else makes an XYZ? Can competitive bidding be obtained on the item? Is professional reference material available so that the XYZ can be further researched? Are others doing the same thing but using another approach? The above questions constitute just some of the necessary background and understanding.

If one states to the administrator that the institution must have an XYZ, an agreement must be reached as to why it has to be that particular XYZ. The original request may have considerable merit, but the XYZ must be studied in greater depth. There are many areas that the pathologist must consider, for example, the advantage or disadvantage of direct purchase, cost of operation, and cost of additional personnel that a new system may require.

New Technology Sources for the Administrator

Through what sources does the administrator learn of the new technology that is available, and how informative and reliable are these sources? One may cite many examples, such as advertisements, journal articles, convention displays, salesmen, staff, experience of others, reading clubs, and clinical engineers, as suitable sources in regard to technology.

It is mandatory that the administrative staff, pathologists, radiologists, etc., jointly participate in the review of new technology. In a joint reading club in one hospital, approximately 200 journals that publish new technological developments are reviewed. This group can look for those technological innovations that are practical for use in a specific hospital and will also meet necessary budgetary requirements.

In general, the advertising media is reliable, but as the hospital industry becomes more business oriented, other resources must be investigated. Proper hospital personnel must be aware of what is under development and what new service products are nearing completion. Only after considering the above can they begin to look ahead and not be concerned only with what is available today. Rapid advances in technology often make equipment that is purchased today obsolete tomorrow. The probability of rapid obsolescence should be a consideration in the decision process to buy and implement new equipment.

Would it not be more desirable for the administration to talk to an engineer who is qualified in the health-care-delivery field? It is logical to assume that one would not talk to an engineer only to discuss the operation of a new device and to a pathologist only to discuss patient care. The engineer and pathologist must work together to improve patient care. So what, then, is the role of this newly emerging professional known as the ''clinical engineer'' in the decision-making process? Of approximately 7000 hospitals in this country, the majority contain less than 150 beds. The number of 150-bed hospitals that have a clinical engineer aboard is very small. Some may share him with other hospitals. The larger hospitals may have their own clinical engineers. But whatever the case, the degree of his involvement and qualifications must be considered. Assume, from a functional point of view, that the pathologist requests a piece of equipment. He might favor an XYZ for different reasons, for example, emotional reasons, the way it is packaged, etc. However, the clinical engineer would evaluate the equipment from the point of view of accuracy, precision, reliability, safety, etc.; far more important criteria. Often we find that many physicians are not comfortable with nor do they understand the implications of this sort of scientific reasoning. There are many pieces of equipment that are being used by physicians that, until recently, have not been subjected to the type of engineering criteria that allows one to improve the equipment's use as a diagnostic tool. More and more physicians and administrators turn to engineers who are knowledgeable in a clinical environment.

Many individuals hear about an engineer working in a hospital environment may think of him as a biomedical, clinical, industrial, or plant engineer. However, attention should be focused on the biomedical engineer and clinical engineer. In either case, they should be familiar with instrumentation from an engineering discipline, as compared to a physician who looks at them only from a functional point of view.

How does a hospital procure an engineer for its staff? On the staff of one hospital, for example, envision a very young and talented individual who is very interested in automated systems. He has paid his way up from repair. As a result of economic considerations, hospitals are forced to operate under a rather tight budget. This, in turn, causes serious impediments concerning flexibility of action. Thus, some may balk at the mention of an engineer paying his own way by repair of instrumentation to reach the position of joint decision maker. Do competent clinical engineers accept the repair role as part of their responsibility in the hospital? It must be understood that certain tasks one performs are, of necessity, done to pay his way. He may not want to do it, and perhaps he should not be doing it, but in a realistic sense the job must be done by him.

Factors to Consider to Evaluate New Available Technology and Determine the Administrator's Recommendations

One of the things that has occurred in examining the broad field of technology and trying to understand the purpose and role of organizations like AAMI is that such organizations have done an excellent job in bridging the gap between the physician and the engineer. Herein, however, an additional problem is posed that has not been satisfactorily resolved. This area involves the relationship of the third component in the health-care triangle who is the administrator, chief executive officer, or health-care manager.

What the administrator can bring to bear on the introduction of medical technology in the community hospital is a rational methodology. Many hospitals do not have engineers available in the decision-making process. In these hospitals, the administrators must bring to bear a methodology that itemizes content and desired goals and asks certain questions in an orderly way to ensure that all necessary areas are considered before launching off in quest of some new resolution of a health-care problem.

Administrators have an obligation to be aware of the areas in which the needs are greatest, areas in which the application of technology can offer the greatest potential improvement. One of the first things the administrator has to do in the area of evaluating data and information and the introduction of new technology is identify the decision-making process. What is his relationship to the board of trustees, and, internally, what channels must decision making go through on route to the administrator? We obviously want and need professional judgment, probably in most instances the judgment of more than one professional. Hence, the engineer must play a vital role.

For example, suppose the pathologist or biochemist requests a new device that will slit blood cells vertically rather than horizontally. Will it serve the needs of its users? The users and the medical staff should be questioned to determine if this service is needed. Is the degree of accuracy that could be obtained through the application of new technology worth the extra cost? Obviously, there are questions of safety to the patient when he comes into direct contact with these new technological advances. What is the implication of the administrative review? Should the hospital also have an equipment review committee, and, if so, who should be on it? There is merit in having such a committee, particularly where, as is almost always the case, the hospital is involved in the area of marginal allocation of resources. Not all needs are going to be met in the course of a fiscal year or perhaps in the course of 2 or 3 years. Thus, the composition of such a committee should include the personnel that use, maintain, and, in turn, make decisions or projections concerning the technological obsolescense of equipment.

With respect to the board of directors, it is hoped that each administrator would have an understanding with his board as to the extent to which decisions could be made to allocate resources, particularly in reference to resources that are unbudgeted or resources that are in excess of budget depending on the cost. It would be unfortunate to be in an administrative setting in which spending $1000 or $2000 beyond the budget would be subject to board approval. Conversely, one can not obligate $75,000 or $100,000 without obtaining board approval. Somewhere, perhaps in the range of $25,000 to $30,000, there would be a level that would merit board approval.

The administrator cannot keep abreast of all the latest technological developments. However, he has to know, for example, what are the legal and safety ramifications. In the state of Illinois, for example, there has been a great deal of consternation concerning the question of serum hepatitis acquired through blood transfusions. Recently, a law was enacted that, as of July 1, 1974, will proscribe the transfusion of purchased blood, except where a physician signs a waiver. Therefore, almost anything that can be done to protect against the acquisition of hepatitis from a blood transfusion is obviously something to which the administrator should be allocating resources. If this is not done, there is a question of legal liability. This has been tested in the courts, and there are law suits still pending. The original landmark suit of Cunningham v. McNeal is still being appealed and remains unresolved.

Cost effectiveness, of course, is very basic. One can easily think of a fairly basic matrix methodology with improvement of patient care plotted along the horizontal axis and cost along the vertical. This approach may improve patient care and decrease cost. It may also decrease cost without affecting patient care, or it may not decrease patient care or decrease cost, etc. There are nine possible alternatives. And probably for all but one or two, the answer is fairly simple. Here we are not just talking about the introduction of major items of equipment but also about the thousands of dollars that are spent on disposable products, for example. One patient-care-products committee has tried to apply this methodology to the introduction of everything from disposable syringes to urinary drainage bags to disposable operating room packs. Such approaches have worked, and from them considerable savings have resulted. The key is the involvement with the people that use this equipment and, where there is a maintenance situation, the involvement of the people that must maintain it.

The cost factors also merit attention. For example, what is the recovery period if an investment in capital equipment were to be made by the board? Would it save manpower or enhance revenue? A recovery period greater than 5 years may require considerable investigation. There are basically two reasons to consider. First, cost estimates can sometimes be fairly spurious. Despite good intentions and research, they can be as much as 100% incorrect. Second, technological obsolescence in the past couple of decades has outstripped functional obsolescence. We do not know whether we will have to invest large sums of money in something entirely new 5 years from now; the way technology has evolved, the period is probably less than 5 years. Anything that cannot recover its costs in 5 years is probably not a sound investment from a financial standpoint. Of course, there may be some very good patient-care reasons to proceed regardless.

Also, there is the question of reimbursement. This is often discussed, and perhaps administrators are looked at as problem describers rather than problem solvers when they talk about their reimbursement problems and the medicare cost formulas. Basically, however, what it amounts to is: Can something be leased rather than purchased and still recover most of our investment? One cannot always get full reimbursement when talking about depreciating equipment over its useful life because, as indicated earlier, the useful life usually outlasts the technological value of the equipment, and one is left with equipment that is useless or relatively so without having recovered our full depreciation expense. Obviously, some of the questions that must be asked are: Does the institution already have any instruments like it? What, if any, will it replace? Are back-up systems readily available? What is the necessary preparation for installation? For example, a new piece of equipment is purchased, and it is found that a $15,000 to $20,000 minor investment must be made.

The lease on a previous piece of equipment may have been canceled, which may leave the institution in a sort of hiatus until the situation can be resolved.

What can one expect in the areas of maintenance, spare parts, and other supplies? For instance, a hospital may have been attracted to a device that was sold by the ABC Medical Instrument Company. Then an attempt was made to procure replacement parts and maintenance and found they were not available. What about the training of technical personnel? Is there some degree of flexibility in interchanging parts? How accurate are the delivery dates? Some companies begin to develop reputations for either making or not making promised delivery dates. Another important area of consideration is the salesman's role in the corporate organization. Will the salesman be available after the equipment is installed, or has his duty been transferred to someone else or a leasing company? Legal precedents have shown that hospitals cannot withhold payment to a leasing company if they are dissatisfied with a piece of medical instrumentation. The leadership, developing, and refining of these methods is one that should be shared. Shared power is more power.

When to Buy or Update

The properly trained engineer is the only one who can give you an answer to this. It's the type of problem wherein a community hospital that does not have a bioengineer should be able to bring in an engineering consultant to look at these aspects of the question as well. This gives a broader choice than just to buy the system or not.

The techniques that have been described above as to how to obtain information and how to arrive at a decision do not seem to cover a different area of problems. For example, assume there are a large number of hospitals in the United States that should do the following with their clinical laboratory: Reduce it in size by about 75%; send out most of their profiling tests to an independent laboratory; and replace most of their large equipment with small stat equipment, distributed at various places throughout the hospital. The administrator should not necessarily rely on the pathologist, especially if he is on a percentage arrangement, as a source of information as to whether or not to make such a change. This would be the time to regroup and look at the manner in which the existing technology is being used. A systems approach should be used, both macro and micro, and both within a hospital and within a system.

There are two diverging viewpoints within this problem area. On the one hand, if the opinions or decisions of the pathologist are not reliable, then you may want to consider replacing the pathologist before anything else is done. In short, money is being paid for advice from an incompetent individual. In such a case, one should seriously consider making a change. However, if the pathologist is competent and can't communicate to the administrator, then dollars are being spent on an incompetent administrator, and the board should make a change at the administration level.

The other point of view shares the opinion that any manager who has run a sizable organization realizes that management's major responsibility is to arbitrate between subsystems. Subsystem optimization will not necessarily result in total system optimization. The key to running an organization is just that. If the position is taken that if your pathologist does not have the ability to take a systems approach larger than his subsystem, then you should fire him, a mistake might be made. Some findings have shown that only 1% of all pathologists operate in this manner. Therefore, if that management criteria for keeping people is used, you will not have much of an organization. What is really necessary is that you procure outside consultants when needed in order to make a decision.

In discussing this area further, findings show that the administrator does not view his organization as a system and therefore cannot expect too much from his pathologist. Perhaps the most significant point to remember is that there continually exists a face-to-face confrontation between the administrator and pathologist. Obviously, this is a necessary relationship. If that relationship is good, the process of determining technological introduction will be much smoother.

What are the other alternatives that are available to these two professionals who are not necessarily the only two individuals involved in a decision? Many other alternatives are available to them. For example, there are hospitals that might refer this to a task force, where more people other than the two parties are involved in the decision-making process. Also, there is the opportunity for an outside engineering consultant to be brought in on a complex or complicated system or project in the event the organization does not have the proper engineering capability. Certainly the most realistic approach is for the engineering consultant or the change agent to be present in the client hospital and directly assist the staff in making the right decision. The role of the consultant should not be viewed as something that is known only to the administrator and pathologist. It should be a group involvement. Thus, this approach would include those in the pathology department, paraprofessionals, and technicians. These individuals are also knowledgeable about technological advances. They have their individual insights in addition to keeping up-to-date in their respective fields. They certainly should have the opportunity to contribute as well. This attitude will allow freedom of exchange of ideas and interchange of action.

One problem area is the consulting fee for an engineer. This is a relatively new expenditure for community hospitals. In California, another problem exists in the form of areawide planning. In San Diego, a 75-member board of directors must be approached for a $100,000 expenditure. Much hospital equipment sells for more than $100,000. If area-wide planning approval has not been granted, but you proceed and purchase the equipment regardless, there is no reimbursement. Area-wide planning has begun to take on awesome structure. It is a very powerful, bureaucratic system that one must face. At the present time, reimbursing agencies cause no problems, as hardware can either be leased or bought.

Who should the engineer or engineering group report to in the hospital? Certainly the level should be high enough so that his recommendations will be seriously considered. For example, in a particular 850-bed hospital, which is part of a medical center, a medical school exists that also includes a department of biomedical engineering. This department provides services to the hospital as well. The chairman of the department of biomedical engineering is on a par with the other medical chairmen, reporting to one of three deans. In other words, an attempt is made to parallel the medical school and other departments. Very briefly, the school has an associate dean for medical science and services, which includes pediatrics and psychiatry, as well as a major specialist in surgical science and services and a department referred to as behavioral and biological sciences and services, which is the umbrella that encompasses biomedical engineering, microbiology, biochemistry, and any others. There are M.D.s and Ph.D.s, and anyone who heads a department is normally one of the two

Staff Acceptance

If this new technology is approved and results in a reduction in staff or job-classifications changes, how should it be handled? These sort of questions lead us into the more complex aspects of introducing technological advancement. Most of what has been previously discussed seems to stem from organizational problems. Where the engineer should be placed in the organizational framework and the relationship between the pathologist and the administrator should be clear in the minds of those involved. When we talk about staff acceptance of staff, we refer to any level of organization of personnel who are involved or concerned with change in the method of procedure that is brought about by the introduction of new technology. There are certain principles that administrators and managers should be concerned and aware of in two basic areas. These include minimizing resistance on the part of people and maximizing the effects of the change itself.

First, in terms of minimizing resistance, there are some principles that must be considered. For example, one must be aware that there are differences in perception of change. The pathologist (the originator), clinical engineer, biomedical engineer, supervisor, and administrator all have their own perceptions, biases, and prejudices concerning the change and the reason why it should or should not be made. The second principle is that administrators should avoid impatience with the present practice. Resistance is often caused by criticisms of what is now being done; consequently, the change process starts in a negative manner, thereby causing many problems in the process. The third principle is the involvement and participation of personnel who are concerned with or involved in the change. This, of course, is one of the most potentially effective managerial techniques available, but it is one that is often misused, if used at all. It is also one that requires considerable tact and diplomacy. A fourth principle deals with the timing of the change. Often, as a result of impatience, good judgment is not used in terms of timing the change or in terms of the situation or climate that exists and surrounds the change. Probably one of the main problems in all organizations, including hospitals, is the deficiencies in communication channels. A final principle for minimizing resistance is to promote an understanding of all aspects of the change. These are just some of the more important principles that an administrator must be aware of in terms of facing up to a change that will undoubtedly affect many people in varying degrees.

Second, in discussing maximizing the effectiveness of the introduction of the new process or procedure, it may be well to cite an important principle, that is, the use of a systematic approach to change. If change is to occur, everyone involved will have some effect on their own destiny in terms of how well the change will occur. Thus, there is only one way to create change, and that is to manage it; this requires a systematic, organized approach.

In turn, the three elements of management (planning, organizing, and controlling) must be supported. Of course, this management process operates against a backdrop of an environment of change that has either existed on a positive or negative basis. As indicated earlier, planning consists partly in asking questions. A technique that is used very often by administrators is to create a balance sheet in terms of the key people who will either support or reject that change. First, on the negative side of the balance sheet are listed the anticipated negative reactions that these people will have regarding the change. These may be looked at from social, economic status, security, and cultural viewpoints. For instance, from the viewpoint of economic status, what will be the implications in terms of remuneration to the people who will be affected by the change? Again, on the negative side, the administrator must ask himself questions that other people will be asking themselves. Some of these questions include: If this change were to apply to me, what questions should be answered about future circumstances? What might he have to fear from the change? What might he reasonably expect to lose as a consequence of the change?

On the right side of the balance sheet, list the anticipated positive responses. Again, ask questions that other people will be asking themselves. Such questions would include: If this change were to apply to me, what might I expect to gain from the change? How might I benefit from the change, and what new advantages may I reasonably anticipate as a result of this change? Thus, by prethinking and preparing the balance sheet, one can plan how to overcome the negative side and how to capitalize on the positive aspects of the change.

Planning includes a first step that is often omitted. This is the establishment of objectives for a change or introduction of a new technique. What are the performance results that we want to attain as a result of this new method? Planning includes preparing and distributing information. A proven principle of good communication indicates that the more media that is utilized, the better the chance that the message will be understood. In communication, a very important element is to obtain feedback during the communication process. Lack of feedback can result in failure to communicate effectively. It certainly can happen between an administrator and a pathologist. It also often happens between the administrator and the engineer.

After a point is explained, an indication can be obtained as to whether the other party was listening, whether the message was received, and whether it was understood. This is the type of feedback needed to remove any obstacles to understanding. Failure to understand is often the cause of many communication problems.

Organizing the process involves identifying the person or persons charged with the responsibility for change and specifying their responsibilities. Finally, controlling the change involves setting target dates for phases of the change; monitoring the change through regular progress reports; showing how the change is complying with the initial objectives; and, as necessary, correcting the implementation of the change and making adjustments.

There is also the problem of what to do about an excess of personnel created by the change or changes in job descriptions or classifications. Very little has been done in studying organizations for mobility possibilities. This should be a routine activity of the personnel administration in any organization. When a major change is introduced that will have serious impact on the number of jobs or job content, there are several alternatives for the administration to pursue. There is, of course, normal attrition, which can solve the problem of a reduction in staff. Sometimes, either because of our importance or for economic reasons, we cannot tolerate that approach. Also, there is the possibility of retraining employees, transferral, or even promotion. Again, because of impatience, lack of funds, or priority in the training area, these alternatives can be discounted as viable. There is one alternative that is often overlooked, that is, looking at overtime work that is still maintained even though a new piece of equipment has been purchased. Also, there is the possibility of expansion into additional work or into other areas of activity. This would create the continuance of employment of older people. For example, a Chicago hospital installed a computer system to assist in radiotherapy planning. Prior to the advent of the computer system, it took an average of 3 hours for a technician to set up a procedure. After installation, the time was reduced to 8 minutes. The hospital expanded its workload by setting up cases for other hospitals and only made a slight reduction in staff. Finally, if all possibilities are exhausted, and termination is the only other alternative, the dismissed employee should receive assistance in securing another position.

If it is assumed that job descriptions are to be written for a new hospital that is not yet staffed, and full discretion is given in placing individuals, where should the early adopter (pioneer type) and late adopter (continuous-follower type) be placed, assuming they are both technically equal? At this level one might introduce the concept of a highly structured job position. However, in this case, this concept is not realistic. A more flexible approach is desirable, such as the organizational approach. New relationships must be discovered, and when one is dissolved, another must be established. The goal is continuously to create groups of people who can complete an assignment in terms of achieving specific objectives to which all members of that group can strive. To a certain degree, this concept conflicts with traditional organizational patterns; thus, it is not certain if raising someone to a higher level and giving him a new title or placing him on a full-time basis is the true answer to an organizational relationship problem. What has been described above is known as matrix organization. Several hospitals are presently being organized using the matrix concept.

In the hospital industry, as in other industries, individuals tend to read the same literature and associate with their own peers. Most changes to the hospital industry must come from outside. Generally, this must be the case because most individuals do not have the time or facilities to make revolutionary changes.

After the introduction of new technology, should there be an evaluation to determine whether projected gains are being achieved? If so, how and by whom? What are some of the principal causes for not achieving optimal utilization of the technology? How can the hospital overcome these deficiencies?

All the elements of the system must be thought out and handled in terms of change and introduction of technology. The introduction of new equipment and methods is only the beginning of the other components of change. Certainly it is a matter of thinking in terms of a systematic follow-up and follow-through. Measurement can only be accomplished with respect to certain initial expectations that have been previously established. Again, as indicated earlier, failure to state the objectives or expectations in terms of performance at the very beginning will make it impossible to evaluate them. The main point is to quantify and document the progress in making the change and the failures that have been experienced as best we can. Then, hopefully, we will learn important lessons out of every change that can be applied to any future change.

What are the areas in which the administrator perceives needs or voids that should be examined by the engineering profession? Without going into the introduction or the background of some of the voids, some important points should come to the mind of an administrator as he views the needs that require attention. Cost and its implications are at the top of the priority list. What can engineering do? First, productivity can be increased, as productivity is a national problem, notwithstanding the many other current hospital problems. Materials handling is another problem area that, broadly speaking, engineering can easily solve. Also, information handling and telecommunications can be vastly improved.

In reference to a very simple mundane area, consider a housekeeping staff consisting of about 300 people. We might ask if there are better ways to clean. For example, can more advanced automated vacuum cleaners be designed that could be carried about and operate solely by batteries.

The modulator patient room is another area that requires consideration. The Palacio del Rio Hotel in San Antonio, Texas, is a modularly constructed hotel that was built in less than a year at a fairly reasonable cost. If we would all cooperate, that is, hospital staffs, engineers, etc., and seriously discuss what new technological advances should be incorporated in a hospital room, then overall costs should be lowered. In addition, it is hoped that new facilities will be constructed at a lower cost with a corresponding increase in their capability. Facilities are presently being constructed to last 40 to 50 years.

Technology is changing every 5 to 10 years. This gives rise to a situation in which a new device is obsolete shortly after it is purchased. Thus, to help solve this, it must be constructed of materials that are inexpensive and will still last for a reasonable period of time. This approach makes it mandatory that the best engineering expertise is used.

In addition, the cost of technological development can be lowered. There are approximately 80 different companies making coronary-care equipment of various types. Suppose all of those companies were incorporated into a smaller number, such as 10. Consider how much savings could be realized in research and development by using this approach. If the market forecasts of each of those companies were grouped together, the total would greatly exceed the actual market potential that exists in the health-care industry today. To the extent there is a disparity, there are probably social costs that are being incorporated into patient costs that could be avoided. In a sense, we have an analogy with the automobile industry. Years ago, dozens of companies were making automobiles. As a result of mass production and standardization, the number of companies was reduced, and consequently the consumer realized a savings.

Another area that merits discussion involves problems of the elderly. Technology can do a great deal to enhance the capability of the elderly to remain outside of institutions. Obviously, in the next decade or two, the number of elderly people will increase; hopefully, they will still have the ability to function to a certain degree outside of the institution. Engineering contributions in relation to the elderly, while not yet spectacular, could have an important social and financial impact on our society. For example, envision a pneumatically operated apparatus that could be placed under the chair of an elderly person. It could help him overcome his problem of rising after being seated for a long period of time. There are similar seemingly mundane innovations that might be designed to help the elderly with the activities that are part of their daily living. For instance, they could receive emergency care on their own just by pressing a button or ringing a bell or another sort of monitor that will bring care when needed.

The disposal of disposables is another problem area; it is very costly, and the ecology problem seems to be increasing. In the area of evaluation of products, consumer's guides to medical products are needed. Also, there are no answers to such questions as: How can the effectiveness of any particular product be measured? How can products be compared that have different costs for purposes of investigating their overall effectiveness to a particular application? These are just some of the many areas in which the engineering field can contribute greatly. We must step back and look at patient care as an end product rather than a by-product of all these subsystems. It is the administrator's job to mitigate, moderate, and, hopefully, interpret these natural tensions that do exist among the caretakers of the subsystems.

Engineers have become more and more concerned with technology and its lack of management. In the hospital field, there are clinical engineers, mechanical engineers, biomedical engineers, electrical engineers, etc. We need the engineer who is a specialist in health-care systems and at the same time is a generalist in the other engineering disciplines. He can be the right arm to the administrator and the coordinator of engineering within the hospital. He would recognize the need for technical skills in many areas and be able to develop a much more coordinated program for utilizing technology in hospitals.

21

METHODS TO REDUCE HOSPITAL COSTS

R. N. Davis

Various scientific disciplines, including management engineering and clinical engineering, have much to contribute to the health-care field. Their work can be shown cost effective in at least three ways:

1. Improved patient care
2. Reduced or avoided cost
3. Improved employee welfare

The effectiveness of management engineering efforts over the past 10 years can be demonstrated both generically and from case histories, and it promises similar impact in years to come from the related discipline of clinical engineering. Achieving full potential is not automatic with any engineering discipline; however, some observations on how to get maximum cost effectiveness are reported.

For example, in the state of New York, the Hospital Management Engineering Program, a nonprofit cooperative engineering program operating under the auspices of the Hospital Association of New York State, was developed to apply management engineering principles to the solution of many hospital problems.

This engineering group varies in size but usually numbers approximately 30 professionals and related support personnel. Over its first 5 years, the program has been active in approximately 120 of the 350 hospitals in the state and expanded in scope from a very narrow industrial engineering identity to its present activities across the entire breadth of management engineering.

Definitions and Background

Several definitions are important in order to properly assess the impact of management engineering in the health-care field. The first of these is the term "cost effectiveness'' used in today's program. Defined simply, cost effectiveness relates the benefits of an engineering application to the cost of that application. Often, cost effectiveness can be expressed as a simple ratio between benefits and cost, although other equally valid measures include the absolute increase in productivity or quality achieved, the reduction in undesirable incidents, or the percentage of total potential actually achieved and implemented.

Cost effectiveness can fall into a variety of forms. Probably the most significant in the health-care field is the improvement of patient care or quality without commensurate increases in cost.

A second type of benefit is cost reduction or avoidance. Obvious examples of cost reduction include productivity increases that result in staff reduction or reductions in supply costs because of more effective systems. In the clinical engineering field, examples might include avoided insurance or liability claims costs. One administrator has found a much more pragmatic way to cost-justify medical engineering by simply incorporating functions like television repair into the total cost center and covering the entire operation cost by the savings from that one item alone.

A final form of cost effectiveness is in improved employee welfare. Examples of this might lie in reduced turnover because of better working conditions, improved safety conditions, and even improved supervisory effectiveness resulting from training or coaching.

A second definition that is important in this discussion is that of engineering itself. Engineering is seen as the design of a facility and/or process that achieves particular objectives. It may further be defined as a process that optimizes some organizational goal or organization's return on investment. In the case of a hospital, the resources are often people and money, and the return is expressed in patient care. Within this definition of engineering, clinical engineering is part of a broader field, including biomedical engineering technicians who are responsible for equipment maintenance and related electrical safety responsibilities.

Management engineering may be defined simply as the design of systems to help managers manage better. These systems could fall into any of the management functions, such as planning, staffing, and controlling, and might relate to any of the management disciplines, such as finance and supervision. It is important to note that management in the health field may just as easily be aimed at managing the health of a population as to managing people or things. In this sense, the medical doctor is a manager, and either clinical engineering or management engineering may be aimed at supporting that function.

A third essential definition is that of efficiency, which may be expressed as a ratio of output (including quality) over the unit cost. Efficiency should not be confused with effectiveness, which is a much broader term relating to how well the total health-care system, or one of its components, is functioning. Unfortunately, effectiveness, like quality itself, may be measured only with great difficulty and in an approximate way. Thus, attention will be focused herein on specific measures that are limited to the efficiency criteria.

Potential for Management Engineering

Management engineering has been shown to have tremendous potential value in the health-care field. This value may be placed at almost any level of the complex system known today. Most activities to date have been centered about individual hospitals or small, closely related groups of hospitals. However, there are also applications in the growing trend toward an overall health-system organizational effort.

In the area of productivity improvement, for example, it has been shown that management engineering can lead to improvements of 15–20% in support departments and of 10–15% in professional and administrative departments.

One of the key reasons for management engineering's great potential is that the management process itself is highly complex for hospitals and usually undermanned. Whereas a similar organization in industry might have 5–15 top level administrative people, a hospital of 300 or 400 beds and 1000 employees may have only two or at most three administrative personnel. In addition, managers of major departments in hospitals have often come up through the ranks without adequate management training to complement their professional specialty skills. For these reasons, management engineering, as a discipline that supports management personnel and develops management tools, has led to quantum jumps in performance.

Possibly the most overwhelming reason for the success of management engineering is the value of involving an objective third party in the hospital management process. The scientific method wherein objectives are defined, constraints identified, and the specific nature of the present situation documented is as valuable in the health field as anywhere else. Thus, the very presence of an engineer can have a significant impact on day-to-day operations as well as on longer-range programs. In addition, the recommendations of the engineer are often helpful either in impartial fact-finding or simply in supporting the recommendations of a departmental manager to top-level decision makers. Thus, the potential of management engineering is significant.

Achievements

Management engineering groups across the country have reported approximately a 5:1 ratio between the savings achieved (in a single year) and the cost of the project, although some programs apparently report the total potential savings that can be achieved with full implementation rather than the actual implementation to date. The Hospital Management Engineering Program has found that implemented savings-to-cost ratios range somewhere above 3:1 across the state. In addition, several programs have found productivity increases in support departments ranging from 8 to 12%, although results in professional departments are somewhat less, ranging from 4 to 6%. A significant indicator of the effectiveness of management engineering is the growth of the field itself. In 1961, there were 30 professionals belonging to the Hospital Management Systems Society, whereas in 1971 the number had grown to 600, a 20-fold increase.

Specific case studies are probably the most accurate way to reflect what management engineering is all about. In one of our first hospitals, for example, work began with a project in the nursing department. The first step was to begin a quality-control program wherein the level of patient care was documented with a simple but accurate questionnaire technique and monitored at monthly intervals while patient-care improvements were implemented. Early in this project, however, those involved became aware of a considerable employee turmoil centered about several management problems. The priorities of the project were shifted so that the engineers met with all employees of the department at their convenience and drew from these discussions a series of actions that resulted in allaying employee fears and improving morale. Once the support of employees both for their own management and for the project had been secured, and a quality monitoring system was in force, the engineers proceeded to begin measuring the workload requirements and identifying roadblocks to effectiveness. This process lasted over a period of 2 years, but the results included a reduction in nursing hours per patient day (achieved through attrition as opposed to firings or layoffs) in a period when the acuity of patient care was increasing in the hospital.

A second case history can be drawn from a somewhat larger hospital immediately outside of metropolitan New York. Work in this hospital began approximately 3.5 years ago; during that period, the hospital had invested approximately $60,000 in management engineering. The first project undertaken was in the business function, with a goal of reducing accounts receivable. Management engineering is often seen as merely seeking productivity increases by staff reductions. In a department responsible for generating revenue and assuring accurate accounting, however, a reduction of one or two people could be disastrous. Thus, the thrust in this project was to iron out the system of charging, billing, and following up so that all patients and third parties were billed promptly and credit losses kept to a minimum. The impact of this first project was marked, reducing the accounts receivable by one-third over a period of about 9 months, during a time when the cost per month was going up so that accounts receivable normally would have risen. Following the improvement in the system, engineering efforts spread into the related area of electronic data processing, in which productivity improvements were made and duplications of effort avoided.

Following projects in several specific departments, the hospital became involved in applying the resource monitoring system to gain control of all labor cost. Using the methodology developed by the Hospital Management Engineering Program, a series of benchmarks were developed for each hospital department based on the specific situation and prevalent medical staff policy. Once these carefully tailored benchmarks had been set, a monthly monitoring report form was developed and trend analysis begun for each department. In this way, the hospital was able to identify areas in which a savings of well over $100,000 could be achieved by focusing on internal management.

The efforts of management engineering in this hospital have now matured to the point that the engineer is directly involved in the annual budgeting process. According to the hospital administrator, the hospital is now saving approximately $280,000 per year as a result of an investment of $60,000. Such a savings represents nearly a 5:1 return on investment, even ignoring the fact that many of the savings are repeating year after year.

A final case study can be taken from a third hospital consisting of approximately 400 beds. The management engineering program began in this hospital about 2 years ago. The initial project was, again, in the nursing department. Quality control was bypassed because the hospital already had a similar system in force. Following the success and implementation of savings in nursing and because of certain financial-improvement objectives, the administration decided to proceed with an overall survey of the situation. After applying the resource monitoring system to all departments, the hospital found that four departments represented a sizable savings potential. In-depth studies were immediately begun in all four departments, and after three months of analysis and work with the department heads, it was clear that approximately $500,000 could be saved. With absolute backing from the administration and the engineers' support, the hospital department heads set to work implementing the recommendations for systems changes and staffing adjustments. For a cost of only $80,000 over a 9-month period, this hospital's savings were $480,000 implemented, or a 6:1 return on investment. The savings are particularly significant in that three out of the four departments were professional departments in which the medical staff actually agreed with our findings and set to work installing our recommendations.

These results are not isolated incidents in the state or, in fact, in any area in which management engineering has existed for over a year. Unfortunately, however, they are not universal, either. Many hospitals are not receiving the full benefit of management engineering even when they are making the investment. This situation has led to an analysis of the factors that seem to influence success of a management engineering project. However, certain principles from this analysis seem to bear equally well on the applications of clinical engineering to the health field.

Observations

Cost effectiveness for any engineering discipline cannot be considered automatic. Possibly the greatest key to success is in applying the scientific method to our own performance as well as to the hsopital process to be improved. We must become effective in defining the needs of the hospital or patient first, then developing technology to meet that need. In cases in which we are simply taking established packages or products with an emphasis on sales, we are giving the hospital second best and will soon begin to reap the problems of such a strategy.

Caveat emptor applies equally to the hospital executive. When money is being spent in medical instrumentation or for management engineering, the hospital decision maker must take the full responsibility to get his money's worth. This means that he must focus on the factors that will bring success in an enterprise and assure that the provider can deliver to the hospital's expectations and specifications.

Research and development is both a necessity and a trap. It is clearly needed in any area as fast changing as the health-care field. Providers must have a commitment to research and development if they are to keep current with the field and meet new needs. However, research and development can be extremely expensive and ineffective. It must be carefully controlled and directed to high-priority areas. There is a related danger to the entire profession where some practitioners are developing and selling inferior technology to what remains a rather naïve public. Unless those of us within our respective professions control our own technology and performance, we will together (and rightly) be classified as a group of frauds.

If clinical engineering follows a course similar to management engineering, one must beware of becoming locked into a narrow or inaccurate image. One problem, of course, is differentiating between the design process of the engineer and the maintenance and operation process of the biomedical engineering technician. There is a highly significant need for the latter function; in some cases, men who are engineers by their degree are performing the function. However, it seems that this definition bears some analysis. In the case of management engineering, we are still suffering from the early days of stopwatch time study and rudimentary methods improvement. Even the present use of highly sophisticated computer algorithms and the involvement in every aspect of the planning process does not seem to change this narrow image.

Management engineers have often had trouble concentrating on learning the hospital field and discovering its peculiarities. Technology can be transferred to a large extent from industrial applications of management engineering but only when the engineer understands the context into which he brings the technology. A similar caution must be applied to clinical engineering.

22
THE CLINICAL ENGINEER'S ROLE IN HOSPITAL PLANNING

R. J. Boston

The clinical engineer's primary function has generally been assumed to be involved with medical instrumentation: selection, maintenance, and training. In this role, the clinical engineer provides both technical and administrative services, such as organizing an equipment maintenance program, supervising technicians, and conducting training programs.

It has further been suggested that the clinical engineer might participate in hospital planning activities. Future planning is becoming a major concern in the health-care field. Society is increasingly demanding that the most modern medical care, involving new medical techniques and technologies, be more widely available. These demands require that all hospitals at least consider expanding and updating their range of services.

At the same time, government, the public, and third-party payers are looking carefully at hospital costs, requiring hospitals to investigate techniques and technologies that can yield cost savings (without a sacrifice in quality of care). Because of these cost considerations, most areas require the development of comprehensive plans, along with the approval of a local or regional planning agency, before a hospital can develop new or expanded services. The specific contributions that a clinical engineer can make to hospital planning and the benefits he can obtain from assisting in these activities should be considered.

The Engineer's Contribution

An obvious contribution that a clinical engineer can make to hospital planning is related to his responsibility for instrumentation. If new or modified instrumentation is involved in any plans being considered, the operation of his department may be affected. Such concerns as ease of operation, extent of retraining of hospital personnel, and amount of required maintenance should normally be directed to him as the person handling these matters. In this role, the engineer is functioning as any other member of the hospital administration whose department is involved in proposed changes; he is specifying how the changes would affect his aspect of hospital operations.

However, an engineer can make a broader contribution to hospital planning, especially when the implementation of new technologies and associated changes in hospital operating procedures are being considered. Hospital planning is normally coordinated by the hospital administrator and his staff, with primary inputs from the hospital's medical staff and department heads. Long-term projects are usually considered and often initiated by the governing board of the hospital. These people usually have medical or administrative background and are not necessarily familiar with current technology.

The engineer is familiar with technology; his profession is to adapt new technologies to solve specific problems. In his training, an engineer obtains the technical background that is necessary to understand different technologies and to evaluate their capabilities in a given situation. Also, and probably of greater importance, he learns how to characterize a problem and how to specify the requirements for a solution.

With this background, an engineer can assist department heads and others in forming their inputs for the planning process. His participation usually falls into one or both of two categories: formulation of the problem and evaluation of equipment. Because of his familiarity with instrumentation and the way in which instrumentation specifications are written, he assists in the formulation of a problem and the development of appropriate specifications for a solution. He can determine that all pertinent parameters are included in the planning and that the parameters used are appropriate for comparison with available instrument specifications.

The second category is the evaluation of the actual capabilities of specific pieces of equipment. The engineer can act as the hospital's representative in meeting with various manufacturers' representatives who are trying to sell equipment. Being both technically sophisticated and familiar with the specific situation in his hospital, he can determine the actual capabilities of an instrument and evaluate how effectively it will perform in the particular environment for which it is being considered. He then reports his opinion to those who would actually be involved with the instrument so they may decide on its suitability for their need.

It is important that the engineer recognize the limits of his expertise and stays within them. Specifically, the engineer is qualified (or should be) to point out potential difficulties in the implementation of a particular technology in a specific hospital situation, to determine whether a particular piece of equipment can actually perform as a salesman promises, and to discuss with the hospital personnel involved whether the specifications they have developed for their problem are appropriate and complete.

However, unless the engineer is intimately familiar with the financial and administrative aspects of the hospital and the details of operation on a department level, he can only assist in obtaining appropriate information on which to base a decision concerning the implementation of a certain technology; he cannot specify the information or make the decision himself. For example, in the case of automatic data-processing equipment, he can assist various hospital departments in the proper and complete formulation of their data needs, but he cannot decide what those needs are. He should also be cautious in making strong recommendations, especially when they might be contrary to those of other hospital personnel directly involved.

One problem in which it is difficult to develop written specifications concerns quality of care. While an engineer should be able to comment on what a piece of equipment can do, it is quite a different matter to discuss its effects on quality of care, primarily because quality can rarely be satisfactorily defined, much less measured. Quality evaluations are currently based on subjective criteria, and despite the need for quantitative measures and substantial efforts to develop them, these evaluations are likely to remain subjective for some time. The engineer should be careful to let those with experience in providing medical care evaluate quality considerations.

Therefore, while the engineer can assist in developing a complete set of specifications for a problem and can evaluate the ability of a particular piece of equipment to satisfy those specifications, he is not in a position to develop specifications himself, and he should not attempt to make final decisions. If he recognizes these limitations, he can avoid making judgments outside his technical competence, antagonizing his co-workers, and having his potential contributions to future planning activities ignored.

Benefits to the Clinical Engineer

If an engineer's role in planning is very limited, should he make the effort to involve himself at all? He definitely should, and for several reasons. First, he has an obligation to his hospital to provide assistance in any way he can. Because of the conflicting demands of society for more services and lower costs, hospitals must tread carefully. They must implement those technologies that could yield significant cost savings or needed health services, and they must avoid technologies that are excessively expensive or marginally effective. A crucial input for avoiding these pitfalls is a detailed understanding of the technologies involved, particularly their capabilities and the potential problems in their implementation. A clinical engineer has the background to provide this input.

A second reason why an engineer should participate in planning activities is because he has an interest in what types of instrumentation are used in the hospital. Since he has the responsibility for maintaining instruments and training hospital personnel in their use, it is logical that he would want to offer an evaluation of instruments from these standpoints before decisions are made to purchase them.

A third reason for an engineer's participation in planning is that as the administration and his coworkers see the value of his understanding of technology, they will increase their confidence in him and probably rely more and more on his judgment concerning instrumentation in their own areas of responsibility. In this way, with increasing experience and expertise, the engineer will be able to play an increasingly significant role in planning for the implementation of new technologies in the hospital. The hospital will benefit by a more thorough evaluation of new technologies, and the engineer will benefit through broader responsibilities and an increasing sense of professional accomplishment.

23

THE CLINICAL ENGINEER AS AN INTERFACE IN THE HOSPITAL

T. S. Hargest

The position of the engineer in the delivery of health care and his relationship to the physician has been, and still is, hard to establish. The number of engineers in medicine is growing steadily, but there is poor definition of the organization pattern; thus, conclusions concerning these relationships and their effectiveness are difficult to ascertain. The analysis is a problem because of the lack of definition in hospital organization, which may place the engineer on any one of the three basic hospital operating staffs, administration, medical, or nursing. In each case, his relationship to the others may depend more on his personality than on the hospital organization structure or his technical ability.

It is important that the clinical engineer recognize these interfaces, which exist in nearly every hospital, and quickly learn how to cope with the problems that are generated by this rather unique method of organization.

The small hospital administrator may be a physician, businessman, or former schoolteacher. However, as the hospital size increases, it is most probable that he will be educated and trained for this position. Since it is unlikely that smaller hospitals will be employing full-time clinical engineers, it is appropriate to consider only those hospitals that would employ a trained hospital administrator who would have under his supervision those department heads usually found on hospital operating staffs.

There are nine reasonably possible positions through which a clinical engineer may interface with hospital personnel (Fig. 1). In each circumstance, his relationship to the other divisions will differ by some degree. Those clinical engineers whose services are acquired as (1) a consultant or (2) on a contract basis usually report directly to the administrator and are not required to meet and deal with the staff on a regular daily basis. Since this is the exception rather than the rule, it is more reasonable that the other situations should be those covered in greater detail.

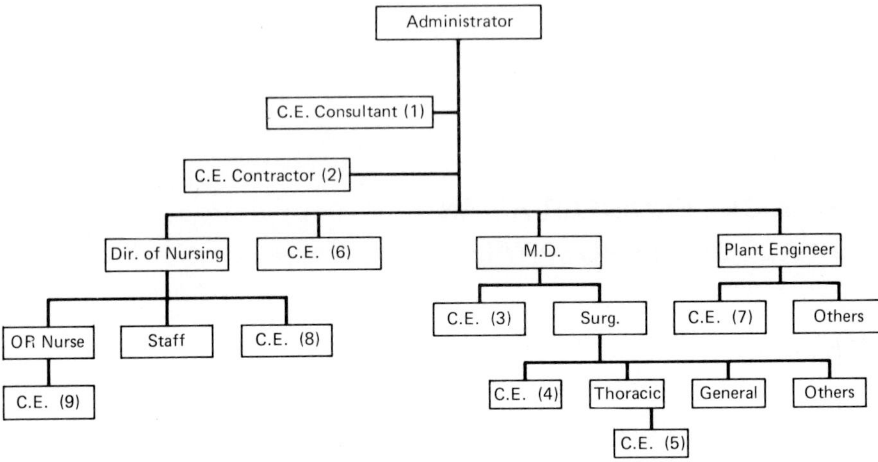

Fig. 1. Sample hospital organization.

In a medical university or teaching hospital in which the clinical engineer is employed for the express purpose of solving problems or assisting with research projects, the desired relationships can probably best be achieved by placing him on the medical staff. His actual position will reflect the scope of his influence. Thus, a clinical engineer who is directly responsible to the director of the medical staff (3) or the chairman of a department, such as medicine or surgery (4), will have far greater responsibility and influence than one employed by a particular division, such as thoracic surgery (5).

In other types of hospitals and those in which the circumstances previously described are not the desired goal, the position of choice makes the clinical engineer directly responsible to the administrator (6).

The table of organization that provides that the clinical engineer be supervised by the plant engineer (7) is the one least likely to have the desired results. Of course, there are those who may disagree with this conclusion; however, there are very good reasons for it. One must recognize that the physical plant engineer has been the person responsible for all hospital equipment in the past. The decision of the administrator or board of trustees to employ a clinical engineer may, whether justified or not, create in the mind of the plant engineer a degree of uncertainty and, in fact, an inferred criticism of his past effectiveness. His ego may be hurt, and he may even feel threatened. This is not always the situation. Certainly, there are plant engineers who will be delighted to see a competent clinical engineer take over the responsibility for those items of patient equipment that are of that degree of sophistication that their maintenance or repair is beyond the capability of the average technician available in most hospitals. Unfortunately, many plant engineers consider the employment of a clinical engineer a danger to their own security. To protect themselves, they do not permit him to function effectively. They feel that every recommendation for a change in policy will be considered a reflection on their heretofore unquestioned judgment. In nearly every case, these conclusions are completely unfounded.

The obvious solution is to eliminate this potential friction by appropriately dividing the responsibility and making each independent of the other but both responsible to the administrator. A reallocation of space and technical personnel may be required so that some of the technicians are supervised by the clinical engineer. This, in turn, may cause the first of several cases of "ruffled feathers," which must be smoothed since it is absolutely necessary that the clinical engineer develop a good rapport with the head of the physical plant. Considerable effort may be required to establish the proper relationship; but unless and until it is accomplished, the clinical engineer will have difficulty in achieving a smoothly operating program.

There are several ways to enlist the support of the plant engineer. The most effective is to utilize his knowledge by seeking his opinion and advice concerning both equipment and personnel. This will indicate to him that his opinion is valued. The clinical engineer should also take time to explain the details of his job and his plans. He should keep the plant engineer advised of the schedule of preventive maintenance and safety checks being instituted and make a continuing effort to reduce possible work-schedule conflicts. The clinical engineer should never suggest or request the assistance of plant personnel without first consulting with the plant engineer. He should also commend highly those things that have been properly handled, thus giving the plant engineer all possible credit when effective interfacing has been accomplished. This will encourage the plant engineer to work with the clinical engineer because he will realize that his efforts are recognized and thus it is to his advantage to be cooperative and helpful.

Once the chain of responsibility has been determined, it is then necessary to establish the relationship of the clinical engineer to the two other primary responsibility groups, the medical and nursing staffs. In most private hospitals in which the physicians are neither full-time employees nor research oriented, as are most medical-school personnel, the contact with physicians is very limited and consists of brief periods when the physician or surgeon makes rounds. This limits the ability of the clinical engineer to establish good rapport with the medical staff and will limit his effectiveness in this direction. On the other hand, such circumstances will increase his daily contact with the nursing staff and should permit him to become very effective in the training and patient-care problems related to their work.

The clinical engineer, fortunate enough to be a member of the medical staff, will find that although his physician-patient contacts are relatively easy to acquire, those with both the administration and the physical plant engineer may be exceedingly difficult.

Generally, the reaction of most employees to the employment of a clinical engineer is "the hospital did fine for years before you got here," and unless support can be developed from within the administrative staff, this attitude may be general enough to make progress difficult at best.

A good approach is to make oneself available to the hospital central supply committee, the group that advises on new purchases. Here, the engineer will come in contact with most of the clinical services and can help point out the apparent strengths and weaknesses of various products from a completely different viewpoint. By so doing, he will develop rapport with these individuals and begin to build the relationships that are so important to his ultimate success.

Recommending new items of housekeeping or patient care to the administrator, being available for comment on possible changes under consideration, and making suggestions that will help on a day-to-day basis in space allocation will build bridges with those with whom he comes in contact. The time expended will pay generous dividends.

Interfacing with the nursing personnel will generate a few unique problems even if one has the support of the nursing director, the administrator, and the medical staff.

One must recognize that the nurses realized long ago that anyone who is relatively happy and/or satisfied with a given situation will go away and leave them alone. Thus, regardless of their personal likes or dislikes, they will pursue such a condition in their relationship with residents, interns, doctors, and most of all, engineers. Therefore, they will generally be helpful and pleasant but frequently forget everything that has been said once the speaker is out of sight. This is probably a defense mechanism that permits them to accept the less necessary demands and requests made by some overbearing supervisor without having their entire day spoiled by that contact. In any case, the clinical engineer will have to prove himself with this group.

He can begin by doing some of the more obvious things that will be of help, such as being aware of what is new in patient care and keeping the nurses informed about new products; protecting their storage spaces when the first renovation comes along and everyone wants to steal that square footage for some other purpose; and trying to be helpful in solving nursing problems, and there are many of these. Some will seem quite simple but always have some hidden snag that makes a solution difficult to find. In addition, the clinical engineer must always be willing to come to the assistance of the nursing staff at any hour of the day or night. As his ability is recognized, and his responsibility increases, the nurse will call whenever she doesn't understand the operation of any device or system, whatever hour it may be. Frequently, it will be less often than necessary, but if the clinical engineer is to achieve that level of confidence necessary to relate well to the nursing staff, he will accept these inconveniences as an indication of their trust in his judgment.

The clinical engineer must also establish an ongoing rapport with the OR supervisor, a nurse who will have more need for, and be less apt to call on, his services. Of all the hospital staff personnel, this individual generally has the least effective in-house support. OR supervisors operate on a philosophy that concedes the inability of the maintenance staff to repair any piece of equipment, consequently, they maintain a great dependence on company representatives.

It is, of course, possible that the clinical engineer might be employed by the director of nursing service to work particularly with nurses or in the operating suite. If so, he could find himself responsible directly to the director of nursing (8) or possibly to the OR supervisor (9). In either of these positions, it is possible to do an effective job as it relates to the operating rooms and the equipment associated with them. Working outside of this area may be quite difficult when in either of these positions since it is unlikely that the plant or medical staff will relate well to such an individual.

Company representatives can be of great value to the clinical engineer. A brief conversation with the nursing staff or purchasing agent will provide a sound basis for the decision to establish a continuing relationship with certain capable company personnel. These men can be of great assistance in acquiring schematic diagrams of equipment, spare parts, and other information that will be of benefit in maintaining the equipment in question.

In certain cases, the hospital may have maintenance contracts with certain companies covering specific items of equipment. The decision concerning the value of the continuation of these contracts will frequently become the purview of the clinical engineer, and he should carefully consider all the problems involved in his determination of whether to continue or to curtail the contract and accept the maintenance responsibility covered by it.

There are other interfaces with which the clinical engineer will deal frequently. For example, there are the support personnel, who may be representatives of the physical plant, housekeeping, dietary team, and orderlies. Here he must be certain not to impose himself, his wishes, or orders without first clearing it with the appropriate supervisor. Creating strained relationships is the last thing that should be done.

The circumstances of contact between the clinical engineer and the various staff members frequently require different approaches.

Certainly one must recognize that the conditions that exist when the nursing staff is being oriented to a new patient-care device differ substantially from a situation in which the device fails to perform satisfactorily in the emergency room.

The clinical engineer must quickly evaluate the immediate conditions and respond in a manner that is fitting. Thus, new equipment orientation and preventive maintenance procedures are usually conducted at the convenience of all parties, whereas patient-care problems or emergencies are handled immediately.

Orientation and maintenance periods should be scheduled and the schedule adhered to as closely as possible. In this way, the contacts become used to seeing the clinical engineer performing his regular duties. Since these programs have been scheduled to provide a minimum of interference with the regular nursing procedures, the clinical engineer's presence will be accepted and his efforts welcomed. This will be particularly true when a reduction in equipment failures has been effected and recognized.

Contacts between the clinical engineer and patients or the relatives of a patient is a situation that requires a controlled reaction in a manner neither familiar nor taut.

The clinical engineer must accept the fact that insofar as the patient is concerned, he cannot assume a position of either responsibility or criticism. There are several rules of conduct that must be accepted by all paramedical personnel in the presence of the patient, and they are quite simple: the first and most basic is that he keep silent. Others of equal importance are: Do not criticize any procedure, and do not make any personal remarks concerning the patient or his condition.

The physician is responsible for the patient at all times under all conditions. His orders are carried out by the nursing staff. *There is no situation or circumstance that would exist that would justify or permit a clinical engineer to interfere in or change the orders or instructions of the physician.*

This does not mean that the engineer, outside the hearing of the patient and his relatives, should not suggest something he feels may be helpful to either the nurse or doctor. It does mean it should be just a suggestion, given as such, and done privately. At such a time, there is no room for argument or discussion unless initiated by the physician.

The reference to comments made in the presence of the patient are made to remind the engineer that an unconscious, dozing, or dying patient can hear, and nothing should be said to cause embarrassment, concern, or alarm.

Contacts with relatives of the patient frequently generate difficult situations. The clinical engineer may or may not know the diagnosis or prognosis of the patient, and even if he does, the relatives may not have been informed. Thus, it is neither the right nor the responsibility of the clinical engineer to discuss the patient or the treatment with relatives. This is the prerogative of the doctor; thus, the comments made to relatives should be innocuous and never reflect an opinion concerning the patient or his care.

Any discussion of interfaces infers a desire on the part of one party to be able to function effectively with others. In the hospital, this will also require an effort to "fit in." One should be recognized for his ability not his appearance. Professionalism is one of the most effective keys to acceptance. Regardless of the "law of the land," long hair, blue jeans, and T-shirts do not produce the accepted picture of professionalism. Those who feel they are obliged to do their "own thing" will find neither a job nor acceptance in the hospital atmosphere. Certainly this does not mean that there are no long-haired doctors. It does mean that those who deal with patients must present an appearance that engenders respect and confidence. Patients generally do not respond well to the casual carelessness that is acceptable today on many campuses and even in some business establishments. Since the clinical engineer will come into close contact with many people of variable backgrounds and opinions, the less controversial his actions the more acceptable he is likely to be. These are facts and the key to successful interfacing.

PART VI

THE ENVIRONMENT OF THE WORK

24

ENGINEERS IN CLINICAL ENGINEERING

M. J. Shaffer

A strong case has been made for more clinical engineers in the hospital and health-care environment based on the amount of instrumentation, the growing complexity of the systems, and the generally inadequate support obtained from vendor-service facilities. It has been estimated that the amount of instrumentation now handled involves approximately 5000 types from more than 1300 manufacturers. Recent publications from engineering societies all maintain that this need for more clinical engineers is urgent and acute.

To meet this need, a scale of one clinical engineer per 250-bed hospital has been proposed for a countrywide total of between 5000 and 10,000 engineers. Based on the regional concept used in Canada and England of between 5 to 10 clinical engineers per 250,000 population, a similar countrywide total of between 4000 to 8000 engineers would be required. Against this alleged need, it seems that the number of clinical engineers presently employed in United States hospitals does not substantially exceed 300, and at the same time, it is extremely difficult to identify any hospitals actively recruiting to meet the shortage. A disparity of this magnitude has to be attributed to some form of unexpected user reaction rather than to miscalculation, and it is suggested that there are two particular contributing elements requiring special study.

First, consider the running costs. Clinical engineering is presently operated somewhat uneconomically as an overhead item. There is no viable product, and the function will have difficulty in developing an active demand until it can demonstrate that it can indeed support itself, perhaps on a fee-for-service basis embracing a number of hospitals. Up-to-date, there has been no widespread adoption of the "shared-hospital" service concept.

The second aspect not often discussed involves an inbred personality difference between the physician and engineering specialists, differences that can render them almost 180° out of phase from each other. For this reason, it is often suggested that physicians with engineering orientation make better clinical engineers than engineers with clinical orientation, the supposition being that the physician–clinical engineers think as the users of the service and so deal better with their peers.

The second aspect will be discussed in detail as it is concerned mainly with a very important characteristic of a clinical engineer. And that is how a clinical engineer can interact effectively and diplomatically with a physician so that health-care delivery can be improved. It is widely recognized that the hospital and health-care field are indeed the physician's domain; he may need engineering assistance, but the type and amount of that assistance is his decision to make. For this reason, neither the physician nor his *modus operandi* should be critiqued, but the engineer who is proposing to participate in the field, to evaluate his general personality and to see whether an interface can be established that is mutually profitable to both specialties should be analyzed.

Considering initially the typical physician, it is accepted that he is a member of a learned profession that has clearly definable boundaries, with his membership recognized by title and uniform. His professional progress is established with specialty-board milestones along the way, each one worthwhile in that those not so qualified can be prevented from practicing the specialty; thus, he has a strong incentive for a continuous lifelong education and for eventual recognition as a "senior" physician. His training and work are crisis-oriented in nature, and there is a steady demand for his services; in consequence, he has a high measure of job satisfaction based on prestige, challenge, working conditions, growth potential, and once he has completed his residency, remuneration.

On the other side of the sheet, the clinical engineer will probably have received his engineering training from the industrial environment in a field that has most undefinable scope, embracing numerous technologies, applications, and products. This enormous breadth and indefinitiveness of scope makes it almost impossible, especially in a fluctuating economic environment, to establish meaningful specialties in which unqualified people can be prevented from practicing. Thus, professional membership, a title, and a uniform have minimal value, and there is little incentive for lifelong education other than for self-satisfaction. In fact, it is not unknown where in many positions higher academic qualifications are disadvantageous on the ground of overqualification. Accordingly, his objective for adequate growth potential is not to become a "senior" engineer but a manager. This in itself usually requires that his allegiance becomes aligned not with his field but with his corporate body (which in itself has a natural tendency to oppose profession-oriented restrictions), and his engineering expertise normally becomes diluted in time by administrative chores. In outlook, his training leads toward deliberate long-term planning to get the best results and to design against foreseeable contingencies; with this training, he can well complement the physician. For these reasons, many engineers do indeed look to a union with the more stable learned professions such as medicine or law, which offer comparatively low job satisfaction as applied to working conditions, remuneration, and prestige, and do show possibilities for establishing definable specialties. Thus, it is imperative that serious thought be given to the interface between the physician if a productive relationship is to be exploited.

Obviously, a first step in any marriage is that both parties appreciate and accept the other's background and *modus operandi*. Much can be gained by being able to anticipate reactions.

A second step can be to set up a clear-cut allocation of responsibilities in which both parties are able to use their expertise as much as possible on a nonconflicting basis; specifically, the physicians could be responsible for defining operational requirements, and the clinical engineers could be made responsible for hardware and software design and reduction to practice. This arrangement should not preclude mutual assistance in the other's responsibility area; however, the assistance would be provided by invitation only.

A third step for consideration is that the organization reporting structure should allow both specialties to manage their own people on the basis that responsibility and authority go hand in hand. This is meant to imply that clinical engineers should not report as individuals to a physician, rather that they should be formed into a self-contained unit headed by an engineer who, in turn, can report to the physician or clinical department. The objective here is to develop both interspecialty and intraspecialty harmony; this step can avoid the somewhat disrupting situation in which, because of the close association between the parties, one group can take sides in judging the technical competence of individuals in the other group and, perhaps not appreciating the technology, can back the ones most plausible and least effective. In line with this, the words "self-contained" used previously can be important when the specialty has two clearly separate subspecialties, such as in clinical engineering in which the hardware and software subspecialties are each dependent on the other but easily fractionated if reporting to different heads.

25

MEDICAL FACILITIES AND EQUIPMENT: SHARED TECHNOLOGY

A. Zara

Efficient management of technology in the health-care-delivery industry is a vital role for the clinical engineer. A general viewpoint can be given regarding a broad approach that can be used even in the smallest community—a shared service.

The Problem

As medical procedures and techniques have advanced, much is required to support new techniques. Medical equipment daily becomes more intricate and medical facilities have become complex systems with needs for control of electric power, air conditioning, communications, and transportation, to mention a few. Costs of these activities have risen, particularly, as safety hazards are discovered or aging requirements are met in maintenance. Attempts to manage the technology in these areas have had to face up to a lack of people trained in the field.

One critical problem has been the continuing scarcity of clinical engineering personnel with the necessary competence. In 1974 it was estimated that there were 3000 hospital engineers in a total labor pool of 1 million engineers. If one contrasts those numbers to the clinical engineering needs of the more than 7000 hospitals in the United States, the scarcity of qualified personnel becomes readily apparent. An important additional factor to consider is the cost for hospitals to maintain full-time departments having needed levels of plant and clinical engineering expertise. It is a major expense. However, positive steps can be taken.

Large hospitals are beginning to hire graduate engineers and highly trained technicians. Medium and small community-type hospitals, which comprise the largest number of hospitals, are becoming aware of the problem and their staffs must be expanded to include a manager of technology. Additionally, part-time personnel, and shared services, or the use of consultants must be considered.

An engineering shared-service, a voluntary, nonprofit group appears to be a viable solution for even the smallest group to render engineering and technical services in accordance with the needs of each institution. Such an agency can through volume, obtain back-up and assistance necessary.

Organization and Functions

Some of the functions can include: (*a*) establishing standards of performance; (*b*) establishing patterns for costing of services; (*c*) augmenting educational capability; and (*d*) coordination in any problem area, particularly where differences exist and in problems that involve many areas under different jurisdictions.

Hospitals, generally, turn to equipment manufacturers and dealers to provide service on much of their equipment. Some indicate that some manufacturers view service after the sale as a necessary evil—and not a major product. The fee for hourly rates is high, and most manufacturers service only what they sell. This can lead to overlap, duplication, or independence on the part of the supplier, which may not benefit the user.

Without continuing engineering personnel, many find that organized preventive maintenance, calibration, and safety programs cannot become firmly established. Also, hospitals may lack proper engineering expertise to choose the optimum or most appropriate type of equipment.

Ideally, hospitals should have full-time clinical engineers on their staffs. However, not all hospitals can or have yet learned how to afford in-house programs or employ full-time clinical engineers. In addition, there is scarcity of personnel with the necessary competence. Thus, shared services are acknowledged as reasonable approaches toward greater economy.

A number of shared clinical engineering service programs have evolved nationwide. Table I is a listing of some major programs. The following chapters provide details on some others.

Types of Shared Services

There are models to hospital shared services in other areas. Blumberg (see Bibliography) has compiled an extensive listing of functions which have been shared by hospitals as shown in Table II. Clinical engineering can fit into many of them.

Each shared service group should have a core of professionals and a number of technicians. Part-time assistance can be used at all levels. The main purpose is multifold:

1. Implementing a cost effective program to train people, procure equipment, and establish procedures
2. Continuing education is a paramount objective of technology management

TABLE I
Listing of Some Major Shared Service Programs

Arizona Hospital Education and Research Foundation, Inc.
4202 East Raymond, Phoenix, Arizona 85040

Samaritan Health Service
1033 East McDowell Road, Phoenix, Arizona 85006

Cooperative Institutional Services Corporation/Shared Biomedical Engineering Service
6255 Sunset Boulevard, Suite 817, Los Angeles, California 90028

Shared Clinical Engineering Service and Training Center
Suite 765, Pacific Trade Center, Honolulu, Hawaii 96813

North Suburban Association for Health Resources
Medical Physics Service
1500 Shermer Road, Northbrook, Illinois 60062

Regional Health Resource Center
Biomedical Engineering Service Team
1406 West University Avenue, Urbana, Illinois 61801

University of Maine
Clinical Engineering Laboratory
Barrows Hall, Orono, Maine 04473

Technology in Medicine, Inc.
3 New England Executive Park, Burlington, Massachusetts 01803

Greater Grand Rapids Hospital Council, Inc.
Biomedical Engineering Department
2096 Waters Building, Grand Rapids, Michigan 49502

Medical Instrumentation Systems—Hospital Shared Engineering Services, Inc.
15133 Kercheval Avenue
Grosse Pointe Park, Michigan 48230

University of New Hampshire
Northern New England Clinical Engineering Center
Kingsbury Hall, Durham, New Hampshire 03842

Hospital Research and Education Trust of New Jersey
Biomedical and Engineering Shared Technology
1101 State Road, Princeton, New Jersey 08540

Emergency Care Research Institute
913 Walnut Street, Philadelphia, Pennsylvania 19107

Carolinas Hospital Engineering Support Services
P.O. Box 4587, Charlotte, North Carolina 28204

Northwest Ohio Clinical Engineering Center
4427 Talmadge Road, Toledo, Ohio 43623

Hospital Central Services, Inc.
2100 Westgate Drive, Bethlehem, Pennsylvania 18018

Shared Hospital Electrical Safety Services
Texas State Technical Institute, Building 19-7, Waco, Texas 76705
Texas Hospital Association, P.O. Box 4553, Austin, Texas 78765

University of Vermont
Technical Services Program
Royall Tyler Annex, Burlington, Vermont 05401

TABLE II
Hospital Activities Subject to Sharing by Several Hospitals

Hospital Administration
1. Combined administration
2. Industrial engineering efforts
3. Legal services
4. Public relations
5. Legislative representation
6. Accreditation
7. Liability insurance

Business Services
1. Data processing-computer
2. Payroll preparation
3. Patient billing
4. Collection Services
5. Accounting
6. Negotiating charges with third parties

Medical Staff
1. Shared Medical Staff
   a. Medical Director
   b. Chief of Clinical Service
   c. Pathology
   d. Radiologist
   e. Others
2. Concurrent Staff Meetings
3. Postgraduate Education

Nursing Services
1. Administration
2. Roster of temporary employees
3. Service manuals procedures
4. Evaluation of procedures
5. Student nurse education
6. Graduate nurse education
7. Practical nurses
8. Nurses aides
9. OR technician training

Regional Planning
1. Developing planning agencies
2. Implementing regional plans
3. Designated services to specific hospitals

Regional Planning, *continued*
4. Hospital utilization committees
5. Bed locator services
6. Planning public transportation
7. Parking
8. Home care services

Medical Records
1. Management of medical records
2. Design of standard forms
3. Statistical analysis

Purchasing and Storeroom
1. Group purchasing
2. Storage of supplies
3. Evaluation and testing
4. Central sterile supply service

Food Services
1. Preparation of meals
2. Preparation of staff meals
3. Shared dietitian

Personnel Activities
1. Administration of personnel
2. Recruiting
3. Job descriptions
4. Negotiating wages
5. Job placement
6. Insurance coverage
7. Health career planning

Other Services
1. Joint laundry operation
2. Housekeeping services
3. Plant maintenance
4. Duplicating or printing services
5. Pharmacy
6. Blood bank
7. Coordination of ambulance services
8. Laboratory services

3. Performance of maintenance and repair procedures with full documentation thereof
4. Maintenance of standards
5. Quality control checks to verify all work done

Most hospitals that use shared clinical engineering services are nonprofit acute care general hospitals. A few clinics and nursing homes and other facilities are

TABLE III
Hospitals Served as Categorized by Bed Size

Number of beds	Percentage of hospitals served
under 50	Less than 5%
50–100	25%
101–200	more than 25%
201–400	33%
over 400	more than 25%

provided services. A W. K. Kellog Foundation sponsored report by Dodson and Latimer (see Bibliography) indicated bed-size characteristics of hospitals which participated in shared clinical engineering programs in 1975. The results are shown in Table III.

The same report also indicated the differences and similarities among shared clinical engineering programs. Pertinent average data between 6 successful programs in 1975 centers is shown in Table IV.

The figures in Table IV can be used to determine the ranges and averages of dollars spent per bed served, per hospital served, and per program staff employed, as well as the average number of beds per hospital served and the percentage of eligible hospitals served. Per bed year, for example the cost (yearly budget plus parts and 1/5 of capital per year) is $58.89.

Costs of shared-service effort include maintenance, repair, and safety and all relevant procedures and backup supplies. There are many ways to fund payments of shared services. Each group must be individualized to cover both start-up and subsequent maintenance.

TABLE IV
The "Average" Shared Clinical Engineering Program

Number of Hospitals Served	24
Number of Beds Served	5,058
Service Staff (Engineers and Technicians)	9
Number of Operation Centers	2
Dollars Invested in Capital Equipment	67,000
Dollar Inventory in Repair Parts	4,500
Yearly Operating Budget	279,996

26

BASIC MODELS

J. H. Tolbert

Shared biomedical instrumentation engineering services have become a recognized means of supplying a biomedical-engineering capability to the community hospital in the various suburbs throughout the United States. There is no question of the value of shared services for hospitals and the fact that shared engineering services reduce the cost for this capability to hospitals. The most common question asked by many hospital administrators and chief engineers is: "What type of shared biomedical instrumentation engineering plan is most adaptable to my hospital, least costly, and will be most successful in establishing an efficient and workable preventive maintenance program?"

There are two basic plans in use today: One is the concept of a central group of technicians; the other is that of individual technicians placed in the various hospitals involved in the plan. In each hospital, an SMI laboratory facility is organized under supervision of the associate administrator or chief engineer.

The first of the two plans, which is the central group or centralized laboratory, involves a private organization to which the member hospital in the plan pays a fee for services rendered. These services involve sending technicians to the member hospitals to perform various types of instrumentation repair and maintenance functions. There are several disadvantages to this plan. First, if a preventive maintenance system is involved that requires that equipment be brought to the central laboratory, which in itself entails transportation of equipment or transportation costs for personnel, the possibility of failure or damage increases. Another disadvantage of this plan is that a technician assigned to one hospital for repair work may not return to that hospital again very soon. The tendency is to have certain technicians specialize in certain types of equipment, and as specialists in that equipment, their services could be in demand in two or more hospitals at the same time. For example, one who has a special ability with ECG machines and is very familiar with them would be in demand; therefore, should failure of ECG machines occur in several hospitals at the same time, a conflict could result. Also, a technician assigned to a member hospital does not have a particular interest in that hospital. Essentially, he is no different than a service technician employed by a manufacturer. Thus, his only interest is the particular machine that he is going to service, and after repairing the instrument, he returns to the central laboratory

An example of this plan is the Biomedical and Engineering Shared Technology (B.E.S.T.) is a clinical engineering shared service of the New Jersey Hospital Association, which provides a clinical engineering consultation service that includes electrical safety, biomedical equipment management, education and training seminars on the proper and safe use of medical equipment, preventive maintenance, and on-call equipment service.

The need for programs in clinical engineering, electrical safety, and biomedical equipment management has long been recognized. Recently, considerable attention has been placed on this from the Joint Commission on Accreditation of Hospitals in the United States, insurance companies, and a number of other national and state agencies.

The B.E.S.T. program is designed to assist hospitals in the following ways:

1. Prepare inventory forms for all biomedical equipment and design a system to ensure regular maintenance and calibration
2. Provide consultation on electrical safety and equipment management, including current and proposed rules and standards of regulatory agencies
3. Provide maintenance and repair service on all types of biomedical equipment
4. Conduct electrical safety inspection in the hospitals
5. Provide prepurchase advice on equipment and inspection of incoming equipment to ensure its compliance with specifications, proper operation, and safety
6. Conduct training sessions to enable hospital staff to recognize potential electrical and safety problems, understand safety as applied to all activities of the hospital, and learn proper operation and utilization of complex medical equipment
7. Provide on-call biomedical services to assist physicians in setting up blood-pressure-monitoring equipment; testing cardiac pacemakers, electrode catheters, and other implantable electronic devices; determining the patient's stimulation threshold; and assist in operation and use of ultrasonic diagnostic equipment, cardiac-output instruments, and other sophisticated medical-electronic equipment
8. Conduct OSHA-type survey followed by comprehensive report and engineering consultation for implementing a program to effect compliance with codes and standards of the regulating agencies
9. Update, redesign, and interface existing instruments to help the hospitals realize a greater economy and utilization of medical equipment

Although many hospitals are placing strong emphasis on the above program, it is believed that the greatest value will ultimately lie in the professional clinical-engineering services. The clinical engineer, in consultation with staff physicians in a hospital, will be able to develop equipment modifications, redesign, and interfacing, which will lead to greater utilization of existing equipment. This will provide customizing of instrumentation to the physician's need, effecting better health-care delivery.

Due to the extremely rapid proliferation of medical equipment and the simultaneous demands of most health-care personnel to obtain the latest state of the art in medical instrumentation, hospitals have become exhibit halls of hundreds of different kinds of devices. The lack of systems engineering and in-house expertise has caused much of this equipment to be grossly under-utilized. Manufacturers often will not advise or help in interfacing their equipment with that of another manufacturer. Too often their solution is to sell the hospital thousands of dollars worth of extra equipment instead of making a relatively minor modification. This is understandable in today's highly competitive market, where the state of the art is changing so rapidly. They cannot spare an engineer's time from the design of their next generation equipment to do special custom projects with perhaps only a one-time application. Hospital-shared services with innovative and experienced clinical engineers who are dedicated to problem solving in the clinical setting is the answer to this dilemma. New Jersey hospitals now have an access to this capability, which is usually only available in the large university medical centers.

The following is a list of the initial modular program: (*a*) full-time BMETs with clinical engineering back-up and support; (*b*) part-time BMETs with necessary clinical-engineering support; (*c*) on-call biomedical services and engineering consultations; (*d*) service contracts on specific equipment; (*e*) engineering project contracts; (*f*) training and educational seminars; (*g*) equipment-control program; (*h*) OSHA survey with comprehensive report and engineering consultation; and (*i*) preventive maintenance and patient safety inspections with comprehensive reports. This program will be expanded to include health physics, radiation safety, and areas of plant engineering. B.E.S.T. is looking forward to a close cooperation with the other shared clinical engineering services.

The second plan involves the establishment of the position of a biomedical instrumentation engineer to act as director of the SMI department in a central contractor hospital. Once he has established his department in the central hospital or base hospital and has trained a technician to perform the repair and preventive maintenance functions, he is then ready to begin working with the member hospitals in a systematic fashion, establishing SMI laboratories in each of the hospitals with their own technicians. The hospital management is aware of what he is doing and his performance. Consequently, there is a strong incentive for him to take an extreme interest in every instrument in the hospital and every aspect of safety related to medical instrumentation. As a result of this plan, the technician is complimented for his initiative and effort. In other words, he has the opportunity to expand, advance himself, and propagate information on biomedical instrumentation engineering.

27

THE NYACK PLAN

I. M. Kane

The Nyack plan, also referred to as the Kingpin Hospital concept, is an example of the second plan. Some of the main advantages of the Nyack plan are (*a*) a low cost to all hospitals in the plan; (*b*) increase in patient/staff safety; (*c*) periodic calibration of instrumentation by qualified personnel; (*d*) reduced outside-vendor repair costs, (*e*) higher return on purchasing dollars; (*f*) immediate attention to instrumentation emergencies within the hospital; (*g*) a higher degree of confidence because of data resulting from preventive maintenance programs wherein sufficient documentation and data retrieval are involved; (*h*) reduction in malpractice liability; and (*i*) possibility of eventual reduction in insurance premiums.

In comparison, the Nyack hospital plan has a greater advantage over the central group plan in that there is no repetition of services; for example, the central group plan is costly since the central laboratory is required to obtain its own malpractice insurance or liability insurance. A small addition in premiums to the hospital's regular insurance is all that is required to cover a biomedical instrumentation engineer within the hospital. However, there is no addition to the hospital premium to cover its own SMI technician. The additional cost of secretarial personnel, utilities, instrumentation owned by the plan, compensation insurance, and the costs of operating a separate business must be paid for by the member hospitals of the central group plan. This is a duplication of effort on their part because within their own hospital they already have available, in almost every case, secretarial time, utilities, telephone, etc., that they are paying for and do not use full time.

The Nyack shared biomedical instrumentation engineering plan is a very direct, and by virtue of its simplicity, effective plan that can best be described as consisting of three phases.

Survey and Problem-Definition Study Period. During this phase, the biomedical instrumentation engineer conducts a fairly rigid survey of the member hospital joining the plan. It is culminated in a confidential, comprehensive engineering report to the administration of this hospital.

Implementation and Training Period. During this phase, the biomedical instrumentation engineer assists the member hospital in interviewing, for technical capability, prospective BMETS. The BMET is trained in hospital techniques, shown the operation of the preventive maintenance system, assists in setting up an SMI laboratory in the member hospital, and is made aware of necessary safety modifications.

Follow-Up, Engineering Consultation, Direction and Education Seminar Continuing Program. Throughout this phase the BMET is checked by the biomedical instrumentation engineer at certain intervals to assure that the program is fruitfully carried out. Data from equipment evaluations are shared, and the biomedical instrumentation engineer is consulted on types of equipment or modifications and is available for investigations in cases of accident. Periodic lectures on safety and safe use of equipment (with visual aids) are given at member hospitals by the biomedical instrumentation engineer.

The Nyack shared biomedical-instrumentation-engineering plan has been in existence for more than 2 years. Membership in the plan has been extended to eight hospitals within a 75-mile radius of the central hospital, encompassing four counties.

The progress made in increasing the mean time between failures of scientific and medical instrumentation has been extremely encouraging. It can be shown statistically that as a result of the preventive maintenance programs installed, the number of repairs has been reduced.

28

THE IMPLEMENTATION OF A MEDICAL ENGINEERING SERVICE

J. A. Hopps, J. Busser, N. Anderson, A. Colombo, D. Djordjevic, C. Laszlo, J. Lenihan, J. Matauschek, J. McCormick, M. Meyers, M. Milosevic, F. Norman, P. Paraskevopoulos, B. Pendic, S. Pocock, A. Remond, R. Thorner, R. Tomovic, B. Van Eijnsbergen, J. Weinman, M. White, T. Williams, and T. Zeren

Any administrative plan for a medical engineering service in health care must reflect a partnership status, recognizing the substantial contribution that the engineer or scientist has made in the advancement of medical diagnosis and treatment. For example, maintenance and repair demands may range from (1) A minimum, providing only for maintenance and simple repair, to (2) A fully integrated service with professional bioengineers and scientists providing centralized and local services for maintenance and repair and research and development (R&D) at any location in which medical research, clinical care, or mass screening procedures are undertaken.

The objective should be to match the level of medical knowledge and practice with an equal competence in science and technology. Such a partnership is necessary to avoid strangulation of medical progress for want of technological back-up.

The ability of a health-care system to undertake R & D in association with medical research is basically a financial matter, sometimes requiring a separate funding channel. On the other hand, maintenance and repair are operating costs and as such are normal budget items for health-care institutions at all levels. It will be apparent that the required scientific back-up will differ greatly between the extremes of (1) and (2).

Where the principal objective is efficient maintenance and repair, the structure is rather simple and the service may be attached to hospital plant engineering services, government services (post office, communications, public works, etc.), military services, or teaching or research institutions with technological facilities.

At best, these are compromise solutions, and all offer some disadvantages, as outlined in previous sections. The present trend to locate extensive instrumentation facilities at the larger medical centers serving the needs of regional hospitals strongly recommends a similar pattern for the administration of maintenance and repair services. While local administration of a small bioengineering unit takes care of routine services, there must also be an access route for technical and professional bioengineering liaison with authority so that the unit is well informed of technological developments, the pattern of common instrumentation failures, and the experience of other units of the system.

This is more simply expressed in the injunction: Do not cut off your technical services for external contacts. It is equally important that communication be encouraged with medical colleagues for the effective exchange of data on the use and maintenance of equipment and that a career structure for technicians, bioengineers, and physical scientists be created, providing incentive for all employed in the unit.

Concurrent with the definition of goals and planning of physical facilities, a policy must be established for the hiring and development of professional and technical personnel. The classification of engineering staff may in certain instances be supplemented to suit specific needs. Sheet-metal workers, machinists, computer programmers, and other skilled personnel may be required in a large unit serving all or a substantial part of the health-care system.

It bears repeating that technical services of a medical engineering nature should be consolidated in a single group for effective administration and maximum utilization of available facilities. It may be realistic, however, to assign members of this group to look after the recurring needs of technologically oriented departments such as radiology in order to achieve a continuity of service and a specialization of expertise. It should be stressed that we do not classify the medical technologist (e.g., radiographer, laboratory technician, etc.) as a staff member. A differentiation between technologists and technicians must be made.

It is most important that a compatible relationship exist between the medical and paramedical staff on the one hand, and the professional and technical staff on the other. Both groups should be active in a continuing program of mutual education. The staff can play an important role in support of complex surgical or clinical investigation procedures, and if they do, they will have a better appreciation of the more mundane "housekeeping" area of their duties. Both branches of the staff should share the responsibility for planning and supervising safety procedures, developing emergency measures, and designing future health-care services. It is also recommended that an interdisciplinary scientific advisory council be formed that could serve as an interface between health services and scientific research and development. Such a council could advise on major policy for engineering activity within the health-care structure, in institutional research, and industrial development.

The Responsibilities of Administration

Medical engineering services, like other departments in a hospital, should be responsible to the administrator. It is important that he be familiar with the extent and limitations of available services and that he make these known to other departments of the institution.

The administrator must allocate funds for operations and have the final authority for the approval of budgets for staff, facilities, training, maintenance parts, and test equipment, and other requirements of the service. He should require a competent accounting of expenditures and should approve capital expenditures for its expansion. It is recommended that he direct the head of the service to prepare a procedural manual that determines the terms of reference for medical engineering activity and that he, with competent advice, ratify acceptable procedures to effect a clear understanding of the operation of the service.

Negotiations for contracted services or purchases are the function of administration but should be conducted after consultation with the engineering staff where applicable. Expertise should be used in planning extension or renovation of facilities or installation of new plant facilities. This type of liaison will prevent minor disasters in planning, such as inadequate radiation protection of radiology and nuclear-medicine installations, indiscreet location of electrically sensitive instruments, lack of monitoring facilities in operating theaters, and ICUs or CCUs, and unsafe electrical systems in the patient-care area.

Patient care is the legal responsibility of the administration. This determines the extent of interface of engineering personnel with the patient in such areas as prosthetics and orthopedics, pacemaker clinics, cardiac-bypass procedures, dialysis treatment, etc. It also underscores the importance of an effective discipline of patient safety, particularly in protection against electric shock or combustion of flammable agents and monitoring of environmental hazards. These are areas of safety that are generally assigned to the medical engineering department of a hospital.

The administrator should insist on periodic reports from the staff of scheduled preventive maintenance inspections undertaken, the volume of repair work completed during the period, and the results of all safety-inspection tours.

The hospital administration should provide an environment and a career opportunity that will provide incentive to the members of the staff. Salary scales should be commensurate with their responsibility and comparable with those prevailing in the region.

The head of a unit or department will be normally the senior medical engineer or physical scientist. He will serve as a consultant on technology, methodology, research and development, and, in advanced health-care institutions, data acquisition and conversion and system analysis and synthesis. He will be responsible for the program of preventive maintenance, the safety of instruments, installations and clinical procedures, the guidance and instruction of maintenance and repair personnel, the scrutinizing of technical-service contracts, and the evaluation of equipment before purchase and its inspection upon arrival.

The responsibilities of the administrator and engineering head, as outlined previously, apply in the case of an institutional engineering unit or department. If the facility is at a national or regional level, it may have an autonomous status. Then the head must assume the responsibilities listed for the administrator, as he is the administrator of a health-system facility. He will report to the proper authority on financial and other policy matters, and the authority may assume control of purchasing and personnel administration. Even so, he will probably require more clerical assistance than would a hospital unit and will need a more comprehensive storekeeping system. These back-up services are vital to the effective operation of the unit and must be provided for at the planning stage. Transportation demands will also be more critical for a unit serving more than one hospital.

Organizing a Medical Engineering Service

The organizational framework for technological services in a health-care system must be planned with two purposes in mind. The facility must be patient oriented and must offer a satisfactory environment that will attract and retain competent staff. It may be complex, with responsibilities for computation, data handling, and design and development, or it may comprise only maintenance and repair services. It should be available to all the medical departments but responsible to the administration rather than to any specific service.

A typical medical engineering department that would provide a comprehensive service in a large health-care institution should include a computer applications group of modest proportions. If the institutional commitment to data processing is great, this group often is split off to form a separate department that may share the technical facilities of the unit.

A more typical establishment has as its central core an engineering and technical-service group whose major commitment is in maintenance and repair services but that may have some involvement in design, clinical design, or health-care planning. The latter activity should be recognized by the administration as more intellectually fulfilling to the professional members of the engineering staff and encouraged, therefore, as an incentive feature of their program. Even in a modest unit serving a small hospital, there is occasional opportunity for constructive input from the staff in planning and development. It should be encouraged as a functional role of the department.

The director of the service should have the status of a department head in the hierarchy of the health-care service. In addition to the units shown on the organization chart, he will require administrative, clerical, and storekeeping staff and an effective transportation service if the department's responsibilities extend beyond the institution in which it is located.

The administrative duties will include the maintenance of records on all hospital equipment from the time of purchase until its ultimate disposal. The determination of service policies is dependent on accurate cost accounting of maintenance and repair procedures, and these costs should be included on the equipment record sheets. It may also be necessary to cost account all operations if the department operates on a fee-recovery basis, charging other health-care departments for services rendered.

The organization should include a library of technical information, manufacturers' literature and users' manuals, copies of safety or performance standards, and periodicals appropriate to the type of departmental functions.

If the unit has any extensive responsibility for the purchase and accounting of spare parts and components, adequate staff must be provided to handle these duties. The effective management of the stores section becomes most important if replacement parts are not readily available locally. In an institutional unit, ordering and stock audit duties may be assumed by a member of the technical staff.

For maintenance and repair services for health-care institutions with in-house engineering departments, the involvement of the engineering staff commences before purchase and continues until the final disposition of equipment, at breakdown or obsolescence. The manufacturer's or agent's services are utilized where available. Complex equipment such as X-ray, dialysis systems, or monitoring installations frequently require such services, and the warranty against failure may be conditional upon the supplier's participation in their installation and in staff instruction. It may be possible at the time of purchase to decide on the need for supplier services if the decision is reflected in the purchase price.

The above indicates a commitment by the medical user in routine maintenance. Generally, this is a very elementary nature—cleaning of electrodes and recording pens, routine replacement of fuses, film cassettes, etc. It introduces a situation, however, that is often encountered when engineering services are organized in a well-established hospital. Medical departments (particularly radiology) may have technical personnel on staff to handle maintenance problems. Should they be transferred to the engineering unit? The decision depends on the use of their time, the requirement for a unique expertise, and the dependence on ancillary services. Many health-care systems have found the retention of departmental technical staff to be compatible with the engineering unit concept. It is important that such personnel have access to the facilities of the medical engineering unit. If the service is located outside the institution, departmental technical staff provide continuity to the routine maintenance program.

There also is an involvement of the engineering unit in hospital safety. The responsibility is shared with the medical departments involved. For example, the unit can provide a radiation-monitoring service, but only the medical staff can enforce its use. Similarly, the medical engineering department has an important function in protection against electrical hazards, but safety in clinical procedures depends on the recognition by medical and nursing personnel of an implemented discipline.

The engineering service has an extensive role in the commissioning of new equipment, commencing with assessment of proposed purchases, provision of required specifications for the equipment, necessary spares, operating instructions and maintenance/repair manuals, and recommendation of the appropriate policy for maintenance to the extent that it might influence contract agreement with the supplier, agent, or manufacturer. The planning of the installation is the next consideration of the medical engineering staff. Specifications should be prepared for special requirements such as services (gas, water, air conditioning, electrical supply); floor loading; radiation shielding; access for installation; patient use; and maintenance and support facilities (film-processing units, remote controls, dressing rooms, etc.).

The involvement of engineering personnel in the inspection of incoming equipment and instrumentation may save the health-care system from unnecessary expense. If the inspection is not an automatic procedure, short shipments, transport damage, or faulty performance will not be detected within the warranty period, and long delays in putting the equipment into normal service may result.

The potential value of staff instruction in technical matters is often overlooked in the health-care system. It is not practical that medical staff and their supporting services should be subjected to extensive technological training, but a rudimentary understanding of the basic principles involved in the operation of instruments and equipment can provide more effective use and less misuse. In the organization of a service, staff should be allocated for this important function. It is equally important that the technical staff understand the rationale for the medical use of the equipment, and provision should be made for their instruction.

The requirement for internal staff training in medical engineering technology, maintenance and repair procedures, machine-shop practices, etc., will depend on the external access to such instruction. Where possible, staff should be selected for their professional or technical qualifications as engineers, electronics technicians, craftsmen, etc., so that additional training is limited to the special requirements of health care. Much of this specialized instruction is available in industry. X-ray equipment and medical electronic instrument manufacturers now offer seminars and training programs on installation, operation, maintenance, and repair. In some areas, community technical colleges offer a wide variety of courses in paramedical technologies.

Irrespective of the training facilities available outside the health-care system, some provision must be made in the organization of a service for the ongoing teaching and updating of staff members as technology develops and the medical instrumentation commitment increases.

Equipping a Facility

The facilities required for a medical engineering service in health care depend on the extent of service to be provided. In a small hospital, the unit may consist of only one staff member occupied in preventive maintenance and simple repair procedures. On the other hand, a large institution or a health-care system may have extensive services and undertake a wide range of activities, including major repairs, construction of instruments or accessories, hazard monitoring, research and development, hospital planning, and consultation. The facilities, therefore, vary from basic tools and test meters to extensive shop equipment and laboratory instruments. It then becomes useful to examine the general requirements for the different areas of operation.

Preventive Maintenance

Such maintenance usually comprises periodic inspection of instruments and equipment, cleaning of electrodes, recording pens and cases, loading of expendable supplies (recording paper, film, ink, etc.), lubricating moving parts, and rudimentary electrical or mechanical tests. For this task, the service staff will require simple hand tools, electrical multipurpose meters, cleaning supplies, basic electrical and mechanical hardware items (wire, connectors, handles, screws, etc.), and the supplier's maintenance manual.

Instrument Calibration

In addition to the preventive maintenance items, the staff will need the necessary instruments for measuring parameters or applying calibration voltages, currents, impedances, fluid or air flows, heat or propagated energy, simulated physiological signals, etc. For electrical or electronic equipment, a signal generator, frequency meter, and oscilloscope with recording camera may be required. The supplier's manuals must include adequate calibration instructions and charts. In some instances, specific accessories for calibration must be obtained from the manufacturer or supplier.

In-House Repair

Service manuals must be provided with circuit diagrams, test and repair procedures, and special instructions. The test equipment for calibration or preventive maintenance must be supplemented with laboratory items such as power supplies, oscillators, signal sources, test loads, and display instruments. Components, replacement parts and modules, wiring supplies, insulating material, and hardware must all be stored or readily available. Portable power tools and hand tools should be available for each member of the repair staff.

Shop Facilities

If the in-house repair service includes rebuilding of damaged parts or construction of ancillary equipment (racks, cabinets, tables, etc.), more extensive facilities are required. These may include glass-blowing apparatus; sheet-metal brakes and shears; drill presses; grinders; milling machines; electroplating supplies; paint spraying and baking equipment; punches; printed circuit supplies; woodworking equipment; and other items appropriate to the repair program.

Safety and Environment Inspection

Leakage current and circuit continuity meters, receptacle testers, and isolating devices are necessary for checking and implementing electrical safety in patient-care areas. Radiation detectors and monitors are required for protection against X-radiation. Conductivity testers are needed to test electrostatic hazard protection. Environment assessment may require instruments to measure temperature, humidity, and high-frequency or magnetic interference signals.

Office Facilities

The basic requirements are dictated by the administrative duties, but in addition to the normal office furnishings and equipment, they must include a comprehensive filing system for equipment records, maintenance and repair operations, programmed overhaul schedules, maintenance and repair manuals, equipment and parts catalogs, trade journals, and reference texts. It is important that the technical library be updated on a regular basis and that adequate staff time be allocated for this function.

Stock-Room Facilities

The effective operation of an in-house service depends on the immediate availability of replacement parts and components, which requires an efficient stores organization with a carefully maintained inventory-control system. The sophistication demanded of such a system will depend on the number of items stocked and the trade-off of staff costs versus automated system expense. A large service will account for 3000–10,000 items. The stock audit system must provide an indication when supplies drop to insufficient levels. Adequate storage facilities—bins, shelving, and space—must be provided. It should also be remembered that the storage of such items as X-ray tubes, films, and some components will require control of the environmental temperature and humidity. If the department serves other institutions or dispatches equipment for servicing by others, it should also be equipped with shipping facilities, including instrument cases designed for safe transit of delicate gear.

X-Ray Testing and Repair Facilities

The medical engineering department should have space allocated for the various types of repair procedures. The X-ray repair shop will require space for temporary connection of the control circuitry, power system, and radiation unit and may need some permanent or portable radiation shielding plus operator protection (gloves, apron, etc.). Dosimeters will be required for calibration of exposures, plus apparatus for testing transformer oil, measuring exposure intervals, etc.

X-ray repairs will include accessory equipment such as examination tables, bulky mechanisms, film-processing equipment, and storage devices. For such procedures, sheet-metal working and woodworking facilities add to the competence of the service.

Meter Testing and Calibration Facilities

The test facilities should include a separate room in which electrical meters can be tested, calibrated, or repaired. For this purpose, standard current and voltage meters should be available with regulated supplies of the various power services necessary for the evaluation of instruments. Replacement components should include meter movements, shunts, rectifiers, cases, and miscellaneous hardware.

Electronic Diagnosis and Repair Facilities

Electronic repairs other than replacement of vacuum tubes, circuit boards, fuses, etc., are best undertaken in an electronics workshop in which suitable test facilities are available. These should include tube and transistor testers, oscilloscopes with suitable time bases and input circuits, high-frequency and low-frequency signal generators, power supplies, battery chargers and testers, test circuit boards, hand tools, soldering irons, multipurpose analysers, etc. If not available from the manufacturers, patch cords should be made up to permit servicing of subassemblies in an accessible position. Test leads should be fitted with connectors compatible with those on the equipment under repair.

Other Facilities

It should be recognized that the engineering department is a service agency and not a warehouse. If one of its functions is to store new equipment awaiting use, storage accommodation should be provided. Consideration should also be given to the allocation of space and facilities for some research and development program and for staff instruction. In one large children's hospital, the R & D section of the medical engineering department has made a substantial contribution to clinical practice in the development of monitoring equipment designed for the needs of the young patient.

A recommended area for a well-equipped facility has been estimated at 200 m^2. It should be provided with adequate electrical and water services and preferably with air conditioning to maintain suitable working conditions.

Staff Training Programs

At present, there is a lack of adequate training facilities in various locations. Furthermore, the training potential in and by industry is not being utilized to the best advantage. Thus, it is apparent that there exists a problem in implementing a training program for medical engineers and technicians.

It should be recognized that the technical training facilities within the health-care system or individual hospital almost certainly will be inadequate to produce efficient maintenance technicians unless they have first qualified in some area of basic technology. The key personnel for a department should be recruited carefully from applicants with certification in electrical, electronic, mechanical, or machine-shop training, and then they should be given the specialized instruction necessary to qualify them for maintenance and repair of medical instrumentation. The extent to which this training should be provided within the system depends on the availability of national or regional facilities and the competency of the supervisory staff. There is some evidence that the hospital service can best serve its needs by giving its clinical training to technicians whose basic training was in industrial trouble-shooting in electronic test departments or semiconductor application laboratories.

In some areas, community colleges and trade schools offer courses in a number of medical engineering areas. A typical 2- or 3-year course offers a period of hospital experience, and the technical graduate usually is well qualified to handle routine maintenance and repair.

Manufacturers of medical instrumentation can play an important role in technical training. Many offer factory instruction or teaching seminars with a nominal or no tuition fee. Such instruction is valuable for the installation and maintenance of complex systems for radiology, patient monitoring, or other high-technology areas. Some of these suppliers also offer field seminars with updated instruction on maintenance and repair procedures. The health-care administration should utilize this training to the fullest extent as it offers unmatched opportunity to familiarize the maintenance staff with detailed service methodology usually not available elsewhere.

Equipment manufacturers can also contribute greatly to the training program by providing competent maintenance manuals. These manuals should include detailed information on the principle of operation, circuit diagrams, exploded assembly drawings, test procedures, and check lists of possible faults and their correction Good manuals are often used as reference texts in technical schools because they stress methodology to supplement academic theory.

The US Army, Medical, Optical and Maintenance Agency has had 30 years experience in training BMETs. This experience is applicable to the needs of trainees as they represent a wide variation in academic backgrounds and potentials, and there is a similar need for self-reliance in an environment in which commercial resources may not be available. The agency conducts training at two skill levels in two separate basic and advanced courses.

The basic course teaches students to maintain and repair mechanical, electrical, and electromechanical biomedical equipment. In the advanced course, they are trained to maintain and repair all other types of biomedical equipment, including diagnostic X-ray apparatus, medical laboratory equipment, and patient-monitoring instruments.

The basic course is structured in four 3-week phases and a final 1-week phase. The first phase involves the student with electrical theory sufficient for the diagnosis of malfunctions in equipment. The remaining phases are devoted to dental, sterilizer, and pulmonary equipment and feature trouble-shooting techniques following instruction on the purpose and use of the equipment. More than half of the instruction period is spent in the laboratory. These three broad equipment headings actually encompass more than 75 items, including centrifuges, suction and pressure apparatus, jet-injection equipment for immunization purposes, radiographic film processors, and many other items. The training includes shop instruction on the use and care of hand and power tools, electrical servicing, and many other functions. In the final week, the student is instructed on management maintenance topics, including hospital safety, identification and procurement of repair parts, maintenance records and budgeting, inspection and maintenance procedures, and shop organization. Training aids are utilized in teaching electrical circuit theory.

The US Army's advanced course comprises seven 5-week phases of comprehensive training, including all equipment and instrumentation not covered in the basic course. Two phases are allocated to advanced electronics, including solid-state devices and digital principles. Following these 10 weeks of electronic theory, the student moves to 10 weeks of equipment instruction. The items covered include electrocardiographs, diathermy apparatus, ultrasonic equipment, patient-monitoring systems, radioisotope devices, pH meters, blood-cell counters, flame photometers, blood-gas analyzers, gas chromatographs, etc. The final 15 weeks are spent in study of diagnostic radiology equipment, including X-ray generators, cineradiography, closed-circuit-television image intensifiers, rapid-film changers, and radio contrast injection apparatus and techniques.

Only students with demonstrated ability are permitted to move directly to the advanced course from the basic course. The others are transferred to patient-treatment facilities for a year of on-site training and are then evaluated before acceptance in the advanced regime. Provision is made for recycling students through periods of difficulty and for advancing those with superior skill or knowledge. There are also supplementary and refresher courses offered to graduates at periodic intervals.

The pattern of training used by this US Army agency has been effective in producing competent BMETs for the health-care system. It was the prototype for a number of civilian courses, including a program sponsored by the US Veterans Administration. In Canada, a similar format is followed in BMET courses offered by some community colleges.

The AAMI has recognized the need for accreditation of BMETs to ensure a standard of performance that will encourage their employment in hospitals. The AAMI program offers an examination to candidates and provides a certificate to those who meet their requirements. Provision of certification gives the BMET status and enhances his career opportunity. It should be considered as an essential feature of any national training program.

The NIH maintains a systems maintenance section in its biomedical engineering and instrumentation branch. This section is charged with the responsibility for the maintenance and repair of a wide variety of medical equipment and supports NIH clinical and research groups with instrumentation development, where necessary. It is organized into electronic and mechanical groups with satellite subgroups to look after the various equipment specialties. The service maintains its own shop facilities and offers some in-house training, although it employs qualified BMETs wherever possible. Instruction is also offered to medical and paramedical staff on the use of equipment. The biomedical engineering and instrumentation branch maintains an equipment supply service, increasing its required commitment in staff instruction and responsibilities for effective maintenance and repair training.

Any in-house BMET training program undertaken by a health-care system must be based on supervision by professional bioengineering staff. The engineer can determine the need for specific instruction and can recommend the types and availability of training courses. He should also arrange for periodic updating of maintenance and repair instruction. The health-care system should be prepared to invest funds for the continuing education of its technical staff. At the outset, it may have to underwrite the specialized training of the medical engineer. The best compromise is to appoint an individual qualified in conventional area of engineering and to offer him graduate training suitable for his job requirements. This is the normal avenue of qualification for the engineer. It supplements the essential, broad-based background of the engineer with the life-science training that he will require in a medical environment. Graduate training is offered by many universities.

The medical engineer should organize his maintenance and repair teams into functional groups and endeavor to improve their expertise in specific procedures. A logical breakdown is to divide the service staff into electrical, electronic, mechanical, and machine-shop groups. X-ray maintenance and repair may account for the greater portion of the department's operations, justifying a separate group for this service. Each group should have a senior supervisor. It is advisable to provide periodic recycling of staff members to extend their competency and provide a nucleus of trained personnel for future expansion of engineering services.

The group supervisors should be responsible for developing maintenance and repair procedures. This includes individual and group instruction, the preparation of service manuals to supplement commercial publications, and the organizing of teaching aids. With the engineer(s), the supervisors should direct and participate in programs of instruction on the operation of instruments for the medical users. Involvement in clinical research or medical procedures will augment their capabilities in a reciprocal way. A two-way exchange of technical and medical knowledge will enhance the engineering service to the hospital or system.

Part of the ongoing training program for personnel of the medical engineering department should be periodic attendance at scientific or technical meetings in which they can exchange information with colleagues, learn of current developments, and inspect new instruments and devices. State-of-the-art seminars on such subjects as hospital safety, patient monitoring, or diagnostic techniques are particularly valuable for the engineering staff. They also offer a useful training for medical staff, presenting an insight into the technology that is an important constituent of clinical practice.

New trends are developing in the education of engineering staff. Training of technical staff is being related more closely to the clinical environment. The biomedical technician student is exposed to hospital procedures and encouraged to consider himself as a part of the health-care-delivery team rather than as a "serviceman.'' Similarly, the graduate student engineer may serve a term of internship in a hospital as part of his qualification. During this service, he may be associated with a surgical team, assess patients in a pulmonary laboratory, assist in clinical investigation, or engage in other patient-oriented activities. This is a far more pragmatic approach than the traditional university training that tended for many years to develop an individual for a research career or for continued university association but did little to produce graduates suited to the clinical environment or to the needs of the medical-engineering industry.

There is an increasing trend toward qualification in both engineering and medicine and a growing interest among medical graduates in acquiring some engineering background. The present technological invasion of medical practice makes it apparent that more effort will be required to teach engineering science to medical students at either undergraduate or graduate levels.

Maintenance and Repair Procedures

Establishing a Preventive Maintenance System

At an early stage in the organizing of a service, an inventory should be taken of all medical equipment and instrumentation throughout the hospital or system. The listing thus obtained will help to determine the requirement for services, and the format of the inventory record can be designed for the specific control of the maintenance and repair routine.

The maintenance and repair service unit should maintain a card or form for each item of equipment or instrumentation. It should contain the complete history of the item, from the date of purchase to ultimate disposal. Included should be total purchase cost, records of maintenance and repair operations with cost accounting of these procedures, and an estimate of probable life expectancy.

An equipment record form could become the key reference for all service functions. However, the maintenance and repair staff will need guidelines for procedure. There should first be drafted a standard guide covering procedure for all operations by the unit; it should document the method of recording work undertaken and materials and time expended and should detail basic principles of selection, inspection, preventive maintenance, and repair. It is in fact the ''charter'' document for the service and should detail the department's operations as thoroughly as required, even to personnel matters, job travel arrangements, etc.

The standard guide should be supplemented by procedure manuals for all but the most elementary items of equipment. These manuals suggest the required frequency of preventive maintenance, procedures to be undertaken, calibration instructions, probable causes of failure, repair policy, etc.

The service staff now has the record of the defective item, a manual for its repair, and a guideline for performance of their task. These aids will be supplemented by instruction and supervision. A schedule for preventive maintenance will assure that routine services are not overlooked.

The Equipment Repair Program

A requisition form for repair services should be available to all "user" services. At the time of failure or apparent damage, the engineering department should be notified and a repair requisition prepared. On the basis of convenience or experience, engineering administration will then decide whether the repair will be attempted on site, in its maintenance facility, or by an outside agent. In the last instance, the engineering department will be responsible for issuing instructions for repair and for the shipping procedure and will inspect the returned unit before placing it back in service. For internal repair procedures, a work order form should be prepared and directed to the appropriate staff (e.g., X-ray group, electronics shop, etc.). On completion of the repair, the details of services rendered should be transferred from the work order form to the equipment record card.

If the department operates on a fee-for-service basis, the engineering department should include a cost accounting of the repair services on the work order form. Even if repair costs will not be recovered, the cost accounting serves a useful purpose in determining the point of uneconomic repair.

It is important that repairs be directed to the area of maximum expertise and that maintenance manuals be constantly updated on the basis of past experience. It is also important, if the department contemplates construction of replacement parts as an in-house function, that the material and time costs be comparable with the cost of external purchase. Such action usually is justified only on the basis of saving time in restoring the equipment to service.

On-site repairs can reduce the out-of-service period and eliminate costly shipping charges. If the work is performed by an engineering department away from its headquarters, some sort of organization will be necessary to ensure that the necessary facilities are available. This organization may take the form of a local repair center or a mobile workshop. The former is only justified at a fairly large healthcare unit, and in such case there probably will be some local service staff to undertake the repairs. The extent to which repair facilities should be provided in individual hospitals depends on their instrumentation demands. The facilities should be recruited for the most prevalent requirements and the less commonly encountered repairs left for the central engineering agency to handle. From this sort of regional structure can develop technological clinics in which repair staff visit routinely to perform necessary service and to update local personnel on operation, maintenance, and repair procedures.

The alternative to the local repair center is the mobile workshop. This can be fitted with the more commonly needed tools and facilities, supplemented by the specific requirements for a particular operation. The mobile workshop can also be used as a circulating clinic offering periodic service and instruction at various centers.

A Policy for Equipment or Instrument Replacement

It is just as important to know when as to how to repair defective instrumentation. There comes a time when repair is uneconomic, but this may not be recognized unless a policy has been determined. The policy depends on two factors: an accounting of the repair costs for each item and a prediction of the time of obsolescence.

There is a diversity of opinion on the desirable cut-off point of repair costs. Indeed, it is impossible to state an invariable percentage of purchase price beyond which further repair is wasteful. Some items have predictable high maintenance costs inherent in their function, and replacement may not eliminate subsequent expenditures. Others may be subjected to unusual damage of a nonrepetitive nature—fire or flood, etc. It obviously is impractical to write off such equipment on a statistical basis if it can be returned to effective operation for a reasonable expenditure.

However, the record of repair costs after purchase does provide a useful index for assessment; where possible, a level should be determined at which a decision must be made to replace or to continue repair service. This level is often set at 50% of the purchase price. It may, in fact, be more realistic to establish the replace/repair level at a given percentage of the replacement price since this may be quite different from the original purchase cost. Not only should the total repair account be examined, but the rate of expenditures should be considered in determining the policy. In general, annual repairs in excess of 10% of the purchase price and produced by normal usage should indicate the need for evaluation of the wisdom of further repair funds.

The decision to replace does not necessarily mean the abandonment of old equipment. It may be allocated to a less demanding service in which limited use or less stringent performance requirement can extend its useful life. Alternatively, it may be kept available for standby use during repair of other units, given to teaching or research establishments, or used as a source of parts for repair of other equipment.

Earlier it was mentioned that a recommendation be made such that the equipment record form should show an estimate of probable life expectancy. This information allows the health-care system to establish a replacement budget. If the equipment is predicted to have a 5-year useful life, funds for replacement can be allocated for the appropriate time. Such action does not mean that retirement of the equipment will be mandatory in 5 years. As that time approaches, the serviceability and functional requirement of the unit should be reviewed. However, unless some attempt is made to anticipate the probable replacement needs, it will be difficult to budget funds for continuous upgrading of instrumentation.

It is difficult to anticipate the ‘‘wear and tear’’ depreciation factor for many items. Knowledge of the probable amount and kind of use is a useful index. The environmental conditions will also affect the operational life. These factors generally are predictable. The state of the art should also be examined from both technical and clinical viewpoints. Equipment using vacuum tubes and conventional wiring is now almost totally replaced by smaller units utilizing transistors, integrated circuits, and printed wiring assemblies. Even if the older equipment is still operable in a few years, will replacement parts still be available? Will the old instruments be compatible in systems using the new generation of equipment? Will safety considerations outlaw its use? Similarly, there must be a projection of the medical demand a few years hence. Automated chemical analysis equipment has been cited in this report as an area of instrumentation that is in a transition state at the present time. The nature of required tests is changing. It is essential that the medical specialist give an evaluation of the useful life before obsolescence.

Purchasing New Equipment

The criteria for selection of new instrumentation were presented earlier, and here we will add only a few comments on implementation of a purchasing policy.

The first step in selecting equipment should be a collaborative study by the medical user and the engineering staff of the clinical requirements and the suitability of available equipment. Let us use blood-flow measurement as an example. The medical staff must advise whether it is for short-term quantitative measurement or for chronic implantation to study flow-rate changes and for large or small blood-vessel studies. The engineer can then determine the appropriate type of flowmeter: perhaps an electromagnetic device for more exact measurement or an ultrasonic flowmeter for ease of implantation and telemetry monitoring. The present selection of equipment for hospital use is at best a hit-and-miss process determined largely by what the medical practitioner has seen or read about or by the perseverance of a salesman! The selector should keep in mind compatibility with other items and consistency with similar equipment already in use. The cost of maintaining spare parts will be reduced if such standardization is possible.

At the time of negotiation, the supplier should be questioned about installation and subsequent service available (and its cost); warranty conditions; user instruction and maintenance manuals; terms of sale and delivery; local access to replacement parts; recommended spares, compliance with safety and performance standards; compatibility with environmental conditions; availability and cost of expendable supplies such as recording paper, ink, or electrodes; and, if necessary, references of present users and applications.

The purchase order should stipulate the conditions of sale based on these negotiations. It should demand adequate instruction and maintenance literature, establish the supplier's liability for installation, user and maintenance staff instruction, replacement of defective or damaged shipments, and the exact terms and date of commencement and expiration of the warranty period. The terms of the warranty may be conditional upon the subsequent service policy and should be established at the time of ordering. If the manufacturer offers factory training on maintenance and repair, it should be contracted for in the purchase order, not at some future time when repairs become necessary.

Inspection of the incoming equipment is part of the purchasing routine. If possible, part of the purchase price should be held back until inspection and acceptance. In any case, the equipment should not be put into service until it has been examined and tested.

A Central Instrument Supply

The US Veterans Administration has reported a rental program in which hospitals lease much of their instrumentation from a central VA agency and return it when it is no longer required. Two benefits from the system are that more equipment is available with more effective utilization, and the individual hospitals can obtain more for their equipment funds in a given year. The VA agency uses the rental fee to buy more equipment. The program objective is to recover 40% of the acquisition cost the first year and the remaining 60% by the end of the half-life of the instrument. Thereafter, a nominal rental fee covers maintenance costs and increased costs of replacement. More recently, a research equipment program has been established that attempts to locate unused apparatus and put it to productive use.

Such a program is applicable to the needs of a complete health-care system. The engineering service could issue equipment on demand and recall it later for reallocation. Any reserve stock would eliminate shutdowns of clinical service during repair operations. An additional premium might be the reduction in purchase price for consolidated ordering by one agency. Space would have to be allocated for storage of unused equipment.

Maintenance and Repair Stores Procedures

The importance of an effective organization to maintain spare parts, replacement components, accessories, and raw materials should be stressed. Any service is just as good as its resources, and the engineering department must often look for these material resources within its doors. The problem is not very different from that of any industrial storeroom except perhaps in the diversity of items that must be stocked.

The stores section can be divided into three categories. The major responsibility will be to maintain an adequate stock of spare parts and replacements for all medical instruments (excluding surgical tools). The determination of stock quantities will depend on price and availability, storage facilities, and limitations on the shelf life of some items. A temperature- and humidity-controlled environment may be necessary in climatic extremes. Special arrangements should be made for the quick acquisition of recurring replacements such as batteries and rotating-anode X-ray tubes. Most of the delay in returning hospital equipment to service can be traced to the time consumed in ordering and awaiting replacement parts that could be delivered in a fraction of the time. Where possible, standing orders should be set up with suppliers, locally or abroad, to expedite this procedure.

The second category of stock is a supply of electrical, electronic, and hardware components, metal, insulating materials, wire, solder, welding, and paint supplies, etc. The hardware should include machine screws of the several standards used by instrument manufacturers—a formidable variety. Also included will be shop supplies, lubricants, cleaning solutions, etc.

The remaining storeroom function will be to keep and account for maintenance and repair tools, drills and bits, wrenches, taps and dies, punches, shears, and all the other items used in a repair shop. These items will be normally for departmental use only, and their accounting may be by a comparatively simple ledger or card system whereby the borrower signs for the tools or equipment when he obtains them.

The stock-audit requirement for the spares, replacements, and components is more stringent and is designed to prevent depletion to a dangerously low level. A reorder point should be established for each item, a continuous tally kept, and immediate purchasing action taken when the stock drops below the reorder point.

The stores section should handle shipping and receiving duties for the biomedical equipment department. For this purpose, and for dispatch of instruments to medical departments, it should have an adequate supply of carrying cases and shipping crates, padded to cushion the contents against damage. The dispatch of transport vehicles on maintenance or repair missions may also be assigned to this section.

Safety-Maintenance Procedures

The equipment maintenance program of a health-care system must include measures to ensure the safety of both patients and staff. The engineering service can expect to become involved in two areas of hospital safety: electrical and radiation protection.

Electrical safety falls into two categories. The first involves the risk of fire or explosion in the presence of flammable anesthetic or other agents. In recent years, an enforced discipline of protection has reduced the incidence of hazard in operating theaters, recovery rooms, and other critical areas in a remarkable way. The approach is twofold. Protective measures are taken to prevent electrical discharges that might ignite gases—or shock the patient or staff. These include high-quality electrical receptacles that are water- and explosion-proof and elimination of extension power cables within the hazardous area. A protective grounding system reduces the hazard from fault currents generated in or conducted through instrumentation. Ground current interruptors are used commonly to open circuits when such faults exist.

There is another facet of explosion protection, important in a dry, temperate environment. It is the reduction of electrostatic discharge hazards. The simple act of walking across a floor can build up a static charge that will be discharged at the first point of contact. Such discharges have produced sufficient energy to ignite flammable gases. The protection is based on the reduction of electrostatic charges by elimination of certain fabrics in clothing and drapes, maintaining a humidity level of about 50%, dissipation of electrostatic charges by use of conductive footwear and flooring, and treatment of fabrics with conductive sprays. These measures control the electrostatic hazard effectively, but the presence of conductive flooring adds to the electric-shock hazard. It has become standard practice to isolate the electrical service from ground in areas in which conductive flooring is installed. It then becomes necessary to monitor the integrity of the isolation with a detector device that will alarm if a fault current reaches a critical level.

The fire and explosion hazard has decreased with the diminishing use of flammable agents, but at the same time the increasing use of electrical and electronic instrumentation and the invasion of the body by implanted probes, conductive catheters, and cardiac pacemaker leads have increased the shock hazard to a critical level. The danger is greatest in patient-care areas in which multiple instrumentation is attached to the patient for monitoring or therapeutic treatment.

The protection against shock hazard involves meticulous attention to the provision of a protective ground system in the hospital service and in power-operated instruments and equipment, isolation of patient leads, and careful sçrutiny of all patient-centered systems to ensure that fault currents cannot flow through the patient's body.

The rationale of electrical protection is very complex. In general, however, the safety maintenance team will require high-impedance meters to measure fault currents and voltages, meters to measure the effectiveness of insultation, and impedance meters to measure the quality of grounding systems and the continuity of equipment grounding. The patient-care areas should be catalogued in their various levels of risk and levels of protection assigned to their equipment and installed services. All instruments should be examined for electrical safety during their incoming inspection and periodically thereafter. The engineering department should be consulted before any new instrumentation system is used in patient diagnosis or treatment.

Radiation protection is associated principally with the radiology and nuclear medicine departments of a health-care service. The onus of responsibility for staff and patient protection rests with the medical user but the biomedical equipment department may be asked to provide X-ray film monitors, geiger or scintillation counters, or other detection equipment. The engineering staff may also be involved in the design of building protection and detection systems.

High-frequency and magnetic radiations are not usually associated with safety hazards in the hospital environment, but they pose other problems that must be countered. Air-propagated or powerline-conducted signals may interfere with the operation of sensitive amplifiers. The solution is to eliminate or reduce the interference signal source if it is local by filtering or shielding the equipment causing it, by relocating the affected instruments, or by shielding the environment in which they are installed and filtering the electrical power system. The engineering department should be competent to supervise noise-meter evaluations and to recommend appropriate measures for abatement of interference signals.

29

HOSPITAL ENGINEERING

W. E. Williams

The world of the hospital engineer has become incredibly complex and is growing constantly. This is to be expected, as the engineer works in the shadow of essentially all of the manifold changes in the health-care field. Not only are hospital facilities increasing in size, but what were formerly simple units have become complex and sensitive health-care systems. Most significantly, engineering is now an inseparable part of medical diagnosis and treatment.

The situation today requires one to examine the hospital-engineering profession. It is never easy to look closely at ourselves, and most of us only do so when forced by a crisis or a confrontation with reality. While the hospital engineer's position is not viewed as one of crisis or anxiety, there is an unquestionable need to examine the goals, direction, and priorities as new health-care systems evolve.

In discussing the role of the hospital engineer and what the hospitals of the United States require, it should be understood that of the roughly 7000 hospitals in this country, most have a capacity of under 200 beds. With regional planning and the trend for small hospitals to become affiliated with larger ones, it seems safe to predict that the most complex equipment will gravitate to the larger central hospitals. In fact, expanding technology makes this changing role mandatory, as the very small hospitals simply cannot afford to provide all the required services to all its patients.

Because these large central hospitals are now able to treat greater numbers of patients, new technical problems have evolved. To help solve these problems, communications will become much more complex, transmission of medical records will have to be revolutionized, more laboratory tests will have to be automated or simplified, computers will make diagnoses, and technicians will have to be trained to handle advanced laboratory and medical equipment. Also, engineering departments must be staffed with more qualified personnel to help in the solution of these newly created, complex problems.

Impact

The impact of the medical engineer in the development of new medical equipment has been immense in the past few years. This has necessarily led to the development of a number of new "allied health" technicians. Unfortunately, this technical phenomenon is simply evolving, unmanaged and uncoordinated. For example, there are technologists in radiology, cardiology, nuclear medicine, inhalation therapy, laboratories, and ECG. All have been trained in very limited disciplines. The majority of advances in medical technology in recent years can be attributed to the collaboration of engineers with physicians.

Hospital engineering departments attempt to handle all of these changes with varying degrees of competence. Some departments have qualified, technical people maintaining and monitoring every facet of technology related to the physical plant and equipment, and, in other instances, this competence is lacking in new technical areas.

If all the technical, practical, and administrative items are examined that relate to the hospital's plant and equipment, it immediately becomes apparent that no one individual can possibly be an expert in all of these areas.

As a result of new health-care systems, developments in plant and medical equipment, intimate contact of new sophisticated equipment with the patient, and the expanding role of engineering in the hospital field, the question must be asked, "What should be the role of today's hospital engineer?"

In some smaller hospitals or those lacking modern, sophisticated equipment, the hospital engineer may unfortunately be categorized as a glorified boiler operator or janitor. However, this interpretation is not followed by most individuals who are knowledgeable in the hospital field. Hospital administrators are now requiring broad practical experience, expertise in the trades and plant operations, and management ability from their engineers. In today's hospitals of appreciable size, finding that the hospital engineer is a graduate engineer is not unusual. Further, registered professional engineers are also emerging in the hospital field.

However, technology has advanced at such a high rate that the average hospital engineer is unable to keep up with this rapid change in technology. One of the unfortunate facts is that very few hospitals have ever planned programs to develop and utilize the technological potential for new and improved patient care. Hospitals have pursued a piecemeal approach and have attempted to fill each vacancy by creating a new job only whenever a new need occurred. More often than not, these specialized new jobs have been created because some department in the hospital has not met the problem. For example, nurse surveillance officers are hired because doctors are not reporting infections. Environmental specialists are added because those who had the responsibilities are not meeting them. Generally, nurses and engineers have not provided for the medical technological needs through their own growth. Superimpose the status of and empire building of physicians in larger hospitals in which technologists are hired to work in the confines of only one service, and the result is the present highly specialized, provincial, fragmented organization of the highly technical, developed hospital. In short, the health-care field needs to begin to manage technology through technical managers.

In broad terms, hospitals have delegated to the hospital engineer the job of providing an efficient, safe, and clean environment for the patient and health-care team. This, of course, includes the plant and equipment that are an integral part of the environment organized to deliver health care. The emerging role of the hospital engineer is to develop the capability to integrate all the technical knowledge of the necessary engineering disciplines into a unified program for the hospital.

The hospital engineer must concentrate on the broad spectrum and have the expertise to relate properly new developments to the health-care field in terms of real needs. He must relate to other engineering colleagues, such as biomedical, electrical, mechanical, and structural engineers, as well as architects, doctors, and others to act as the coordinator of the physical plant and equipment technology. Expressed more succinctly, the hospital engineer must become the manager of technological development for the hospital.

While an understanding of technology is important, the management of this technology through qualified people is an equally important responsibility. For many years, hospital engineers have managed departments that included technical people such as electricians, refrigeration and air-conditioning mechanics, and other skilled trades. The addition of medical technicians to the engineering departments of hospitals is common. Thus, the engineer has to a large degree been harnessing technology within the hospital.

However, symptoms indicating that the overall management of technology in hospitals is inadequate have become quite evident. Perhaps the best known is the furor over electrical safety. Those looking for a cause and others with some personal gain in mind have exploited and exaggerated the magnitude of this problem. A good grounding system is not especially new or complex. A typical example of what is new is the need to be aware that implanting devices within a patient has created a new dimension requiring more sensitive protection. Most hospital engineers who are aware of these new advances are developing programs to increase their overall competency, particularly in critical areas. Nevertheless, that the emergence of these new areas has become such an issue is evidence of the need for better technical management in hospitals. Considering the variety in size and development of different hospitals, there are obviously different needs with respect to the qualifications of the hospital engineer. However, the trend is clear.

Hospital-Engineering Functions

The hospital engineer should be a generalist, a technical manager, and a leader who is capable of directing those responsible for the provision, operation, and maintenance of the physical plant and its equipment. He should give engineering advice when equipment is purchased to assure that all equipment, including electronic devices, are compatible with hospital systems, are standardized where possible, do not have a high-maintenance-cost history, and will meet specifications both functionally and from a safety point of view. He should work with medical engineers and other qualified individuals in the engineering field to achieve the above goals. Also, he should act as the hospital's coordinator and adviser with architects and engineers on design construction projects.

In addition to the above responsibilities, today's hospital engineer should (*a*) provide tools, work areas, competent supervisors, engineers, technicians, and tradesmen willing to work together to provide planned maintenance, calibration of equipment where needed, and routine maintenance to preserve the capital investment; (*b*) assure that any violation of fire and safety codes relating to the physical plant and equipment are corrected and that safety programs are implemented; (*c*) supervise construction or alteration work done by hospital personnel or outside contractors; (*d*) be responsible for the operation of mechanical electrical systems, including electrical distribution, emergency power, oxygen and vacuum, plumbing, communications, and the environmental systems (these environmental systems include internal air temperature and quality control, air pollution, and solid waste disposal systems); (*e*) be responsible for programs designed to educate subordinates; and (*f*) conduct appropriate training of other hospital-staff personnel.

Finally, the engineer should comprehend clearly the psychological and social impact of everything under his control relating to patients, staff, and the outside public community. Generally, technical people have not always been sensitive to the psychological problems they have created.

Beyond the basic responsibilities previously presented, which logically fall under the purview of a competent hospital engineer, there are other areas that need to be considered if technological advances will benefit the public efficiently. Technicians must be taught to operate more than one piece of equipment, should watch monitors, and work with the health-care team. New communications systems should be developed. Also, better coordination by health-care technical resources is needed.

30

FUNCTIONS OF A HOSPITAL CLINICAL ENGINEER

J. O. Wear

The complete clinical engineer could be called the "new Renaissance man." He could be well versed in all engineering disciplines. In fact, one might begin with clinical engineering and make the classic disciplines of engineering subdisciplines under this one name for health-care delivery. Since it is very difficult to educate or train a complete clinical engineer, one must subdivide clinical engineering into various subspecialties such as electronic engineering, mechanical engineering chemical engineering, and industrial engineering. At the same time, a clinical engineer can be an individual with a background in one of the physical or life sciences but with experience and training in engineering techniques. This type of subdividing allows the clinical engineer to assume different rolls.

The term *clinical engineering* has been used to distinguish among those engineers who work in direct health-care delivery from those who work in research and development. The R & D engineers are more appropriately termed biomedical engineers. The clinical engineer works in the real world with patients either directly or indirectly. He may work for a hospital, as a consultant to two or more hospitals, or within a medical-university complex in which he is closely affiliated with a university hospital.

The majority of the clinical engineers work mainly in a hospital environment. In this environment, they have firsthand exposure to problems that arise in the delivery of health care that can be solved with the application of engineering techniques. Only in this environment in which they maintain close contact with patient and observe the interrelationship among the medical staff and patients, equipment and facility, can they understand all the ramifications of the problems within the hospital. Here they can work with the medical staff to assure that any solution they arrive at is not a sterile solution and also that it would not adversely affect patient care while it solves a problem in the delivery of health care.

The smaller hospitals, those under 200 beds, generally can not afford the full-time services of a clinical engineer. Most smaller hospitals require the full-time service of this individual, but there will always be a certain number of hospitals that cannot utilize a full-time clinical engineer. However, hospitals having as few as 10 beds do require certain services of the clinical engineer, and to give maximum patient care, these services must be provided. As in any other field, whenever a full-time individual is not required, either part-time or consulting services can be utilized. In clinical engineering, this can be broken into two different types of consulting: first, a shared service, or the use of engineering expertise among several hospitals on a regional basis, and second, the independant consultant.

Several shared engineering services to provide clinical engineering to smaller hospitals have been initiated throughout the country, and such services appear to be an excellent method for smaller hospitals to obtain quality clinical engineering support. This shared service occurs when a larger hospital furnishes the base of operations, and they provide services to the smaller surrounding hospitals, or it may be established as an entirely different, nonprofit entity that is supported by a state or regional hospital association.

The independent consultant in clinical engineering is becoming more widely known as the problems of hospital safety receive increasing attention. Unfortunately, today there is very little quality control over the individual doing this type of consulting. Some of these individuals are not clinical engineers; they are engineers from some other discipline and do not have a knowledge of a clinical setting. On the other hand, there are many qualified consulting engineers who operate similar to those affiliated with shared services except they operate for a profit.

The last base of operation for the clinical engineer is the university. In general, bioengineers in universities are research oriented and do not have a clinical background or an interest in the clinical setting. But in those cases in which they are affiliated with a medical center at the university hospital, they can be very effective in clinical engineering, generally operating similar to the clinical engineer in the hospital.

Maintenance and Repair

The area of maintenance and repair of medical instrumentation is one of the first areas in which the clinical engineer works in a hospital. The reason for this is that it is an area in which cost reduction and savings can be achieved in order to pay for his technician's salaries and the cost of establishing a clinical engineering laboratory. Direct cost can result from the reduction in service contracts. Of course, these cost reductions will be supplemented by less downtime and better utilization of the instrumentation.

The clinical engineer is not a medical-equipment repairman or even a biomedical equipment technician. His role is one of supervising and maintaining a maintenance and repair operation; in other words, he is a maintenance manager. He is responsible for hiring BMETs and medical-equipment repairmen, supervising their activities to assure that the maintenance of the hospital instrumentation is performed efficiently as possible. Frequently, this will require very good supervising skills to assure the best utilization of the talents of the technicians.

In establishing a maintenance and repair facility in a hospital, the clinical engineer must be a competent maintenance manager. He must consider the current workload, expansions, type of equipment being brought in to the shop, and the type of individuals that are required to maintain this shop. He must give consideration to the parts that he needs, sources for them, and what kind of spare parts he will have to keep in inventory since this will be part of the initial setup operation.

In establishing the repair and maintenance program in a hospital, the clinical engineer must establish a method of record keeping and a preventive maintenance schedule. He must also consider lifetime and replacement of instrumentation since most of this is not readily available. He will develop many of these on his own. One of the best sources for this type of information is the lifetimes and the preventive maintenance schedules already developed by the Veterans Administration. Information on these can be obtained from the Chief, Clinical Engineering, Veterans Administration Central Office in Washington, D.C. In these records, he should have a history of each instrument, which will allow him to develop better lifetime preventive-maintenance schedules and maintenance cost.

In the maintenance and repair of hospital instrumentation, the clinical engineer must study cost effectiveness. Cost effectiveness is an area that the hospital administrator understands and in which he is willing to spend money to save money. It is frequently a better selling point than improvement of patient care since cost effectiveness is real and can be shown, whereas improvement of patient care is sometimes indirect and nebulous.

Cost effectiveness can be viewed from a direct standpoint of saving on service contracts and less total repair costs due to preventive maintenance. Unfortunately, this is not very evident since most hospitals do not have reliable past records to compare against. If good records are kept initially, then some improvement can be shown over time as the program develops. Another direct savings may occur in the longer lifetime of instrumentation However, obsolescence must be considered, for even though an instrument has been maintained in good working condition, it may still have to be replaced in a relatively short lifetime due to obsolescence. In a private hospital in which services, such as X-ray and clinical laboratory, are charged out, downtime can be looked at from cost effectiveness since this is real money. Also, the indirect cost should be considered, which means improvement of patient care—possibly shorter stays in the hospital due to equipment constantly being in operation and tests being performed as needed, the salaries that are saved as a result of less downtime, and the indirect benefits of the overall increased effectiveness due to instrumentation functioning properly all the time.

Another very important aspect of the maintenance and repair program is instrument calibration. Again, this is an area in which some calibration equipment standards do exist, but frequently they do not. Therefore, the clinical engineer will have to develop both standards and methods of calibration. This calibration can be built into a preventive maintenance program, which will allow testing to assure that the instrumentation is functioning within proper limits. Improvement in this area can be sold on the basis of assuring patient care and because this type of program is required for hospital accreditation. This calibration program should include areas of the hospital such as instrumentation in the clinical laboratory, X-ray, and monitoring equipment.

New Equipment

A very important part of the clinical engineers's function relates to new equipment that is purchased for the hospital. The clinical engineer is involved in the selection, receipt, inspection, and installation of this equipment.

The selection of new equipment is a very important role the clinical engineer can play since most physicians are not familiar with instrumentation from a design and specification viewpoint. Also, the instrument salesmen are at times not totally familiar with what their equipment actually can or cannot do. At times, a salesman can and will take advantage of the physicians' lack of knowledge in this area and sell a hospital instrumentation that either will not fully meet the hospital's needs, is of poor quality, or for which there is no maintenance and service support. The clinical engineer can discuss with the physician or other medical staff the need for instrumentation and what medical criteria it must meet. He can then look at the instrumentation from this viewpoint, as well as engineering specifications, and the support the company can provide in the area in which the hospital is located.

One important area of consideration with all instrumentation is how it will be utilized. One decision that must be made is whether or not the instrumentation is really needed or whether there is other instrumentation available that will do the job as well or better at a lower cost. At the same time, the clinical engineer should be aware of the state-of-the-art so that he can advise the hospital as to whether or not the instrumentation they are considering will still be current and not be obsolete within 6 months. With the rapid development of medical instrumentation, this can be a major problem. Frequently, companies will try to sell instrumentation that they will be superseding within a few months due to some significant breakthrough either in the field of electronics or the field of medical instrumentation.

Another area that the clinical engineer must examine closely when considering new equipment is the safety factor, especially when it is interfaced with the existing instrumentation. Of course, all companies will declare that their instrumentation is safe, but it has been found that much of the equipment will not meet current safety standards that are already established, especially in a field of leakage current. Also, some medical instrumentation and equipment has been found to be completely unsafe and does not do the job that it is sold to do due to faulty engineering designs. Many of these have been reported in the last few years in the publication entitled *Health Devices*. The clinical engineer should be able to look at the medical use and the medical setting and assure that the instrument will be safe in the setting. One of the problems that has arisen with much medical instrumentation is that it has been designed to do a job without the designers being aware of the setting that it is to be utilized in and/or the condition of a patient that it is to be used on.

The clinical engineer should require a demonstration of all equipment before it is purchased. In many cases, companies will place instrumentation for a 30-day trial period so it can be evaluated. During this time, the clinical engineer should be in charge of the evaluation to see that it is properly evaluated as a piece of instrumentation. He should work closely with the medical staff to see that it also meets the medical criteria. The clinical engineer then becomes the interface between the company and the physician since he is in a position to effectively communicate with both parties.

Whenever new instrumentation is received by the hospital, it first should be inspected by the clinical engineer and his staff. This is necessary to ensure that it meets the bid specification, company's design specifications, and all pertinent safety requirements. Studies have shown that at least 30% of all instrumentation purchased by hospitals does not meet either company design specifications or bid specifications. This initial inspection will also allow a clinical engineer to be sure that his shop receives a manual, his people learn how to operate the equipment, and that a maintenance history and inventory on the piece of equipment is established.

The installation of medical instrumentation in the hospital should be at least partially, if not fully, supervised by a clinical engineer. This is especially true in ICUs in which the interface with the facility can have a major bearing on safety. There must be very close coordination with other hospital personnel, especially other members of the engineering department, such as electricians, plumbers, and architects.

The involvement of the clinical engineer with new equipment does not assume that he is solely responsible for these items but instead that these are part of his job. Naturally, the equipment selection should be done by a committee of which the clinical engineer is a member, together with the purchasing agent and various members of the medical staff. This does not necessarily mean that he is the only person that performs all the inspections and physically oversees installation. Some of the inspection can be done by technicians on his staff.

Patient Safety

The clinical engineer has a major responsibility with regard to patient safety. The area of electrical safety has received much publicity and has been responsible for many engineers entering the hospital field. However, it should be stressed that patient safety relates to physical, psychological, and radiation safety as well as electrical safety.

In electrical safety, the clinical engineer is responsible for making inspections of ICUs, operating suites, and other less sensitive areas of the hospital. In the area in which there is an electrically susceptible patient, the clinical engineer is responsible for inspecting for leakage current levels. Since this is an area in which there is some uncertainty as to what the actual levels should be, he is also responsible for evaluating standards and deciding what his hospital will utilize as their standard. In addition to leakage current, there are many other electrical hazards in a hospital that can result in macroshock that must be inspected periodically by the clinical engineering staff. These include such simple things as frayed cords, improperly wired outlets, and disconnected ground wires. As hazards are found, they should be corrected by the clinical engineer and his staff whenever possible; whenever they involve facilities, recommendations should be made to the proper personnel in the engineering department. The clinical engineer should assure that the proper corrections are made, and once they are made, he should check again to assure that such corrections have solved the problem. The electrical safety is another area in which records on each instrument and test measurements must be maintained. This could be very useful in protecting the hospital in a legal liability case so that the hospital could prove that it had tried to the best of its ability to assure that its instrumentation was safe.

Physical safety is another area that the clinical engineer must consider; and it is frequently ignored since it involves more common sense than engineering practice. In intensive-care areas in which several pieces of instrumentation may be connected to a patient, extension cords are frequently used and strung out around the patient area, or just the cords, hoses, and tubes are strung to the convenience of the individual making the connections.

Also, consideration frequently is not given to the possibility of staff members carelessly tripping over cords and tubes and other simple hazards, which would be dangerous to both the patient and staff. The clinical engineer and his staff should make inspections for these potential hazards and recommendations for corrections. In fact, the clinical engineer's staff should make all the corrections that they are capable of, such as reducing or increasing the length of cords and hoses.

A very real area of patient safety that is frequently not given enough serious consideration is psychological safety. This is an area for which the clinical engineer should develop an understanding since it requires an understanding of the patient and how he feels in a hospital situation. This, then, has to be related to the instrumentation and the physical environment that a patient is in. Solutions to these problems are generally of either an architectural or engineering nature. The noise level in an intensive-care area is frequently very high, and the least the clinical engineer can do is to ensure that his technicians working in the area do not increase the level any more than is necessary. Also, he can make recommendations as to how the noise can be absorbed or how procedures might be accomplished with less noise. Perhaps the clinical engineer can examine this overall system of intensive care and make recommendations as to how work can be scheduled so as to reduce the number of people and instrumentation in the area at the same time, which would result in reducing the noise level. Also, the clinical engineer must be certain that various systems with alarms function properly so that there are not many false alarms that would be very disturbing to the patient.

The clinical engineer must instruct his staff on how they approach a patient and how they approach instrumentation problems surrounding a patient. This has to be done so that the patient has confidence in the care he is receiving and does not get the impression that he is being monitored or his life is maintained by equipment that is faulty and undependable. The clinical engineer and his technicians must be certain to remember that whenever they are in a patient-care area, the patient is of primary concern, not the instrumentation. They must also learn to give the patient assurance about the instrumentation and, whenever possible, explain how it is utilized and its functions, especially when the patient inquires.

Another area of psychological safety that should be considered at the time of purchasing new equipment is the appearance of the equipment. It should be pleasing to the eye, efficient, and fit within the general area in which it is to be used. Although this may seem trivial to a patient, it may be very critical, especially when he is in a very guarded condition.

Many of the larger hospitals have radiation-protection officers who are also considered clinical engineers.

As more and more nuclear-medicine techniques are being utilized for diagnostic tools, the safety of both patients and staff from radiation effects becomes more important. The problem has become more acute with the increased use of X-ray equipment and newer legislation that applies to such equipment. Such items as microwave ovens also come under the scope of radiation safety. Here the clinical engineer may have a physics background rather than a classic engineering background, but still he is a clinical engineer.

The clinical engineer may also be a person who is known as a safety engineer in many hospitals. His interest in safety within the facility may refer to the staff to as large a degree as it does to patients. This will include fire safety, safety from falls, explosions, and other such occurrences that are due to an unsafe facility or an unsafe practice within a facility. More patients are injured from falls in hospitals than any other accidents. If the emphasis in the position is on the safety of the staff only, if patients are not considered, and if the individual performing the job performs only these functions, then he should not be considered a clinical engineer. It would appear that in most hospitals safety of the patient is as important as the safety of the staff. If there is a possibility of a staff member falling, then there is a greater possibility of a patient falling.

Training

Training is a major part of the clinical engineer's job, especially when he is the only clinical engineer in a hospital and the position has been recently established. The clinical engineer is involved in training the BMETs and medical equipment repairmen on his own staff, other hospital staff, and patients. These training responsibilities may be those he will perform himself; or, he may design curricula, and the work will be accomplished by technicians under his supervision.

The biggest training job the clinical engineer has is continuing the education of his BMETs and medical-equipment repairmen. These individuals must be continually updated in basics, electronics, and mechanics, as well as the basic principles of instrumentation that the hospital purchases. This can be an especially large area of concern if the technicians do not have a biomedical background and if the entire operation is new to the hospital. In this case, the instrumentation must be thoroughly understood before service contracts are canceled and the shop assumes the servicing of this instrumentation. In some cases, there will be medical-equipment repairmen who will want to learn a sufficient amount to qualify them as BMETs. The necessary training will have to be set up by the clinical engineer. Much of this training can be accomplished through videotapes, correspondence courses, and educational institutions, but the clinical engineer will have to decide what programs will meet the hospital's needs and in what areas he wants his individuals trained.

Training the hospital staff as to the operation of instrumentation and its safety is also a responsibility of the clinical engineer and his staff. Once the BMETs are trained, they can do much of this training. This training may be formalized or may be done on an informal basis. Whenever there are a high number of service calls in a particular area of the hospital, the technician may find that operators are improperly utilizing equipment and can informally show them how to use the equipment in these areas. On the other hand, whenever a new piece of equipment is brought into the hospital and is to be used by several operators, a formal training session may be held on the use and daily preventive maintenance of the equipment. As new operators are brought in, these may be trained informally by a technician spending half an hour or so with the operator.

Training intensive-care personnel in safety and daily preventive maintenance of their equipment is a procedure that the clinical engineer should be sure to establish at a very early stage in his program. This will develop confidence in the nursing and medical staff in the utilization of the monitoring equipment. This will also allow them to properly utilize the equipment and to detect any defects.

The early detection of faulty instrumentation in these areas may reduce maintenance and at the same time assure that unsafe equipment will not be used. Intensive-care personnel must be thoroughly familiar with the basics of electricity and why electrical safety is important in an intensive-care area. The training of these personnel has to be a continuing program since there is a high turnover rate in these areas.

Another area in which the clinical engineer can be of major benefit in patient care is the training of patients who are utilizing such devices as dialysis units, pacemakers, and various prosthetic devices. The patient should be taught something about how the equipment is designed, what its function is, as well as how it is utilized. If a patient has more understanding of the equipment, he will have more confidence in it and will also probably take better care of it. He will also be in a position to recognize malfunctions and see that they are corrected. In this training role, the clinical engineer will work with the medical staff as part of a training team. The use of the engineer in this training should give the patient more confidence in the equipment on which his life, or some particular function of his life, may depend.

Development and Modification of Equipment

The area in which the engineer uses his best engineering skills is the development and modification of medical instrumentation equipment. This is not a research area, but instrumentation that has been newly developed must often be modified for a particular case, a particular individual, or some particular function for which a physician wishes to use the equipment. The first concern of the clinical engineer is to be certain that the modification can be made without altering the overall function of the new equipment or interfering with the overall system.

In the development of instrumentation or modification of existing instrumentation, the clinical engineer should apply research developments and not attempt new research in the clinical setting. He should be up-to-date on the latest developments in biomedical engineering as well as in his engineering specialty. He should also be able to draw on the many sources in the literature to discover what has already been done on a particular problem that he is working on and then apply new research to the solution of the clinical program.

Whenever a development of instrumentation is required or even a major modification, the engineer will design what is needed. In making his design, he must consider what medical criteria are needed, as well as what kind of specifications the device must have; must it be autoclaved, must it have a 1 or 10% tolerance, must it be operated by unskilled personnel, must it be portable, and with what will it be interfacing in the hospital setting? Once he has made his design, he may have his technicians or an outside firm develop a prototype.

Once a prototype has been developed, it should be tested and evaluated by the clinical engineer to determine whether it meets all the design specifications. If it is to be utilized on human beings, then a consideration of animal experiments should be analyzed before it is utilized on a human being. This, of course, will depend on what the instrumentation is designed for and what effects could occur if it malfunctions or does not perform as designed. After the clinical engineer has assured himself that the development or modification will perform as expected, then he should work with the physician and supervise its utilization in the clinical setting.

This modification of equipment may frequently occur when different manufacturers' equipment is being interfaced together to develop a system of instrumentation.

Administration

In addition to the administration of a maintenance program for the hospital and the various record keeping that accompanies it, as well as supervising various operations under his department, a clinical engineer may be an administrative engineer doing operation research for industrial engineering. This is an area in clinical engineering that is frequently not considered, although it is a very important aspect and can relate both directly and indirectly to patient care.

The hospital is an archive of records on many patients and many procedures. The most important record of a hospital is the medical record that is kept on each patient. This record includes the physicians' notes, the nurses' notes, patient's temperature, medication, X-rays, laboratory tests, and anything else that may indicate something about the patient's condition. The medical record is utilized by the physician in his diagnosis and treatment and is referred to again if a patient is readmitted to the hospital. Therefore, it becomes a record that is kept for a long period of time, and the storage of these records becomes a problem. In addition to mere storage of records, it is also desirable to be able to retrieve information from these records for future use on individual patients and also for statistical surveys that might aid in projecting future hospital needs.

The medical record is becoming increasingly computerized so that information can be retrieved, and in some hospitals the medical record is kept to a large degree on a real-time computer basis. In this area, the clinical engineer should become involved in both the hardware and the software of developing a system for maintaining and utilizing these records.

The clinical engineer is also involved in the legal liability of the hospital in respect to instrumentation, the performance of personnel, and the safety of the facility. This involves making statistical studies in such areas as infection and other problems in the hospital that are not engineering problems but can be solved using engineering techniques. In this area, a clinical engineer works with attorneys, physicians, and other administrative personnel for the hospital. His stays, with regard to potential problems or possible problems in the hospital, could reduce the legal liability of the hospital in certain areas.

The operating research and industrial engineering tools of the clinical engineer are utilized in looking at the cost of the hospital. Hospitals have been criticized about their increasing daily room rates, and frequently the hospital has difficulty explaining how these increases come about or how they could have been prevented. In many ways, a hospital is an inefficient system, and its efficiency can be improved by engineering studies. However, any engineer studying a hospital system must consider the patient and the care of the patient. These are not studies that can be made by any engineer who only views the hospital as a business. Although the hospital is a business, its primary concern is patient care. The major cost in patient care is employees, and many of these employees, of course, can be utilized more efficiently or even be replaced by instrumentation. But if any of these steps are recommended, consideration must be given to what is happening to the patient during this time. Only a qualified clinical engineer is capable of considering all these aspects.

Patient Care

The clinical engineer is involved as a part of the medical team in patient care. This is reflected either directly or indirectly, in all the previous sections. In addition to his responsibilities in many other areas, the clinical engineer has specific responsibilities in clinical areas. In a large hospital setting, he may be specialized in a clinical area such as surgery, nuclear medicine, neurology, cardiology, and the clinical laboratory.

In the clinical laboratory, the clinical engineer works in an indirect patient-care area since he does not have direct contact with patients. However, he can have a major effect on patient care from this area. As the clinical laboratory is becoming increasingly automated, the engineer is required for interfacing different pieces of equipment and doing so with either a dedicated computer or a shared computer. The entire clinical laboratory is a system with considerable materials handling, and the engineer can look at different methods to improve the handling of these materials. There are also many scheduling problems since a definite amount of routine work must be done and then superimposed on this emergency analysis. All of this results in a complex operations research problem to make maximum utilization of equipment and personnel. Quality control is another important factor in the clinical lab that requires engineering expertise.

Nuclear medicine is an area that utilizes a clinical engineer. Again, much of his work is indirectly related to patient care, although patients are brought directly into the nuclear-medicine area. Much of the nuclear-medicine measurements today are being analyzed by computers, so the clinical engineer is involved in interfacing the equipment with small computers or shared systems. He may also be involved in developing the overall system and keeping the system operating both from a hardware and software standpoint. Therefore, he could be working full time in nuclear medicine. This type of clinical engineer is also responsible for radiation safety since this is where the largest amount of radiation occurs. He is also involved in improving the measurements from nuclear-medicine instrumentation, analyzing areas such as positioning, culminating beams, and increasing the intensity of the instrumentation. This clinical-engineering position may be filled with a person with a background in physics, but still much of the work is performed using engineering skills.

Another area in which the clinical engineer functions is radiology. In many respects it is similar to nuclear medicine. One of the differences is that radiology is found throughout a hospital and requires considerable instrumentation. In most cases, it has not been computerized yet, although computerization will certainly become a reality and will require more and more engineering expertise. In radiology, the engineer has the opportunity to use his knowledge to improve the X-ray and its diagnostic qualities and also assure the safety of patients and staff members.

The area in which the clinical engineer's presence is readily apparent is his involvement with monitoring equipment. Here he has a direct relationship with the patient. For example, he may work with cardiology in ICUs for surgery, medicine, and cardiac care. These are areas of the hospital that have become heavily instrumented in recent years and in which most of the safety concern arises. It is an area in which the engineer must consider the instrumentation as it interfaces with the facility and the patient. He must consider electrical, physical, and psychological safety. The clinical engineer working in this situation must have a basic knowledge of the physiology of the heart and the electrical impulses that are generated. He must be able to read an electrocardiogram as well as other allied health personnel can. Also, he must be familiar with emergency equipment in this area, such as the defibrillator, and be prepared to utilize it should the case arise in which he is the only person available who can do so. In some hospitals, the clinical engineer and his technicians may actually be manning the monitoring equipment. In other cases, they may only perform safety checks and provide maintenance.

The clinical engineer, especially one with an electrical background, has the opportunity for considerable involvement with the intensive-care and cardiology personnel, even in the area of research and development, an area in which most people will think of a clinical engineer as being part of the medical team.

Another critical area in the hospital is the operating suites that relate to the recovery room and to the surgical ICU. The operating suite is a location in which the clinical engineer may actually be scrubbed, dressed out, and on standby during major operations, which is especially true when an implant or open heart surgery is being performed. In this role, he and his technicians may actually operate equipment such as the heart-lung machine. In any case, both will be on standby to assure that everything is working properly, or if something does malfunction, that it is repaired as soon as possible. Also, the operating staff may be told that the instrumentation cannot be repaired and the operation must be terminated as expeditiously as possible. This is an area in the hospital in which many engineers do not feel at ease because this is as close to patient care and the balancing of human lives as he can come. Here he works very closely with a surgeon in applying new instrumentation and new pieces of equipment and devices, such as catheters, pacemakers, heart valves, etc. Much of this involves material engineering as well as mechanical or electrical engineering. Even though these devices are well tested before they are used on patients, each patient is different, and there is always the possibility of some malfunction. Hopefully, the engineer is in a position to provide advice and consultation that may make an operation successful that might otherwise have to be terminated because of some simple malfunction. Engineering skills may also be used to overview the entire operating suite in the program area and recommend possible changes in material movement and in personnel utilizations. Any recommendations in this direction must be very carefully considered and very closely discussed with the chief of surgery so that the overall picture is considered. Sterilization is a problem that must be considered by the engineer in this area since infection during operation can be fatal. It has been found that the classic 10-minute scrub is not sufficient to remove bacteria from the staff's hands. Such simple factors that have normally been accepted practice must be examined and reviewed by the clinical engineer.

The hemodialysis area is another area in which the clinical engineer can make a contribution. As previously mentioned, it is an area in which the clinical engineer can work in the training of patients in the use of the dialysis equipment. He can also work in the training of the staff and technicians in maintenance and utilization of this equipment. The clinical engineer can also work with the physician to develop better procedures, to evaluate equipment, and to decide which is the best to use in the hospital or in the home. His technicians will be responsible for making surveys of homes in which dialysis units are to be placed and assuring that these are properly installed. His technicians will make regular rounds to provide preventive maintenance and repairs on this life-supporting equipment in both the homes and hospitals.

Prosthetic aids constitute another major area within the clinical engineer's domain in which some improvements can be made to modify prosthetic aids for individual problems and fitting. There are many repairs and adjustments that can be made by the clinical engineer's technicians. Again, the engineer can work with the patient in showing him how to use the prosthetic aids and how to make minor adjustments on some of them.

Cardiac catherization, as it becomes more prevalent in many hospitals, could require a large amount of the clinical engineer's time. The clinical engineer and his technicians must maintain all the instrumentation that is used in a catherization laboratory and the actual involvement in the cardiac catherization. It is highly desirable that a clinical engineer or his technicians be available at the time of cardiac catherization to solve any instrumentation problems and also to monitor for possible problems involving instrumentation.

Other areas in the hospital in which the clinical engineer might become involved on a specialty basis and to which he may even be fully assigned, depending on their size, are pulmonary function, audiology, and neurology. These areas of the hospital involve a considerable amount of instrumentation and require technicians to operate and maintain the instrumentation. The technicians are generally specialized, for example, pulmonary-function technicians and EEG technicians. In some areas, these technicians might work for the clinical engineer and might also perform maintenance and calibration of equipment in addition to being operators. The clinical engineer is also utilized in this area to aid in interpreting data from instrumentation and determining whether part of the data is artifacts. He also helps in the best utilization of the instrumentation.

From these above examples of the clinical engineer working directly or indirectly in patient-care areas, one sees that there are many functions of the hospital that the clinical engineer can cover. Obviously, all such areas cannot be handled by any one individual and will require specialization by clinical engineers, especially in the large hospitals. In all cases, the clinical engineer will have to work very closely with the medical staff, especially if he is not trained in a given area.

31

A LARGE INSTITUTIONAL MODEL

J. Cavallari

The instrumentation service of the department of medical physics performs the clinical engineering functions at Memorial Hospital for Cancer and Allied Diseases in New York City. Memorial Hospital specializes in cancer detection, diagnosis, and treatment, and stresses research in its laboratories. It performs treatment by surgery, radiation therapy, and chemotherapy. Historically, the department of medical physics has provided some services to the entire center, including the Sloan-Kettering Institute for Cancer Research; some services throughout the hospital; and some to specific departments, such as radiation therapy, diagnostic radiology, medicine, and surgery. The instrumentation service has been primarily concerned with electronics and electrical engineering design and maintenance and construction services carried out by the medical physics department for various clinical departments in the hospital.

When the division of medical systems planned and acquired a large computer to automate its clinical laboratories, the instrumentation service participated, with assistance on design and construction of electronic interfacing. Also added to the clinical engineering responsibilities of this service was that of electronic safety for the hospital.

The instrumentation service is divided into four sections: electronic maintenance, electronic design, diagnostic low-voltage X-ray maintenance, and electronic safety. The service also provides supervision for the physics instrument shop and consists of engineers and technicians, as well as machinists responsible for electromechanical design and maintenance, fabrication, and installation.

Electronic Maintenance

The electronic maintenance section, a four-man group, consists of a section head, one engineer, and two technicians. They have the primary responsibility for maintaining all the radiation-related equipment in the department of radiation therapy and the nuclear medicine service. The equipment includes (*a*) a 6-MeV linear accelerator; (*b*) three cobalt teletherapy machines; (*c*) a 22-MeV betatron; (*d*) three radioisotope scanners; (*e*) a gamma camera; (*f*) a pulmonary-function analyzer (including a small dedicated computer); (*g*) two portable isotope scanners; and (*h*) all isotope uptake monitoring equipment in clinical labs and teaching laboratories.

In addition to maintenance of radiation-related equipment, the group maintains the interface equipment used between the biochemistry laboratory and the on-line IBM 1800 computer of the Division of Medical Systems.

Although not their primary function, this section also performs design and is now relocating and redesigning a radioisotope scanner. This particular unit was originally built in 1964 and includes out-of-date and unreliable electronics and data-storage components. When it was necessary to dismantle the scanner because of new hospital construction and to move it to a new location, the electronic package was redesigned. Modular components were substituted for integrated nucleonics; a paper-tape, data-storage unit was replaced by an incremental magnetic tape deck; and all auxiliary circuits and cabling were updated.

Electronic Design

Electronic design is the responsibility of one electrical engineer, whose primary assignment is to assist physicists supporting the department of radiation therapy. As a result of his design, devices have been built that have increased the safety and accuracy of radiological monitoring and calibration equipment. One example was the design of a redundant, independent dose-rate integrator for the hospital betatron. This device has two separate and complete dose rates and monitors, including two monitor chambers. If the primary monitor fails, the second, which is set to run slightly slower than the primary, will shut down the betatron.

New designs are initiated under the condition that if the device does not exist, and there is a need, there will be an investigation as to the feasibility to design and build it. Other designs are initiated when it is necessary to customize commercial equipment to users' specifications. An attempt is always made to create the least maintenance burden by using a straightforward approach where less sophisticated techniques were employed.

Another project was the design of the biochemistry-computer interface for the division of medical systems. This consisted of input/output control terminals located at laboratory analyzer stations. These boxes allowed lab technicians to enter fixed data, see a digital display of the sample under analysis, and receive an audiovisual alarm when a message comes over a line printer or CRT display. A decoder/distributor centrally located in the laboratory decodes a 16-bit computer word, which selects a control terminal, determines if the terminal is in the input or output mode, and gives message status and output data. If the data is in the input mode, this is routed to the data-input channel of the computer. Analogue-retransmitting potentiometers were incorporated in the SMA-12, which performs 12 analytical tests.

Two flame photometers and four colorimeters were similarly supplied with potentiometers, along with 10 bridge amplifiers (with reference power supplies) designed to output the computer multiplexer.

The design engineer utilized the support of the electronic maintenance section and the instrument shop to fabricate and install the equipment and cabling, although the actual cable pulling was completed by the hospital electricians. As mentioned above, the electronics maintenance section now maintains the interface equipment. Both the electronic maintenance and design sections occupy the same well-equipped electronic laboratory of about 600 sq ft.

Diagnostic Radiology Maintenance

This is a two-man group, a senior and junior engineer, responsible for the maintenance of all the radiological equipment not only in the department of diagnostic radiology but also for the entire center, which means service is provided for both clinical and research machines. They have a shop and storage area located in the department of radiology, which includes 15 routine rooms, 6 portable units, and a special procedure area. In this area, there are four special procedure rooms (myelographic, vascular-angio, neuroangio, and pneumoencephalographic) in operation. A fifth room for lymphangiographs is being installed. Service is provided for nine other radiographic rooms used for research, teaching, radiation-therapy simulation, and treatment planning. The senior engineer also teaches the fundamentals of X-ray circuitry to technology students and provides technical support and advice to the department of radiology and the physicists performing X-ray calibrations.

Instrument Shop

The instrument shop is a four-man shop consisting of a supervisor and three instrument makers who provide hospital-wide service ranging from simple tasks, such as the sharpening of surgical tools, to the fabrication of a complicated gamma, camera-light pipe.

Their shop occupies 1100 sq ft, which includes two vertical and two horizontal milling machines, several precision and general-purpose lathes, drill presses, and grinders. Because the shop produces many precisely designed radiation shield and collimation devices, a well-equipped lead-pouring facility is also included. The shop has a welding facility used for soft soldering and brazing. Other areas of the instrument shop are allocated for design and drafting, layout stock (both raw materials and fastening components), and storage of mobile tool carts for emergency on-site repairs. The staff works from either detailed drawings or general verbal descriptions of instruments.

Mechanical safety devices are another area of involvement for the shop. When a manufacturer installed a large angular-ring device, which is used to prevent collisions of the cobalt machines with patients being treated in beds, it was noted by one of the technicians that 110 V were present on the metal surface of the ring. In addition, the mechanical sensing of a collision was very insensitive. The facilities of both the electronics and instrument shops were combined in redesigning this ring to increase its sensitivity to both horizontal and vertical forces and to remove this potentially lethal shock hazard. As illustrated above, many duties of the instrument shop and the electronics maintenance section overlap because of the electromechanical characteristics of much of the equipment serviced.

Electrical Safety

The electrical safety program at Memorial Hospital, or more precisely the medical-equipment phase of the program, was officially started with the assignment of responsibilities to the instrumentation service for safety of all electronic apparatus and to the engineering department for electrical wiring. An electronics safety engineer was added to the staff for this purpose. Future plans include expanding this section, with both electronic and mechanical technicians, to repair and calibrate the wide range of medical equipment that is normally serviced in a general hospital by a clinical-engineering group.

A new, 600-bed hospital is planned that will utilize the most modern electronic techniques for patient treatment, care, and plant operation. As a result, a very active ongoing program of new equipment evaluation is being carried out, with technical support supplied by other members of the instrumentation service. A purchasing document has been formulated that outlines to the potential suppliers the expected performance, workmanship, safety, and documentation necessary for hospital acceptance of new medical equipment.

Costs

The budget for the instrumentation service is about $250,000 per year, which includes salaries, operational inventory, equipment, and overhead. Each section head prepares a monthly report based on daily records of the amount of time to be charged to each cost center or department. These section costs are combined into one monthly report. Finally, these monthly costs are combined with the remainder of the medical physics budget to form an annual budget report of charges for medical physics services to each hospital cost center.

The value of a group of this size is readily justified in several ways. First, the equipment maintained has a total cost of about $2 million at present and will increase significantly when equipment responsibilities are increased at the completion of the new hospital. Outside full-service maintenance costs would be over 10% of the $2 million figure, or more than $200,000, depending on the age and complexity of the equipment. The hospital receives not only maintenance coverage for complex equipment but receives this coverage promptly on an essentially instantaneous basis not possible with outside service groups. It also benefits from the design and fabrication capabilities of all the sections. Many devices, such as the radioisotope scanners and the betatron, have been either completely designed by the hospital physicists or so extensively modified that it would be virtually impossible to obtain a service contract from an outside organization.

Finally, the value of the instrumentation service is measured by Memorial Hospital's specialization. Outpatient treatment and diagnosis represent a large portion of equipment time, and long downtimes are costly, both medically and financially. The linac, betatron, nuclear medicine, and diagnostic X-ray machines may be characterized as large, immobile, and nonmodular. Service, therefore, must be performed onsite by highly specialized personnel, and a quick fix through substitution of components is not normally obtained.

Future Plans

The future plans of the instrumentation service include expanding the service to clinical laboratories and initiating a bioengineering group. These include:

Clinical Laboratories. Servicing automated equipment in the hematology laboratory (coulter counters) and biochemistry laboratories.

Bioengineering. Some clinically related investigations have already been completed by the instrumentation service. These were the feasibility study of an artificial larynx design and measurement of intrathoracic pressures during a cough. Although not specifically formulated, projects related to the hospital mission are (*a*) pulmonary-function studies; (*b*) measurement of cardiac output; (*c*) long-term cardiac monitoring; (*d*) electrode-artifact studies; and (*e*) elimination of RFI in patient monitors and automatic IV units. A bioengineering facility is envisioned having the capability to perform analogue simulation of physiological systems and to evaluate patient/nurse data entry systems.

Teaching. A shortage of trained biomedical technicians exist, especially those with experience in radiation equipment. Only one nonmanufacturer school exists in the United States that teaches diagnostic radiology maintenance. Preliminary studies have begun to establish such a program at Memorial Hospital.

Safety Program. The electronic safety program will expand with the hiring of mechanical technicians to service medical equipment such as the heart/lung machine, respirators, OR tables, and hemodialysis machines. The safety section itself will maintain and calibrate all the electronic equipment in the ORs, recovery room, CCU, pediatrics, and other high-risk areas. An important program is under way to update medical electronic equipment to meet existing electrical safety standards.

32

SPECIALIZED SERVICE GROUPS*

A. Zara

The medical engineering department, at Massachusetts General Hospital (MGH) in Boston, has found that an engineering service must give support to all areas of the hospital: clinical, administrative, and research. Technology, in the form of new devices and more complex systems, is playing an increasingly important role in the health-care industry. Engineers and technicians must keep abreast of technological advances and become part of the medical team.

Considering the variety of sizes, composition, and methods of administration of hospitals, there is no optimal format for providing engineering services. The medical engineering group at MGH operates on a fee-for-service basis and justifies its existence by providing essential services more efficiently and at less cost than an outside organization could.

The medical engineering department is an autonomous hospital department that maintains all clinical electronic and electromechanical equipment, offers research services, and conducts its own bioengineering research program.

The medical engineering department makes purchase recommendations based on detailed evaluations of equipment; takes responsibility for initial inspection, deployment, and installation of new equipment; and performs daily operational tests and regular preventive tests on existing equipment.

The department also contributes technical support to most MGH research that involves engineering, including a variety of multidisciplinary projects. With the Harvard Anesthesia Center Bioengineering Unit, MGH has worked on researching and applying quantitative diagnostic methods of neuromuscular transmission, using magnetic fluids for noninvasive blood-flow measurements, developing self-powered implantable electronic devices (telemetry and stimulators), and developing

*The editors wish to thank S. Aronow and J. Cywinski of Massachusetts General Hospital and R. Swanson of the Veteran's Administration for use of their input to this section.

hardware for new methods of treatment and diagnosis in cardiology, anesthesiology, and surgery.

The engineering service of the Veterans Administration's department of medicine and surgery is developing and implementing a biomedical engineering program to meet the immediate and future needs of clinical engineering support for VA hospitals. There are two aspects of the program: individual hospital needs and regional hospital needs.

Under the program, VA engineers interact with physicians and provide professional assistance, technical review, and broad coordinating support to technicians and repairmen in the electromechanical maintenance sections. By performing in this manner, the engineer is free to concentrate on the complex professional aspects involved with the complete spectrum of biomedical instrumentation technology as it relates to his hospital or medical district. The spectrum covers biomedical equipment reliability, quality, and safety for patients and clinical personnel.

Biomedical engineering technicians function in the electromechanical maintenance section, maintaining, repairing, and inspecting equipment and supervising medical-equipment repairmen and electronic technicians. It is anticipated that 90% of the total biomedical equipment workload will be maintained by this group. The other 10%, it is estimated, may be accomplished through VA supply depots and commercial-vendor contractual support.

The various levels of expertise are expected, in large measure, to be attained through in-service training where possible. Technical skills are expected to be developed by upgrading in-service personnel where possible. Additional skilled and semiskilled personnel will be recruited where necessary from outside the VA system. Junior colleges and technical schools can be expected to provide the fundamental knowledge and skills for incoming personnel.

In addition to the VA's biomedical engineering program, the VA central research instrumentation program has developed a BMET training program. This program will lead the BMET trainees to a level of skill commensurate with AAMI's certification requirements. It is expected that the program will expand its training opportunities to include engineering training as well as advanced technician training and other hospital technician skills.

Sinai Hospital of Baltimore, Maryland, has developed a full-service clinical engineering group within the 500-bed hospital. This group is within the hospital's department of engineering and maintenance. The group has demonstrated that the clinical engineering technician is indispensable where maximum-quality patient care is required. The input value provided by the clinical engineering group in developing clinical, architectural, and engineering criteria for the construction of a modern CCU is one of the chief accomplishments of the Sinai organization. The clinical-engineering technicians are selected very carefully. Selecting and training technicians comes under the supervision of a graduate biomedical engineer, who is assisted by the hospital engineer and the hospital's medical and nursing staff. Education and experience in electronic trades and graduation from civilian or military electronics programs form the initial basis for selection. The technicians are continually exposed to in-service training and, as they progress, help teach other technicians, nurses, and medical staff.

A sharp delineation of the group's responsibilities is essential. There is a sharp differentiation among the clinical application of monitoring facilities as well as relevant inspection, maintenance, repair, and development. Recruiting and training technicians to work in areas in which nurses and interns previously had spent much of their time was possible with this type of delineation. The technicians work under the supervision of a biomedical engineer.

At the Medical University of South Carolina, there is a hospital engineering support service that provides all types of engineering support to hospitals on a shared cost basis. Their program anticipates the involvement of administrators, physical plant engineers, and physicians of each participating hospital, as well as mechanical, biomechanical, electrical, and electronic engineers in areas of direct patient contact.

33

COST EFFECTIVENESS OF A MEDICAL ENGINEERING DEPARTMENT

J. E. Jacobs and J. A. McLaren

Northwestern University established an interdisciplinary program in biomedical engineering at the undergraduate level to complement its long-standing graduate program in biomedical engineering. Student response to the program has been such that approximately 40% of the undergraduate body within the Technological Institute is enrolled in the interdisciplinary biomedical engineering option. Through the extensive student advisory program, it was learned that a major portion of these students were anticipating applying for admission to medical schools. While the acceptance into medicine of the upper 20% of the graduating class was almost certain, the remaining 80% of the students would understandably be forced by circumstances to establish rewarding careers in other health-related areas. In anticipation of this, the curriculum of the interdisciplinary biomedical engineering undergraduate program was designed so that the student had to complete a series of courses leading to a major in one of eight identifiable options. These are, understandably, all health related.

The student, following his sophomore year, spends alternate periods in industry and receives on-the-job training as he completes the requirements for a BS degree. Under the cooperative education option, 5 years are required to obtain a BS degree. When working in certain institutions, qualified students may, on graduation, obtain a combined BS/MS degree, reflecting the necessity of spending an additional year to obtain the degree under the cooperative education option.

With increasing enrollment in the interdisciplinary biomedical engineering option of the Technological Institute, considerable difficulty occurs in finding cooperative engineering positions for the students desiring that option. This is due to the fact that the industrial community involved in biomedical engineering is relatively small compared to industries involved in the more traditional engineering disciplines. It has long been recognized that a biomedical engineering department can make immeasurable contributions to a hospital. With the increasing awareness of the need for maximum utilization of existing equipment, development of improved safety standards, and 24-hour operation of equipment, the existing mechanisms for providing these services in many hospitals leave much to be desired. A cooperative program with hospitals would be beneficial to both the student and the hospital.

In view of the interrelated needs, the Northwestern Biomedical Engineering Center hosted a meeting for administrators of Illinois hospitals to discuss the effectiveness of the biomedical engineer in the hospital environment. In connection with this meeting, a study of the cost effectiveness of the biomedical engineering department at Evanston Hospital, a member of the McGaw Medical Center of Northwestern University, was presented.

Details of the Biomedical Engineering Department

The biomedical engineering department at Evanston Hospital employs four people at a personnel budget of approximately $50,000. It has available to it a supply budget of approximately $10,000 and an equipment budget that runs approximately $2000 per year. For the purpose of assessing indirect costs, approximately 400 sq ft are assigned to the operation. The major functions of the department include (*a*) equipment maintenance; (*b*) preventive maintenance and electrical safety programs; (*c*) specification and evaluation of equipment; (*d*) research support and consultation; (*e*) equipment fabrication and interfacing; and (*f*) training and education programs as appropriate. An analysis of the effort of the group indicates that 83% of the total departmental time is spent on electronic maintenance. To arrive at the size of the department, an analysis was made of the existing maintenance. It was found that approximately $59,000 per year could be obtained for the department by not renewing existing service contracts. One should recognize that this is an actual cash flow and does not reflect the intangible benefit of the availability of in-house expertise and immediate response to service calls by the biomedical engineering department. Thus, it was found that through careful analysis of the existing hospital cash flow as it relates to maintenance of equipment currently in the hospital, funds could be made available to support the biomedical engineering department.

Since the department still must buy parts and occasionally obtain outside assistance, the savings as compared to the cost of the contracts amounts to approximately $5000 per year. However, many other devices not covered by contract are serviced essentially free to the hospital. In other words, the total spectrum of the function of the biomedical engineering department is supported by the money previously spent for a portion of the equipment maintenance activities.

The principal advantages to Evanston Hospital from in-house maintenance are

1. Fast response times. Often a device can be made operative without disrupting patient flow; night and weekend emergencies can also be resolved speedily.

2. More freedom of purchasing. Since they can maintain most of their own devices, the choice of devices is not limited to organizations with large service centers.
3. Around-the-clock, on-call emergency coverage, which has essentially already been paid for.
4. The in-house capability to provide a preventive maintenance program. It is well known in industrial organizations that preventive maintenance programs result in extended life of the equipment with inherent lower cost per year. This is a factor that is often overlooked by hospital administrators and is, in fact, ignored, as evidenced by the increasing trend toward leasing facilities.

Role of the Biomedical Engineer in Hospital Administration

It was apparent from discussion with the administrators of hospitals that have established biomedical engineering departments that they regard the head of that department as a key figure in administrative long-range planning and day-to-day operation of the hospital. This is not surprising when one realizes that the modern hospital is becoming more dependent on effective utilization of the technology related to modern health-care systems. Understandably, a major factor in the assimilation of this technology is an effective evaluation of its impact on the existing hospital operation. This is an area in which the hospital administrator has little background and could do little about before the availability of graduates of biomedical engineering programs. In fact, many of the administrators admitted that before the availability of the modern biomedical engineering department, they were essentially at the mercy of the vendors regarding equipment to be purchased and installed in their organizations.

Four points can be summarized:

1. The modern hospital uses many complex electrical and electronic devices in the delivery of health services.
2. The conventional method of entering into service contracts with vendors is expensive, fraught with delays, and extremely fragmented.
3. The medico legal responsibility of the hospital increases markedly with the acquisition of electronic equipment and the need to ensure safe operation.
4. The acquisition of a biomedical engineer and the development of in-house capability for electronic management is cost effective, broader in the scope of its services than multiple contractors, and safer for the patient.

34

EFFICIENT USE OF PURCHASED EQUIPMENT

L. Goodman

Can equipment still be used after a specific need has been satisfied? The answer may be found in a shared-equipment facility or equipment pool. The biomedical engineering and instrumentation branch of the NIH has created a NIH scientific equipment rental program. The program is applicable to a great extent to any hospital in the 500-bed and above category. However, hospitals below that size could easily have an interhospital program that would be capable of paying for itself.

Many hospital associations are beginning to think in terms of shared clinical engineering services, which also are offered by private contractors, and it seems reasonable to consider shared-equipment services. The interesting facet is that the program seems to work not by having first bought the equipment and then waiting for an interested user but by the programs taking on and maintaining, in good working order, equipment that was originally purchased for a past need. Innovations of this type would seem to answer many high-cost equipment problems at very reasonable charges at the same time that they pay for themselves. The NIH equipment data pool is based on equipment used for research. There is no reason why equipment for clinical use should not fall into the same category.

The NIH Scientific Equipment Rental Program

The division of research services operates a scientific equipment-rental program for the NIH Intramural Community, based primarily on loans from a pool of refurbished instruments. The program is implemented by the biomedical engineering and instrumentation branch (BEIB), division of research services. It is responsive to a federal property-management regulation that states government policy for ensuring utilization of laboratory equipment.

The pool is composed of equipment that has general utility in research work but is not used sufficiently by particular laboratories to warrant permanent possession. Pool equipment is maintained by BEIB and made available to all intramural NIH programs on a completely optional rental basis. Users are charged a nominal fee to make the program self-supporting and viable.

The program offers

1. Ready availability of a variety of scientific instruments in good working condition
2. Reduced delay in implementation of ongoing and new programs
3. Reduced capital investment in equipment costs, especially for short- and intermediate-term projects
4. Reduced burden on laboratory research and technical staff for procurement and care of equipment
5. Extension of instrument life via more thorough programs for preventive maintenance
6. Opportunity to test and evaluate newly developed instruments in the laboratory setting with little or no direct capital investment
7. More complete centralized information on equipment performance, reliability, and maintenance costs
8. Improved utilization of laboratory space

Program Operations

The equipment pool consists primarily of equipment declared as excess or voluntarily contributed by investigators. New equipment is added with funds accrued from rental revenues.

Pool equipment is maintained under the custody of BEIB, and a special code-number series is established for purposes of identification and record keeping.

Billing and accounting procedures are managed according to routine BEIB fee-for-service (revolving fund) activities.

A reserved fund, derived from rental revenue surplus, is used for purchase of equipment and accessories to prevent obsolescence, increase inventories, and provide for refurbishing additional used acquisitions. Generating the fund from user charges provides a convenient and equitable mechanism for distributing costs according to relative demands.

Program Policies

The program is primarily intended to serve the relatively short-term needs of NIH investigators.

Pool equipment, in good condition, is rented to intramural program users normally for periods of less than one year; extensions can be arranged where justified.

The user is charged 3% of initial purchase cost *per month, or any part thereof, for the period of loan.*

Where on-site assembly or disassembly of equipment is involved on delivery or removal, costs for labor and material, at regular fee-for-service rates, are borne by the user.

BEIB bears the cost of refurbishing equipment returned to stock.

BEIB maintains loan equipment in good operating condition and provides replacement parts and labor.

Costs of any special modifications or installation of permanent accessories are borne by the requesting user at regular fee-for-service hourly rates, plus materials. Where the user has purchased an accessory not available in the pool, he has the option to retain possession. Requests for major modifications, which would destroy the basic utility of the instrument, are negotiated and financed on an individual basis.

Costs of installation of expendable accessories are borne by the user at regular fee-for-service hourly rates, plus materials.

In cases in which equipment has been damaged because of user abuse or accident, the user bears full costs of repair at regular fee-for-service hourly rates, plus materials. If equipment has been damaged beyond repair or lost because of user's negligence, disposition of the case is determined by a board of survey as required by existing regulations; the user institute bears full cost of replacement.

BEIB responsibility extends only to provision of equipment, maintenance, repair, and instruction in proper operations where necessary. BEIB does not provide laboratory technicians, nor does it operate a common process facility.

Up-to-date inventory lists of pool equipment are maintained for examination and distribution as required.

The program is intended to serve NIH intramural operations in the Washington metropolitan area. Special arrangements must be made for areas outside this region.

The intent of the program is to provide instruments for short-term rental. Pool equipment is not subject to permanent transfer.

35

INSPECTION OF NEW EQUIPMENT

M. Shaffer

Recent estimates suggest that approximately 40–50% of the instrumentation received by the George Washington University Medical Center contains some fault. Some of the reasons given for this situation include installation, checkout, and operating errors due to inadequate reference manuals. For these reasons, it has been suggested that clinical engineers provide thorough inspection procedures for any incoming instrumentation. If any faults are detected at this point, the purchaser should contact the manufacturer and withold acceptance until the necessary repairs are made. If the manufacturer provides adequate reference manuals, it may be possible for the engineering staff to correct minor defects before the device is put into operation.

While the percentage of faulty instrumentation seems high, a recent survey of the electronic instrumentation received during a 3-month period at the George Washington University Hospital showed some anomalies on receipt in 36% of the units and in 42% of the units after a 2-month shakedown period. These anomalies were attributed to deficiencies in packaging and transportation handling (25%), instrumentation quality control (65%), and other (10%).

These results were somewhat unexpected. It was presumed that the majority of failures would be due to inadequate packaging and rough handling. However, in most cases, the packaging was good, as evidenced by the low figure stated previously.

It is believed that the high quality-control-incidence figure can be attributed to both the nature of the hospital instrumentation market and the production techniques largely forced on the manufacturer. Quite obviously, the market is highly competitive, as approximately 1200 manufacturers market about 5000 different types of instruments. In this limited market, the successful manufacturer is one that can provide what the user wants at an acceptable price, thereby implying the need for production-line methods with relatively unskilled labor. Such methods require that the instrumentation has passed properly through the development stage. Thus, each step in the manufacturing process is adequately described, normally in an enormous amount of paper work, which includes parts lists, component drawings, layout and assembly drawings, wiring running lists, performance specifications, test procedures, and quality-control standards and specifications.

This *modus operandi* can involve considerable time and cost to set up and begin production, and subsequently applied on an economic basis only to high-demand, standard items. Unfortunately, from the manufacturers' aspect, the users of hospital instrumentation are professionally dedicated to extending the state-of-the-art, and new improvements and applications have to be constantly developed. The ensuing changes well affect every one of the production-line documents and so must be well tested and the design frozen before any attempt is made to incorporate any changes in the production line.

In many cases in which the type of change does not make it worthwhile to revise the whole documentation and production-line process, the instrumentation is often made as special units under the direct supervision of the engineering department. However, engineering salaries are high in relation to customer dollars, and any time spent in developing such special units must be kept at a minimum. Many changes may thus be attempted without the benefit of prototypes, evaluation programs, and criteria against which the quality-control specialists can properly judge acceptance. Quality control is then based only on appearance. It may also be that these special units are sold to the user with the misconception that a hospital represents a ready-made test environment more rugged than any synthetic situation that could be implemented in an engineering laboratory. The realization that these units may work or be made to work with limited cash flow in this available test environment can be all too inviting. To compound the problem, the engineers at this point may be reassigned to other endeavors; consequently, the technical writers and field representatives are assigned engineering responsibilities they are probably not qualified to assume.

Thus, the hospital should approach the first production unit with caution, seek the opinion of others, and check the equipment on delivery. The present survey and rationale support further suggest that it is advisable to approach with even greater caution the units made by special procedures.

36

DESIGN FACTORS FOR INTENSIVE CARE AND SURGICAL UNITS

A. D. Lewis

Technological change is transforming the concept of hospital functions. If the hospital is thought of as merely an assembly of complicated components, it can overwhelm designers. A hospital should be an environment that inspires the doctor and the patient. The more complicated a building is, the less responsive it is to the people who work in it. The reasons are that the health field is unlike most other fields, a good example being manufacturing, in which an architect could assume that his client has all the answers regarding its functions and operations, including time and motion studies. However, physicians do not know all the answers because their work is constantly changing. As a direct result thereof, the hospital remains the most complex of the common building assignments.

Medicine, as we all are becoming increasingly aware, is becoming more and more dependent on the physical sciences and engineering. This interdependency is evident from the statement, often made, that "the safest place for a patient to be in a hospital is in the operating suite." This confidence is attributed by medical personnel directly to the technical competence of the OR staff. Regrettably, this confidence could be largely dispelled should a comprehensive analysis be made of the planning, design, and maintenance cycle relative to operating suite and surgical ICUs. Increasingly complex technical problems plague and further compound existing difficulties encountered in designing the operating suite and surgical ICU. Due to the complexity of these problems, contradictions in technical support requirement parameters may have evolved and been incorporated into designs.

A case in point could be the collocation of the recovery and surgical intensive-care functions in one room. Reasons given for this situation are, generally, to reduce staffing and equipment support requirements. Problems created by the situation are: the possibility of increasing cross-infection due to, *inter alia,* an inability to maintain a positive pressure in the surgical ICU relative to zero pressure required in the recovery room; the different requirements for air-volume changes and temperature/humidity control; and in the indescribable increase in ambient noise levels in the surgical ICU (Noise Criteria: NC 25–NC 30) emanating from the recovery room (NC 30–NC 35). It is clear that the problems generated by compromises in design consideration cannot be overcome by the technical competence of the medical staff. What is needed to preclude this situation from occurring in the future is integrated planning and design through the interrelationship and increasing requirements for direct communications between medical personnel and engineers. Without this interrelationship and communication, very little progress can and will be made in meeting the needs of today and the future through technical interactions/support of the disciplines involved.

Significant Design-Factor Considerations

In order to derive general design-factor considerations and to apply these factors in the design and evaluation of operating suites and surgical ICUs, it is considered necessary to know, in addition to administrative, operational, and flow (patient, staff, material, communications, etc.) procedures, the people involved (type, age, and socioeconomic backgrounds of the patients, physicians, nurses, technicians, medical and engineering support personnel, etc.) and in the case of hospital personnel, their functional activities (examining, treating, walking, testing, repairing/maintaining, logistical supporting, etc.). Research aids are needed to evaluate the interrelationships and interaction of a myriad of variables for a particular design and the evaluation of the design, once constituted.

In this regard it should be noted a new type of psychology, architectural and engineering psychology, is emerging. It applies the behavioral sciences to the design of facilities, including operating suites and surgical ICUs. This type of psychology allows the design professions to focus on the patient and his/her individual needs for medical care as the central concern in surgical health care. Until recently, most planning and design decisions have been made intuitively by hospital personnel, engineers, architects, and hospital consultants who have "pseudo-represented" the requirements of the recipients of health care in the operating suites and ICUs. It is currently widely recognized, however, that intuition, while considered essential to any complex decision-making process, is by its very nature inadequate for successful operating suite/surgical ICU design. Planning and design-team composition is therefore of paramount importance. As indicated in Table I, composition of the team is dependent on the functional areas in question.

Perusal of Table I will indicate that the proposed membership of the planning and design team includes four disciplines not normally identified: lighting and biomedical/clinical engineers, the acoustical consultant, and the microbiologists. They have been included as members of the team for very important reasons. In an effort to support this viewpoint, each of their functional areas will require general evaluation.

TABLE I
Planning and Design Team Principle Members

Member	Operating suite	Surgical intensive care unit
Administrator	X	X
Chief of major surgical services	X	X
Head of anesthesiology	X	X
Director of nursing services	X	X
Director of central sterile services	X	optional
Nurse supervisor of operating suite	X	optional
Nurse supervisor of ICU	optional	X
Hospital consultant	X	X
Architect	X	X
Engineer(s)—hospital, lighting, biomedical/clinical, etc.	X	X
Other staff/functions—(as required) acoustical consultant, microbiologist, etc.		

Parameters utilized in the planning and design of operating suites and surgical intensive-care units can be summarized by the following:

1. Facilities and equipment to minimize shock and trauma while providing physical comfort and emotional support to the patient
2. Preventing infection
3. Safeguarding patients and personnel from technological hazards
4. Operating the units efficiently in order to permit maximum time for patient care
5. Operating economically to hold down costs
6. Coordinating with other hospital departments and services, thereby promoting the smooth functioning of all aspects of patient care

Illumination and Color

It is evident that one element that must be taken into account in the design of operating suites and surgical ICUs is light. We know that the appearance of any object depends to a great extent on the light in which it is seen. The lighting in the OR is considered by many as the most important in the entire hospital. It is evident that the reason for this is the importance of the work being accomplished therein. Excellent technical documents currently exist on the techniques needed to illuminate the operating suite and the recovery room, mainly "Lighting for Hospitals (IES)," "IES Lighting Handbook," and the "Westinghouse Lighting Handbook," to name a few.

Although illumination requirements of the surgical ICU are similar to that of the recovery room from the level and quality of illumination viewpoint, there are several additional factors that must be taken into consideration because the lighting of the surgical ICU (some units contain open bay, cubicle, rooms and/or a combination of each) is an important matter. General room illumination (30 footcandles [30 fc] during the day, reducible to 1–3 fc at night), convenience lighting for the patient, nurses observation lighting (2 fc), examination light (100 fc) and night light (0.5–1.0 fc at floor level) should be provided. The examination light should be positioned so that any and all parts of the patient's body can be illuminated by the light. Portable examination lights, either attached to the wall or bed, or patient convenience lights have been and continue to be utilized. They do result in possible disadvantages, depending on the type of patient involved and possible emergencies that may arise, of being in a position that may interfere with the medical staff. Since in the case of surgical intensive-care patients extended periods of time, often many days, are expended confined to beds, certain additional refinements in illumination, beyond that extended to patients in the recovery room should be provided.

The generally accepted approach to this situation is to provide a 2 by 4 recessed fluorescent fixture (with radio frequency interference [RFI]) filters to reduce RFI directly over each bed, controlled by a dimmer. Selective illumination is thereby provided without disturbing other patients. Since we are discussing surgical intensive-care areas, additional lighting should also be provided for examination. This illumination can be provided by either recessed, movable (preset to areas to be examined) incandescent lighting or quartz lighting, located either near or as part of the fluorescent fixture. The fixtures should be controlled by timers because they may be inadvertently left on by medical personnel upon completion of the examination of a patient. Patient discomfort due to illumination during examination periods should be reduced to the maximum extent possible. Attention is invited to the fact that light reflected off a surface material onto a patient often causes a change in the appearance of said patient. The possible situation should not be overlooked, especially when television is utilized for monitoring purposes. However, the traditional concern of the architect and engineer, who design the artificially lit interiors of the areas under consideration has previously been from a visual and aesthetic viewpoint.

The environment in these areas is pronounced as being successful if the areas provide illumination that meets established standards (including quantity and quality). However, there is currently abundant evidence that environmental lighting exerts important effects on human health, far beyond the requirement for vision. Environmental lighting has been shown to affect humans directly from interactions in cells and blood near the surface of the body and indirectly from nervous impulses generated by light. Light has several effects on bodily functions. Only a few dozen are currently known and understood. Hence, architects, lighting designers, and engineers might be well advised to be conservative about introducing great deviations from "natural" light. There appears to be reason enough for the planner/

designer to carefully reexamine the particular environment he may be creating in critical-care areas. It may be that, as in the case of air pollution, many of the by-products of the health-care planner/designer efforts are not fully recognized until such time as they gradually build to proportions that jeopardize the very existence of a patient. In essence, before we design the lighting/fenestration systems for the operating suite and surgical ICU, we must take into consideration the necessity for providing lighting requirements in these areas not only from a visual-identification viewpoint but from a technical/medical supportive one as well. Would the OR staff function more efficiently if the illumination in certain sections of the suite contained lighting that improved their physical well-being? Would the health of a patient situated in the surgical ICU be improved through the utilization of lighting affecting their body functions? Further study is obviously required in this area.

There is a definite interface between lighting requirements and color since the color we perceive depends on the object being viewed, its surroundings, the lighting, the eye, and the brain. One area receiving more and more attention is the impact of color on patients confined in ICUs and being held in preoperative holding areas. Studies have determined that patients are emotionally responsive to their surroundings, and color is one of the chief factors that determines what those surroundings are like. It has been readily recognized that psychological problems can cause physical ones. Because a patient is already suffering from some type of ailment, it is considered essential that his psychological state of mind either contributes to his eventual recovery or at the very best does not make the situation worse. Furthermore, experimentation indicates that patients express stress when surrounded by an unfamiliar environment (the surgical ICU and preoperative holding area) and when confronted with unfamiliar people (medical personnel) and instrumentation.

Tests with colors indicate that the warm colors (the red end of the spectrum) are psychologically warm and stimulating. In essence, the reds, oranges, and yellows act as stimulants that can *raise* blood pressure and pulse rate. At the other end of the spectrum, the cool tones of blues and greens were found to be equally objectionable. In the past, blue has normally been associated with unhappiness and depression. Psychosomatically, the feeling could aggravate a patient's physical condition. The color green, while generally considered a relaxing color, is all too often associated with institutions (hospitals) and therefore could be depressing. Studies indicate that both blue and green colors can *reduce* blood pressure and pulse rate, a situation that could be dangerous. Actual studies are currently in progress in the use of blue-gray (cool tone), a pure gray, and a glazed terra-cotta (warm blue) to offset the impact of color on the patient. Although the grays in bold patterns may be a logical solution to the problem, additional research is needed to determine whether standard color patterns could be modified through variable lighting methods, thereby providing the physician with yet another health-care tool.

The need for fenestration in ICUs has been well documented. A case in point could be that natural light in a recovery room would be highly desirable. In the event a 24-hour recovery room were utilized, natural light would probably become a requirement because of its similarity to a surgical ICU. The patient over a period of time, generally three days, becomes disoriented ("intensive care syndrome"). Therefore, an ICU patient should be able to view the outside or be so bedded as to be aware of it, thus providing him with the concept of day and night and the passage of time.

Acoustic Noise Problems

Although the annoyance caused by the same noise varies considerably, the threshold of tolerable sound is considered lower for ill persons.

In one survey, approximately 50% of the patients indicated that they were not disturbed solely by human noise, and the other half attributed this to maintenance and equipment. Some of the noisiest areas in a hospital are the recovery room and ICUs, and the patients in these areas may be affected by possible hazardous effects of noise. People made most of the noise in both the recovery and ICUs, and sleep in these areas is difficult. Until such time as sufficient research is accomplished to prove that noise-induced physiological alterations are harmless, physicians should consider noise to have possible detrimental effects.

Measurements in the coronary and the medical-surgical ICUs, which are expected to be among the quietest places in the hospital, may be found to be consistently above speech and sleep-interference levels. Average noise levels in the medical-surgical ICUs are just above 65 dB. This is extremely high since the recommended noise level should normally not exceed an ambient noise level of 25–30 dB in ICUs and 30–35 dB in the recovery room.

To aid in the achievement of acoustically well-designed operating suites and surgical ICUs, certain basic considerations, from an acoustical viewpoint, should be utilized, including controlling the type and level of background noise within the area in question, reducing the level of noise and vibration produced by operation of installed building equipment, and reducing the level of sound transmitted between spaces. To overcome noise problems, the acoustical consultant would recommend that, whenever possible, functional areas/spaces that emit or produce high noise levels should be located remote from quiet spaces, both horizontal and vertically. Furthermore, noise-generating areas should be grouped together and surrounded by noncritical buffer space.

However, since in some instances the functional relationship between medical spaces may preclude this arrangement, special sound-isolating construction systems may be required. Table II contains a recommended degree of isolation between space types within typical medical facilities and is a useful tool that should be utilized in the planning of operating/recovery areas and ICUs. A possible constraint on the location of central sterile supply relative to the operating suite and surgical ICU becomes a factor because of their interrelationship (due to the high volume of material flowing to these two areas). Where possible, some type of vertical relationship often becomes a planning and design requirement. It is therefore obvious that

TABLE II
Degree of Sound Isolation between Space Types Within Typical Medical Facilities in Noise Isolation Class (NIC) and Impact Insulation Class (IIC) Ratings

Space types	Chutes/mech. shafts	Mech equipment spaces	Storage	Maintenance	Waiting areas	Corridors	Lockers	Conference	Gen. office spaces	Private offices	Food prep and washing	Laboratories	Exercise and therapy	Dental OR	Exam and treatment room	Nurseries	Labor	Operating/recovery	Consult/interview	ICU and CCU	Tub and shower	Dayroom	Toilet	Patient bedroom
Patient bedroom	55	55	35	55	50	45	50	45	45	45	55	45	55	55	50	55	55	45	45	45	50	50	50	40
Toilet	40	45	30	40	40	40	35	45	40	45	45	45	40	40	45	50	40	45	45	50	35	40	40	
Dayroom	45	45	30	45	40	40	30	50	45	45	45	50	40	45	50	50	55	50	50	50	40	40		
Tub and shower	40	45	30	40	40	40	30	50	45	45	40	45	40	45	45	45	45	45	45	45	35			
ICU and CCU	45	55	35	55	40	40	35	40	45	40	55	50	55	45	45	55	55	40	45	40				
Consult/interview	50	55	35	55	45	45	45	50	45	50	55	45	55	50	45	45	55	40	50					
Operating/recovery	45	55	35	55	40	45	35	45	45	45	55	45	55	50	45	50	55	45						
Labor	45	55	35	55	50	50	40	55	50	55	55	50	55	50	50	55	50							
Nurseries	50	55	35	55	40	40	40	50	45	50	55	50	55	50	45	40								
Exam and treatment room	45	55	30	55	45	45	45	50	45	45	55	45	50	45	45									
Dental OR	45	55	35	55	45	40	35	50	45	50	55	45	50	45										
Exercise and therapy	35	50	30	45	40	35	30	55	50	55	45	50	35											
Laboratories	50	55	35	55	40	35	35	50	45	50	50	35												
Food prep and washing	35	45	30	45	40	35	35	55	45	55	35													
Private offices	50	55	40	55	40	45	45	50	40	45														
Gen office spaces	45	50	35	50	35	35	35	50	35															
Conference	50	55	40	55	45	50	45	50																
Lockers	35	45	—	40	35	30	—																	
Corridors	35	45	—	45	—	—																		
Waiting Areas	45	50	30	50	—																			
Maintenance	35	40	—	35																				
Storage	30	35	—																					
Mech equipment spaces	35	—																						
Chutes/mech shafts	40																							

the acoustical consultant does have an important role to play in design of operating suites and surgical ICUs.

Interesting studies have been conducted utilizing a cousin to noise, music, to provide a nonstressful environment for the patient. In theory, at least, a preoperative patient will arrive in the operating suite at the precise moment that the OR and surgical team is ready. However, since this rarely occurs, patients are often brought to the operating suite earlier. This is done in order to attempt to manage more definitively the logistical support aspects of the preoperative period to offset the situation, and therefore a holding area/room is often established. Since this area/

room should be a nonstressful environment, the provision of carefully selected music pleasing to the patient is currently under consideration. Even more interesting studies have been conducted on patients located in intensive-care-type units. Since these patients are often frightened by this environment, some means of diverting his or her attention is currently being evaluated. Exactly how musical sounds calm, depress, or stimulate the nervous system is currently not known, but evidence does indicate that certain types of music are recommended, however, and that music should be provided to the patient by a localized pillow speaker. This can be utilized as an additional tool/aid in patient care.

The Infection Hazard

Although hospitals exist to treat illness, it has been determined that they often act as reservoirs of infection. When accurate surveys were conducted, results have indicated that a substantial number of the patients acquired some type of infection during their stay in the hospital, infections they did not have upon admission. It would be interesting to determine the number of extra patient days that have resulted because of postoperative sepsis. As previously indicated, one of the primary parameters that should be utilized in the planning, design, and operation of operating suites and surgical ICUs is prevention of infection. Regretably, the rate of hospital infections has not decreased over the last 30–40 years (this in the face of advances in methodology and the introduction of antibiotics), and the type of organism causing the situation may have changed. Apart from the added suffering, inconvenience, and in a limited number of instances, death, the cost of these extra patient days caused by cross-infection bears heavily not only on the patients themselves but also increases funding support required from medical insurance companies, with attendant increases in insurance premiums. Although the annual cost of hospital-acquired infections is difficult to estimate, there are indications, and they are conservative ones, that these costs may well run into the billions of dollars per year. This, coupled with increasing tendency for litigation to arise from improper practices relative to cross-infection control, dictates the need for increased action in this area. It should also be noted that there is currently an absence of widely accepted intrahospital standards for microbial populations in hospitals.

In the past, the main emphasis has been on the careful adherence to aseptic practices such as hand washing, housekeeping, sterilization, and the careful application of air conditioning in hospitals, especially in surgical and intensive-care areas. Increased emphasis has been placed by the designer on limiting cross-infection through the control of microorganisms in the environment, predicated on an understanding of the means utilized in their growth, reproduction, and transmission. Special studies have been conducted on the infection hazard of such special-care areas as the recovery room and intensive-care-type units.

The prime vectors in cross-infection, are the personnel who work in these units. No data are available to demonstrate the effects of architectural design units on infections that occur in these units. Traditional design of intensive-care-type units (recovery and medical-surgical intensive care) is basically that of an open ward, with only one or two isolation rooms. The open-ward approach has been, and continues to be, justified by medical personnel and the planner/designer on the basis that this type of layout provides good surveillance and ready access to all patients. Ongoing studies no longer tend to support this design approach for various reasons, including the limited amount of potential control over cross-infection possibilities. The open ward design fails to:

1. Eliminate or control the microorganisms by keeping them out of the environment (including air quality and quantity and patient control)
2. Kill the microorganisms via germicidal application techniques
3. Reduce them via disinfection and sanitation (disinfection of sinks, equipment, and floors)
4. Create an unfavorable environment for their growth
5. Disrupt or eliminate the means of transmission. (Hospital personnel movement, limited space availability per bed, air movement, and pressure differential requirements, etc.)

Current thinking on the matter indicates that sacrosanct dogma relative to cross-infection is being challenged.

It has been realized that the risks of airborne contamination, as currently measured, does not necessarily correlate with incidences of infection in patients. This concept has upset many theories that tend to equate a high rate of airborne bacteria with a high infection hazard. New concepts for contamination cross-infection in the 1970s are evolving predicated upon:

1. The emergence of gram-negative pathogen as the principal offending organism in nosocomial infection, in lieu of staphylococcus
2. The relative importance of airborne versus contact contamination (exogenous-staff-to-patient and/or patient-to-patient, or endogenous-emanating from the patient's own body functions relative to the wound or the respiratory tract of the patient himself.)

Many gram-negative organisms are not virulent unless they attack patients in a setting of debilitation following injury, severe illness, or a major surgical operation. Under such circumstances, these organisms colonize the throat of the patients even though they are not able to colonize healthy hospital staff.

Interestingly, those who propound the theory that gram-negative pathogens are the culprit (these organisms thrive in moist areas such as wet or sweaty hands, wet sinks, and floors and would not survive for long in small droplets in the air) indicate that emphasis seems to be, although rather slowly, from control of airborne contamination to that of control contact contamination. It is obvious that this situation leaves the planner, designer, and medical operating personnel in a difficult situation. Where should emphasis be placed relative to limiting the possibilities of cross-infection in the future designs of recovery and surgical ICUs? Should air quality and quantity (laminar flow-surgery, etc.) continue to receive major attention, or should more efforts be devoted to the contact contamination problem? If, in fact, airborne contamination is not of principal consideration, then the question arises as to the utilization of airborne contamination as a basis for installing individual cubicles/rooms in recovery and surgical ICUs. Would the installation of air curtains around the beds in these areas be more effective? If airborne contamination continues to be a deciding factor in critical-care areas, then why do we continue to design air-flow systems with return air registers located in room ceilings? The air flow in this case is normally from the ceiling down across the patient, possibly the floor, picking up possible contamination with the air movement and then flowing back up to the ceiling. If while performing their normal functions medical personnel penetrate the upward air flow, could these personnel then become possible carriers? Lastly, can pressure differentials be maintained when patient cubicle/room doors remain open (unless we use air curtains)?

The key to successful planning and design of operating suites and surgical ICUs is

1. Protecting and supporting the well-being of the patient, while promoting the smooth functioning of all aspects of patient care
2. Not second-guessing the medical profession relative to advances being made in the surgical areas
3. Being alert to changes in concepts as they are occurring and sensitive to the direction in which the evolutionary process may take the evolving "art" in the future
4. Continuous communication among all members of the team
5. Holding down not only design/contamination costs but also ensuring economy of operation of the units in function

REFERENCES

American Hospital Association, Hospital Engineering Handbook, American Hospital Association, Chicago, Illinois

ASHRAE, Guide and Data Book (latest), New York, New York

AHRAE, Heating, Ventilating, Air Conditioning (latest), New York, New York

B. J. Brengande, Modular Units Offer Design Flexibility, Hospital, October 1, 1975 (Vol. 49)

Carrier Air Conditioning Company, Handbook of Air Conditioning System Design, McGraw-Hill, New York, New York

P. S. Chancy, Psychology, Hospital, June 1, 1973 (Vol. 47)

L. Cromwell, F. J. Weikell, E. A. Pfeiffer and L. B. Usselmans, (1973) Biomedical Instrumentation and Measurements, Prentice-Hall Inc. Englewood Cliffs, New Jersey

Department of the Air Force - Design Manual: Criteria for Design and Construction of Air Force Health Facilities

Department of the Army, TM 5-838-2 - Acoustical Control (Draft), Chapter V, October 1974

Department of the Navy (NAVFAC) - Design Manual: Hospital and Medical Facilities

Department of the Navy (NAVFAC), DM-1 - Architecture, Architectural Acoustics (Draft) Section 4, 1975

E. M. Dewan, Rhythms, Science and Technology, January 1969
W. Faulkner (1972), Architecture and Color, John Wiley and Sons, Inc., New York, New York
HEW, The Surgical Suite - Functional Programming Worksheets, Rockville, Md.
IEE, Lighting for Hospitals, IES, New York, New York
K. E. Johnson, The Use of Color in Medical Facilities, Spectrum number 3, Pittsburgh Paints
H. Laufman, M.D., The Infection Hazard of Intensive Care, Surgery, Gynecology and Obstetrics, September 1974, (Vol. 139)
A. D. Lewis, P. E. (1973), Proposed General Planning Guidelines for Intensive Care Type Units, WHO/PAHO, Washington, D.C.
A. W. Munster, M.D., Combating Hospital Infections: New Concepts for the 70's, Hospital, November 1, 1975 (Vol. 49)
NFPA No. 76BT (May 1973) Electricity in Patient Care Facilities (Tentative Standard for the Safe Use of), NFPA, Boston, Mass.
NFPA No. 76A (1973) Essential Electrical Systems for Health Care Facilities, NFPA, Boston, Mass.
NFPA Handbook of the National Electric Code, McGraw-Hill, New York, New York
NFPA No. 56A (1973) Inhalation Anesthetics, Boston, Mass.
A. P. G. Peterson and E. E. Gross Jr. (1963), Handbook of Noise Measurement, General Radio, Concord, Mass. (seventh edition)
J. C. Sell, Mechanical Needs in the Operating and Delivery Suites, Hospital, November 1, 1974 (Vol. 48)
D. A. Simmons (1972), Medical and Hospital Control Systems, Little, Brown and Company, Boston, Mass.
Stone, Marraccini and Patterson, Report on the Surgical Suite - Peninsula Hospital and Medical Center, October 1, 1975
The Trane Company, Trane Air Conditioning Manual, Mcgill Graphic Arts, St. Paul, Minnesota
C. Tsung, Electrical System for Hospitals, Progressive Architecture, September 1971
VA, Planning Criteria for Medical Facilities (M-7), Washington, D.C.
R. Wehili, et al (1972), Hospital Bedrooms and Nursing Units. A System Approach for Building Technology, NTIS, Springfield, Va.
R. J. Wurtman, M.D., Biological Considerations in Lighting Environments, Progressive Architecture, September 1973
R. J. Wurtman, M.D., Biological Implications of Artificial Illumination, A paper presented at the National Technical Conference of IES, September 1968, Phoenix, Arizona

37

THE CLINICAL ENGINEER IN ANESTHESIOLOGY

M. Shaffer

This specific application involves fluid mechanics as its prime field of expertise, with electrical/electronic engineering in a back-up role, both to support the gas machines for giving the anesthetics, the monitors for determining the physiological consequences incident to the anesthetic state, the procedures for fluidic and electronic safety, and the record keeping. (Appropriate malpractice suits of the kind preventable by clinical engineering will be described for identifying, from experience, the areas in which attention can best be focused.)

Basic Instrumentation

Anesthetic gases are supplied to the patient by means of a gas machine. In the gas machine shown diagramatically in Figure 1, oxygen and nitrous oxide gases are held in tanks under pressure and are supplied through reducing valves, fail-safe and needle control valves, flowmeters, and vaporizers to the patient breathing system. The hospital central oxygen and nitrous oxide gas supplies may be connected into the machine through one-way valves for normal operation, the cylinders then being in reserve for emergencies. Fittings and valves are available for other gases. The vaporizers are needed for use particularly with ether, halothane, or methyoxyfluorane anesthetics, which are stored in reservoirs on the machine as volatile liquids and must be vaporized prior to administration. In the old-type vaporizers, the energy to supply the latent heat of vaporization was derived from the ambient air, the temperature of the gas was consequently lowered, and the vapor pressure and concentration applied to the patient were affected. This difficulty has been overcome in some recent designs by the incorporation of thermostatically controlled heating (1).

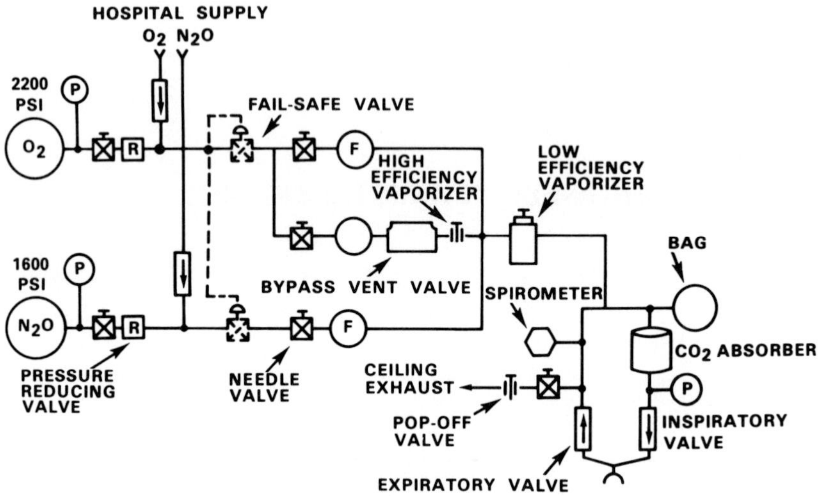

Fig. 1. Anesthesia machine and patient breathing circuit.

The patient breathing circuit can be arranged for three modes of operation. In an open-loop configuration, the gas supplies provide all the anesthetic gases required, and the patient exhales directly to atmosphere; this arrangement is not only uneconomical but exposes the OR personnel to the anesthetic gases not absorbed by the patient. A closed-loop configuration allows the patient to continuously rebreathe the anesthetic gases, the exhaled carbon dioxide being withdrawn by a carbon dioxide absorber cannister containing calcium hydroxide and either sodium or barium hydroxide; in this arrangement, economy is a major factor since gas is needed only to replace that absorbed for metabolic requirements. However, gas concentrations are harder to control. The third configuration, shown in Figure 1, is a semiclosed loop arrangement in which some of the exhaled gases are exhausted from the circuit through a pop-off valve, and the amount of rebreathing varies inversely with the rate at which fresh gases are added. A spirometer, shown in the figure, is provided to measure the patient's tidal volume and, in conjunction with the breathing bag, enables the anesthesiologist to control the depth of inspiration. The output from the pop-off valve may be kept out of the OR atmosphere by means of a room exhaust system. Some anesthetic gases are explosive but have particular applications; cyclopropane is advantageous for old or shock patients due to its rapid induction and its ability to maintain blood pressure; ethylene, also explosive, has characteristics similar to those of nitrous oxide but has the advantage of greater potency.

Apart from maintenance and proper operation of this equipment, the clinical engineering contribution to the dispensing of anesthetic gases should be directed to the adoption of proper precautions, particularly when using the gases of the explosive variety. Some explosions have occurred in operating rooms, although these cases are not now prevalent. The potential danger can be assessed from a case in

Chile about ten years ago when a cyclopropane cylinder was partially filled with oxygen by mistake (2). The temperature of the cylinder valve, which was of incorrect size for oxygen, became elevated when the valve was opened, and an explosion occurred either through friction or static charge; in this case, two patients, two anesthesiologists, and two surgeons died from burns and organic lesions, one surgeon lost his left arm, and two nurses each lost one leg.

Most general anesthetic techniques depress respiration, and a ventilator is usually maintained in the OR to assist the patient's breathing when needed. The principle of operation of a ventilator can be followed with reference to Figure 2, in which

1. The air valve is opened to push the piston down against the piston-return spring a preset distance and then closed
2. The oxygen valve is opened to push the piston down a further preset amount and then closed
3. With the desired gas concentration now in the chamber, the inhalation valve is opened, and the piston-return spring pushes the piston back up to provide a flow of gas to the patient at a rate established by the flow-control system

Most general-anesthetic techniques depress not only respiration but also circulation, and most hypnotic and analgesic drugs cause cerebral depression. The anesthesiologist will therefore monitor the patient's vital signs throughout the procedure to follow the depth of anesthesia and assess the patient's well-being. This can be done to a limited extent without instrumentation by watching breathing patterns, reflexes to surgical incisions, and eye signs; the latter can, however, be considerably affected by atropine and other drugs; a finger on the temporal artery provides convenient information on the patient's pulse.

Monitoring

More positive indications and long-term trends to determine slow response reactions to the anesthetic will be obtained from instrumentation. General status of

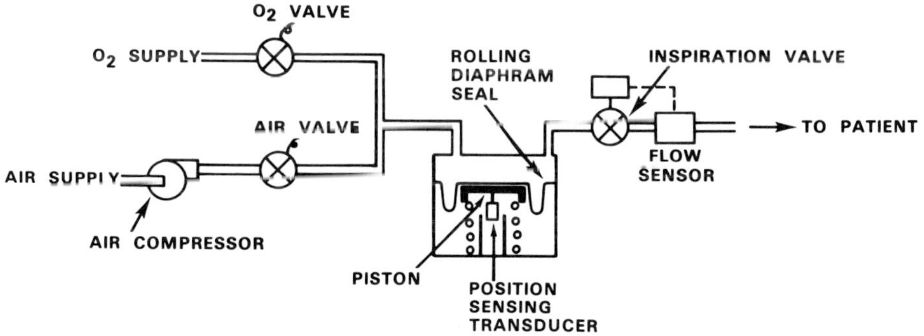

Fig. 2. Simplified diagram of a volume ventilator.

the cardiovascular and metabolic systems can be monitored from the electrocardiograph, 17.9% of patients developing arrhythmias during anesthesia and 0.9% of patients developing serious arrhythmias (3). Almost half of all these arrhythmias are ventricular in origin, indicating an irritable myocardium prone to ventricular tachycardia or fibrillation (4). Heart rate and heart sounds, the arterial, central venous, and pulmonary artery wedge pressures, and the cardiac output are all indicative in the determination of circulatory response to anesthesia. With reference to Table I, which lists the anomalies and applicable indicators used in anesthesia monitoring, it will be seen that arterial, central venous, and pulmonary artery wedge pressure measurements are all indicators of myocardial depression, hydration, hypovolemia, and hypertension; partial pressure of expired carbon dioxide may indicate hemorrhage and pulmonary embolism. Concerning adequacy of ventilation, the patient's general status is indicated by minute volume, blood gases, and

TABLE I
Anesthesia Monitoring—Anomalies and Indicators

Anomaly	Indicator
1. *CARDIOVASCULAR*—General	ECG, heart rate, heart sounds, arterial, central venous pressures and pulmonary artery wedge pressure, cardiac output
Myocardial oxygenation	ECG
Myocardial depression	Arterial and central venous pressures, cardiac output
Cardiac arrhythmias	ECG
Hydration	Central venous and pulmonary artery wedge pressures
Hypovolemia	Arterial, central venous and pulmonary artery wedge pressures
Hemorrhage	Expired carbon dioxide pressure
Air embolism	Central venous and pulmonary artery pressures, doppler
Hypertension	Arterial and pulmonary artery wedge pressures
2. *PULMONARY*—General	Minute volume, blood and expired gases
Hypoventilation	Arterial carbon dioxide partial pressure
Pulmonary vascular resistance	Pulmonary artery and wedge pressures
Cyanosis/hypoxia	Arterial oxygen partial pressure
3. *METABOLIC*	
Hypothermia	ECG, temperature and blood gases
4. *NEUROLOGICAL*	
Spinal sympathetic and stellate ganglion blocks	Pulse, arterial pressure and skin temperature
Cerebral depression	Minute volume, EEG, arterial oxygen partial pressure
Hypertension	Intracranial pressure
Muscle relaxation	Muscle activity

expired gas concentrations. Developing hypothermia can be indicated well in advance by artifacts on the ECG. In the neurological area, spinal sympathetic and stellate ganglion blocks are monitored by pulse, arterial pressure, and skin temperature measurements. The electroencephalograph (EEG) is indicative of cerebral depression; Martin, Faulconer, and Bickford (5) have shown that as the anesthetic concentration in the arterial blood increases, the EEG frequency decreases, and the amplitude increases; administration of more anesthetic leads to brief electrical silence—the "burst suppression phase"—and eventually to complete suppression. The EEG is, however, an unreliable indication with such anesthetic agents as fluoroxene and isoflurane.

A considerable amount of monitoring equipment is available to monitor these parameters, as shown in Table II. The cardiovascular functions can be monitored by cardiotachameters, electrocardiographs, stethoscopes, blood-pressure monitors, and thermodilution or dye dilution monitors. The pulmonary-function indications can be obtained from respirometers for gas flows and pneumotachometers and impedance spirometers for respiratory patterns. Gas analyzers to monitor inhaled and exhaled gas concentrations are available using the paramagnetic properties of oxygen, infrared energy absorption qualities of carbon dioxide, acoustic resonant properties of nitrous oxide and oxygen, the ultraviolet light absorption properties of halothane, and the delay of gas flows in gas chromatography. The recent reduction in cost of the mass spectrometer makes this instrument an economic gas analyzer for pulmonary monitoring by the anesthesiologist.

TABLE II
Anesthesia Monitoring—Equipment

1. *Cardiovascular*	4. *Blood gas*
Cardiotachometer	*Analyzers*
Electrocardiograph	Electrode
Cardiac output meter	*Oximeters*
Stethoscope	Ear
Blood pressure monitor	Cuvet
Blood flow monitor	Reflection
2. *Pulmonary*	5. *Relaxation*
Respirometer	Stimulator
Impedance Spirometer	
Pneumotachometer	6. *Central nervous system*
	Electroencephalograph
3. *Gas*	
Analyzers	7. *Metabolic*
Paramagnetic	Thermometer
Infrared	
Acoustic	
Electrode	
Chromatograph	
Mass spectrometer	

Blood gases are measured by oxygen, carbon dioxide, and pH electrodes, with the arterial carbon dioxide partial pressures determined by Astrup titration and Siggaard Andersen curves. A blood gas analyzer together with a flame photometer for measuring electrolyte imbalance may be set up close to the ORs to provide the anesthesiologist with his data rapidly if the normal laboratory facilities are remotely located. Oximeters are used to provide additional information on the amount of hemoglobin and the degree of oxygenation of the blood.

The relaxation of the patient is a particular measure of the depth of anesthesia and may be determined by electrically stimulating a motor nerve and observing the resultant muscle activity. A needle electrode can be employed near the ulnar nerve for this indication.

Thermometers are used to measure the patient's temperature at the rectum or esophagus. General anesthesia depresses the thermoregulatory function so that the body tends to adopt the temperature of the environment, a temperature that is deliberately dropped in the case of induced hypothermia or unavoidably increased by the use of surgical drapes and lights (1).

Oxygen fuel cells and other gas monitors may be fitted on the gas machine to detect leakages. There is a need for monitoring. The equipment used does not have to be the latest or best type; the standard to be adopted is that which is set by similar hospitals in the locality under similar conditions.

One case published at the end of 1975 is particularly applicable. In *Schoenick* v. *San Dimas Hospital* (6), a 20-year-old woman undergoing dilation and curettage went into ventricular fibrillation and cardiac arrest when the surgeon injected epinephrine while the anesthesiologist was administering the anesthetic intravenously. The arrest was not detected for 20 minutes, the monitor being incorrectly connected. In this case, the patient suffered 80–90% brain damage, and the physicians settled before trial for $750,000.

In the second case, *Mooring* v. *Alexian Brothers Hospital* (7), the patient was admitted for dental surgery, root canal therapy, and extraction of abscessed teeth. The anesthesiologist testified he monitored the patient's blood pressure every 2–3 minutes during intubation attempts; however, the circulating nurse testified she did not see such monitoring. The oral surgeon also contradicted the anesthesiologist, stating his belief that the ventilation had been inadequate. The patient suffered cortical blindness secondary to brain damage, due presumably to a hypoxic episode during the surgery. An award of $1.1 million was made against the hospital and the anesthesiologist.

The location and arrangement of any monitoring equipment in the operating room will involve operating convenience and electrical and hazardous gas considerations. The anesthesia area is one of high congestion, and the monitoring equipment is usually mounted well away from the sterile field and the hazardous gas area; this is often done with the monitor preamplifiers mounted in a large-scale oscilloscope on a wall of the operating room or with the monitor preamplifiers in a remote-control room, in which case the amplified signals are returned back to the OR wall-mounted oscilloscopes for display. The latter arrangement is advantageous since calibration of the preamplifiers can be done outside the OR; it is disadvantageous, as the former configuration is also to a lesser degree, in having low-voltage lines, from the patient to the preamplifiers, that are long and susceptible to electrical interference from electrosurgery and other such surgical machines. Remote-control room configurations servicing a number of operating rooms have been known to induce electrosurgery interference from the originating room into the displays in the other ORs. The new type of numeric display and storage oscilloscope monitors, capable of displaying either waveshapes or trends, should preferably be located within reach of the anesthesiologist for direct selection of the display modes desired. This configuration has the advantage of keeping the low-level inputs short and the interference at a minimum. It also has the effect of reducing the number of interconnections between the patient and the display, each an item of concern.

Hazards

In pursuing the objective of better health care at lower cost, it is evident that any deviation in the use of the anesthesia equipment from the standards defined by the appropriate hospital regulations can create not only hazardous conditions but also the seeds of suspicion and loss of confidence.

The clinical engineer must be very aware of these regulations, specifically the National Fire Protection Association and Occupational Safety & Health Act regulations as they apply to inhalation anesthetic, electrical, and performance hazards in the OR.

Considering first the inhalation anesthetic regulations, the main requirements of the National Fire Protection Association regulation NFPA-56A, applicable to all anesthetic areas, are listed in Table III; the electrical requirements include the need for isolated power systems, line isolation monitors, and equipotential grounding. The main requirements for the anesthetic areas in which flammable anesthetic gases are used are listed in Table IV; the electrical requirements include the need for conductive floors and explosion-proof fittings. In this case, the hazardous area extends up to 5 ft above the floor, and any portable electrical equipment below that height must be either explosion proof, operated on potentials of less than 8 V, or be in an approved enclosure under positive pressure. The only exception to this is the electrosurgery equipment, so long as the equipment is not used on the head, neck, oropharynx, and body cavities, and the patient is draped so as to create a barrier against escaping gases. It is specified also that the switches and control devices of all portable equipment should be kept at least 2 ft away from the flammable gases.

In the event that flammable gases are never to be used in an anesthetic area, and if signs are clearly posted to this effect, then the conductive floor required for all anesthetic areas need not be installed, and the requirements for the flammable anesthetic areas given in the above paragraph do not apply.

If flammable gases have to be used in an emergency in this nonflammable gas area, this may be done, but four rules must be applied:

TABLE III.
National Fire Protection Association Main Requirements for All Anesthestic Areas

	NFPA reference
Humidity greater than 50%; temperature 65°–75°	56A-31
Supply and exhaust system for windowless locations controlled by smoke and combustion sensors	56A-31
Storage rooms outside vented for N_2O or O_2 greater than 2 liters	56A-32
Explosion-proof fittings unnecessary	56A-375
Electrical wall switches at least 5 ft above floor	56A-32
Isolated power system, line isolation monitor, and equipotential grounding	56A-334/5
Conductive high-resistance patient straps	56A-336
Portable appliances to be grounded and enclosed to avoid shock hazards from spillage; photographic lighting to be totally enclosed	56A-351
Anesthetic apparatus subject to approval and labeling	
Equipment introducing current to patient will have its output isolated from ground	56A-377
Scheduled inspections and written reports, no unapproved equipment introduced	56A-377

1. The patient table, gas machine, and the anesthesiologist should all be interconnected by wet sheets or other conductive material.
2. Electrically conductive accessories should be used on the gas machine and the table.
3. The administration of the gas will stop immediately in the event of a ground fault alarm.

TABLE IV
National Fire Protection Association Main Requirements for Flammable Anesthetic Areas

	NFPA reference
Hazardous area up to 5 ft above floor	56A-15
Conductive flooring in operating room and cylinder storage	56A-412/462
Receptacles, fittings etc. per class 1, GP.C., division 1 (unless if portable and under 8 V)	56A-442
Electrosurgery equipment not to be used on head, neck, oropharynx, or body cavities, or within 2 ft of the anesthesia system; patient should be draped	56A-452
Accessories including masks, tubing, bags, belts to be conductive	56A-464
Furniture to be conductive, no paint	56A-469
Dress to include conductive shoes, no silk, wool, etc.	56A-472

4. The reason for the emergency will be noted by the surgeon and the anesthesiologist in their records.

National Fire Protection regulations FPA 76B-102, 76B-207, and 76B-A4013 apply to the electrical hazards, including macroshock, microshock, and static-electricity hazards in the OR, with the specific details of equipment maximum leakage currents, equipotential grounding, and line isolation monitoring given for "extreme risk" patients. *Andrepont* v. *Ochsner*[8] is just one of many cases in which the gaseous mixture in an anesthetic machine exploded due to a build-up of electricity, the grounding being inadequate. To avoid this kind of hazard the engineer should ensure that at least four sets of measurements are conducted regularly in the OR:

1. Grounding of floor, namely, the resistance between the wall outlet ground contact and a 2½ in diameter 5 lb plate on the floor 3 ft away
2. Resistance of conductive flooring between two of the plates on the floor 3 ft apart,
3. Resistance of fixed equipment between the equipment and one of the plates on the floor 3 ft away,
4. Resistance across each caster of portable equipment, using one of the plates insulated from the floor under each caster in turn.

The maximum resistances allowed are between 25,000 and 10,000,000 Ω, except for the caster resistances, which must be under 250,000 Ω each.

Concerning performance hazards, these can be reduced by ensuring the equipment is in good order, calibrated, and the data displayed are indeed accurate. They can also be reduced by the training of the staff in the operating procedures applicable both to the use and abuse of the equipment. Cleanliness of a gas machine, for instance, is hardly a clinical engineering responsibility, but it can affect machine performance, and as such should represent a challenge to technology. In *Dierman* v. *Providence Hospital* (9), the patient was admitted for a tonsillectomy and removal of a wart from his nose. During anesthesia, an explosion occurred in the patient's oral and nasal passages, presumably due to the use of a hot electric needle and an improperly cleaned anesthetic breathing tube. The hospital was unable to show the gas was indeed free from contamination. Such a case as this can be cited with benefit in the training of staff.

Anesthesia record keeping constitutes a current challenge to the anesthesiology-oriented clinical engineer. At present, a multiform record is normally maintained by the anesthesiologist in real time to cover

1. The preoperative visit with the patient on the eve of the operation in order to review status and determine the anesthetic agents to be used
2. the surgical procedure, including the gas flow and vital-signs charts, and the catheters, anesthetic agents, relaxants, and intubations used
3. the recovery-room course, including the vital-signs charts
4. the statistical data

Some hospitals keypunch the statistical data on to cards for data processing to obtain anesthesiology departmental and personal statistics. These statistics may cover the numbers of patients handled by age, procedures, regions of operation, anesthetic techniques, preanesthetic and postanesthetic complications, the average times per procedure, and other such information. The departmental statistics are needed as background support for hospital accreditation; the personal statistics are becoming increasingly important as evidence of the anesthesiologist's experience at the time of recertification by the new professional standards review organizations.

It is evident from inspection that the real-time record is often indecipherable and a poor record, the subsequent punching of the statistics cards is wasteful, much of the data are duplicated in the OR supervisor's log, and there is room for considerable improvement. Automated methods are being attempted, but little receptivity has been achieved, primarily due to two prime factors: the anesthesiologist's lack of enthusiasm for the use of a keyboard, and the inadequacy of most available systems to meet operational requirements. Continuous operation is essential, and no equipment failure may be allowed to interrupt service in more than one OR; yet seldom are standby facilities incorporated for such contingencies. The Federal Rules of Evidence for United States courts effective July 1, 1975 (10), emphasizes the importance of the requirement for continuity, specifying in effect that it may be presumed a matter, normally done and normally recorded, was not done if it was not so recorded. Applying this to anesthesia records, it can be concluded that in the event of a record-keeping interruption, all anesthetics given during the interruption may be presumed to have not been given. It might be suggested that in the event of such an interruption by an automated record-keeping system, the anesthesiologist revert to his manual form, however such a suggestion is not normally well received.

The experience and authority of knowledge gained by the anesthesiology-oriented clinical engineer in the management of fluid dispensing and physiological monitoring systems render it a small step from the OR to the ICU in which similar equipment is in use. The association of responsibilities can best be appreciated by reference to the case of *George Rose* v. *Hakim* and *Ho,* (11) which was settled out of court, and to the companion case of *George Rose* v. *Washington Hospital Center,* which was settled by jury trial. In this instance, George Rose was admitted for tonsillectomy and adenoidectomy, suffered cardiac arrest for 2½ minutes during surgery, and on discharge was suffering from brain damage and cortical blindness for life. The case against the anesthesiologist and surgeon was settled for $270,000. In the case against the hospital, it was found that the attending physician in the recovery room ordered that the patient be kept at 90°F; however, in the ICU, the telethermometer of the hypothermia machine was reading 4.6°F low, there was no thermometer in the unit capable of reading below 94°F, there was no resuscitator available, the heart monitor was not connected, and the ventilator hose developed a kink whereby the patient was without oxygen for an estimated 10 minutes. The patient was awarded $294,777, and the jury found the surgeon and anesthesiologist in no way to blame.

TABLE V
Typical List of Anesthesiology/Surgery Equipment in an OR Suite

OR #	Function	Data acquisition							Other
		ECG	EEG	PRESS	SCOPE	ANESTHETIC machine	ANESTHESIA ventilator	Electrosurgery	
1	Neurosurgery	1	1	2	1	1	1	1	Microscope Physiostimulator Neuronerve stimulator Microcoagulator Bipolar coagulator Cold light headlamp
2	Thoracic	1	1	3	1	1	1	1	Temp and dye sig. processors AC fibrillators (2) Fiber optic surgeons light Heart lung pump console Aortic balloon pump
3	Eye	1			1	1	1	1	Microscope Portable operating light Ophthalmoscope RF diathermy unit Amoils cryo ophthalmic unit TV recorder and display
4 5 6	General (Each)	1			1	1	1	1	
7	OB-GYN	1			1	1	1	1	
8	Orthopedic	1			1	1	1	1	Automatic tourniquet
9	OB GYN and neurosurgery	1			1	1	1	1	Automatic tourniquet
10	Plastics and urology	1			1	1	1	1	Automatic tourniquet
11, 12	In and out	1			1	1			Uterine aspirator Automatic tourniquet Photocoagulator
1,2	Cysto (Each)	1			1	1		1	Urological table Fluoroscope

continued

TABLE V, *continued*
Typical List of Anesthesiology/Surgery Equipment in an OR Suite

		Data acquisition							Other
OR #	Function	ECG	EEG	PRESS	SCOPE	ANESTHETIC machine	ANESTHESIA ventilator	Electrosurgery	
	(Central)								Fiber optic surgeons light Defibrillator Fluoroscope film processor
—	Laparoscopy cart								CO_2 tank and controller Coagulator Fiber optic surgeons light
—	Bronchoscopy cart								Fiber optic surgeons light
—	Central control and storage								Mobile X-ray Ultrasonic doppler flow detector Portable ECG scope Portable ECG/press scope Two channel recorder Fetal heart detector Telethermometers (2) Autotransfusion pump Phaco emulsifier Tonometer Defibrillator Controlled water warmers (2) Fiber optic ''luminator''
	Facilities								Sterilizers 1 General purpose 6 Washer/sterilizers 1 Sonic Ground Fault Alarm/ isolation transformer system and tester

TABLE VI
Potential Activities of a Clinical Engineering Organization

1. *Support medical research*
   - Basic research
   - Evaluation testing
   - New equipment design
   - Model shop operation
2. *Provide consultation and engineering services*
   - *Planning*
     - Proposed systems
     - Facility, equipment, and interface diagrams
     - Manufacturing and test specifications
     - Cost estimates
     - Operational, maintenance, and data storage/retrieval plans and procedures
   - *Purchasing*
     - Sales literature files
     - Sales quotations
     - Buying decisions
   - *New installation*
     - Contractor liaison
     - On-site installation and checkout support
   - *Training*
     - Scheduled nurse/technician training courses
     - Educational seminars
   - *Evaluation*
     - System performance
     - Statistics
     - Cost effectiveness
3. *Provide operation, maintenance, and calibration services*
   - Routine alignment and calibration
   - Preoperation preparation and checkout
   - Routine performance/safety checks
   - Equipment operation
   - Failure repairs
   - Incoming quality control inspection and test
   - Spare parts
   - Schematic, instruction book, and reference library
   - Operational improvements

In a similar case involving ventilators and the physiological monitors, *Chidester* v. *Stanford University Hospital* (12), a Guillain-Barre syndrome patient became quadriplegic after his ventilator failed. On investigation, the cardiac monitor printout showed a slowing of the pulse for 5 minutes followed by cardiac arrest for 4 minutes. The audible alarm of the monitors had been disconnected because of their tendency to false alarm. Key systems are now provided on some equipments to prevent the unauthorized disconnecting of alarms.

The scope of work required of the anesthesiology-oriented clinical engineer in the field of gas dispensing and physiological monitoring systems can be summarized most simply as the selection of good equipment, integration of the equipment and the using staff, management of preventive and corrective maintenance, training of the using staff, and above all, help to avoid irregularities.

Anesthetic equipment was the forefather of electrical safety at ''static electricity'' level. But it has gone further. Because the depth of anesthesia has involved vital signs and monitoring equipment, and since its inception is a total commitment, the anesthesia department could assume responsibility for all monitors. With this competence, an anesthesia department can support other departments, such as surgery, in their electrical-equipment problems. Table V lists some anesthesiology/surgery equipment in an OR suite for which maintenance is needed. With an expanding work scope, a decision must, of course, be made whether it is advisable to keep this work scope under anesthesiology or under administration as a core function in any specific institution.

Future Anesthesiology activities may include:

Electroanesthesiology, automation of the anesthesiologists' record, and integration of this data in an overall patient-information system. In these, clinical engineering activities are needed, such as listed in Table VI.

REFERENCES

1. Leonard, P. E.: Medical Engineering in Anesthesiology, published in Medical Engineering; editor Ray, C. D.: Year Book Medical Publishers, 1974.
2. National Fire Protection Association Quarterly Report, January, 1964.
3. Walts, L. F., Lebowitz, M., and Dillon, J. B.: A means for recording force of thumb adduction. Anesthesiology 29:1054, 1968.
4. Michenfelder, J. D.: Electrocardiography for the Anesthesiologist. Lecture No. 124, 19th Annual Refresher Course Lectures. Read at the Annual Meeting, American Society of Anesthesiologists, Washington, D.C., October 19–23, 1968.
5. Martin, J. T., Faulconer, A., and Bickford, R. G.: Electroencephalography in anesthesia, Anesthesiology 20:359, 1959.
6. Schoenick v. San Dimas Community Hospital, Cal. Sup. Ct., Los Angeles Co., Docket EAC 16259, May 16, 1975.
7. Mooring v. Alexian Brothers Hospital, Cal. Sup. Ct., Santa Clara Co., Docket 306220, 1975.
8. Andrepont v. Ochsner, L.A. App., 84 So. 2d 63, 1955.
9. Dierman v. Providence Hospital, 31 Cal. 2d 290, 188 P. 2d 12, 1947.
10. Federal Rules of Evidence in U.S. Courts, HR 5463, Public Law 93-595, Rule 803 (7) approved January, 1975.
11. Rose v. Hakim, D. C. Dist. Ct. 335 F. Supp., later op 345 F. Supp. 1300.
12. Chidester v. Stanford University Hospital, Cal. Sup. Ct., Santa Clara Co., Docket 223,960, 1970.

38

THE CLINICAL ENGINEER IN SURGERY

L. C. Sheppard

Solving clinical problems in surgery challenges the engineer to be innovative in the application of technology. Sound engineering practice dictates the use of proven methods to effect durable solutions. Clearly, the greatest strength the engineer brings to health-care delivery is the facility to assess problems lucidly and devise pragmatic answers. Analytical ability, technical competence, and direct involvement are the characteristics needed.

A Model Application

Because of anticipated increases in surgical case loads and a growing shortage of nursing staff, work was begun in 1964 to investigate the feasibility of employing a computer-based system to automate the measurement and charting duties and certain therapeutic interventions in the care of patients following open intracardiac operations. During the first phase, the ICU procedures and operations were intensively analyzed. Therapeutic measures and their indications were identified. They were formally structured so that decisions could be made and interventions controlled logically, based on numerical measurements applied within the framework of rules and limits. The objective was to relieve the nurses of time-consuming routine not directly related to patient care. The purpose was to focus on mechanizing clinical tasks that were repetitive and well defined so a computer system could be used to reduce the work load (Table I and Fig. 1).

Having performed the system analysis, established objectives, and defined the problem, the next step is to formulate technologically feasible solutions. The scope of this model project was constrained to postoperative cardiac surgical patient care, but the problem-solving techniques employed are applicable to clinical engineering

TABLE I
Repetitive and Well-Defined Clinical Tasks

Signal source	Derived parameter	Measurement method	Units
Electrocardiogram	Heart rate	Surface electrodes	per min
Intraarterial pressure	Systolic	Strain gauge	mm Hg
	Diastolic		mm Hg
	Mean		mm Hg
Left atrial pressure	End expiratory	Strain gauge	mm Hg
Right atrial pressure	End expiratory	Strain gauge	mm Hg
Rectal temperature	Average	Thermistor	°C
Chest drainage	Cumulative	Load cell	ml
	Hourly rate		ml/hr
Urine output	Cumulative	Load cell	ml
	Hourly rate		ml/hr
Indicator dilution curve	Cardiac output	Densitometer	L/min
	Cardiac index		$L/min/m^2$
	Stroke volume		ml
	Stroke index		ml/m^2

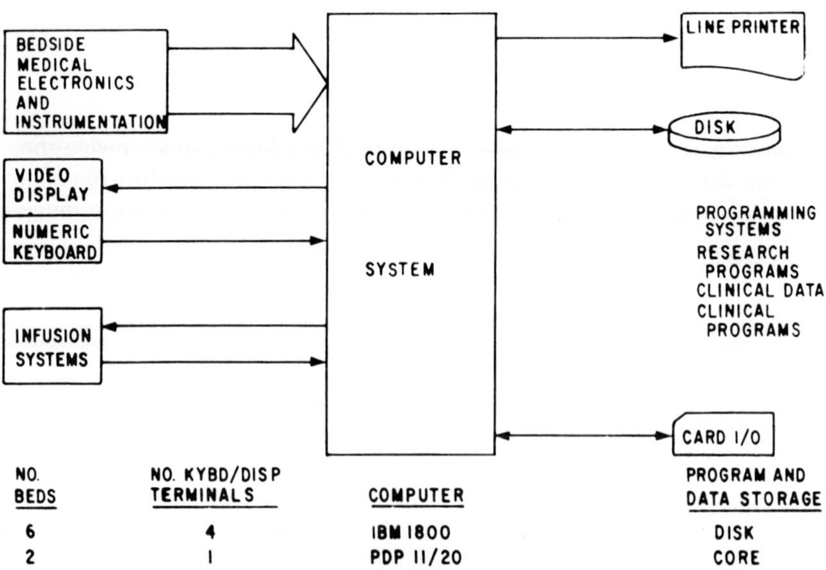

Fig. 1. Schematic diagram of an automated medical charting system.

in general. This discussion of the system that evolved provides insight into the underlying principles that were applied and is thus a useful model for clinical engineers to consider in their surgical work.

System Design Concepts

Detection of the physiological signal is the first of several crucial steps essential to the derivation of clinical data. The electrodes, cannulae, sensors, and sampling devices must be positioned with great care to obtain measurements with acceptable consistency and accuracy, for these elements couple the patient to the monitoring system. Failure to properly prepare and maintain this interface severely diminishes system performance, producing measurements of questionable reliability. Careful technique in the application of the signal-acquisition devices is most important because the overall system performance is in the balance.

The next stage encompasses consideration of the electronics modules that amplify and process the signals from the electrodes, thermistors, pressure transducers, densitometers, and other sensors. This and subsequent phases of signal manipulation are so interdependent that the design possibilities are practically infinite. Initially, preamplifiers that presented raw or filtered waveforms were used. As improved electronics are introduced, one can convert to analog preprocessing to filter, follow peaks and troughs, and calculate rates prior to computer processing.

The ECG signal fidelity, for example, is dependent on the careful site preparation and proper electrode placement to develop an acceptable impedance at the electrode/skin interface. R-wave detection for average heart-rate computation is an integral part of the preamplifier. The surface electrodes are also used to measure respiration rate from the fluctuations in transthoracic impedance phasic with respiration.

Intravascular and intracardiac pressures can be obtained with indwelling cannulae connected to tubing that provides fluid-filled columns to transmit the hemodynamic pressures to strain-gauge transducers for conversion to their electrical analogues. Continuous flushing devices must be used to maintain patency by providing a slow infusion of heparinized physiological solution. Analog preprocessing of the waveforms can provide the derivation of peak systolic, diastolic, and mean arterial pressures. Intracardiac pressures obtained from small plastic cannulae placed in the right and left atria can be measured in patients following cardiac surgical procedures. By this means, cardiac function and the need for therapeutic intervention can be assessed readily. Arterial and venous blood are sampled manually and analyzed for determination of blood gases. These measurements can be transmitted to the computer by keyboard entry.

Measurements associated with fluid balance, electrolyte balance, and metabolic requirements include chest drainage and urine output by load cell weighing systems, blood infused with computer-controlled calibrated pump, manually entered intake and plasma potassium, base excess calculated from blood gas measurements, and core and extremity temperatures measured by rectal and surface thermistors.

Direct delivery of care by closed-loop feedback control of therapy through the maintenance of left atrial pressure by blood infusion has been performed automatically in over 6000 cardiac surgical patients by us since October of 1967. Computer-programmed rules are utilized to actuate computer-controlled infusion pumps when left atrial pressure measurements are not at desired levels.

Regulation of mean arterial pressure in hypertensive patients by computer-controlled infusion of hypotensive agents has been performed in a number of patients during the first 24–48 hr following surgery.

It is imperative that electrically safe practices be followed in the CICU to avoid subjecting the patient to microshock hazards and noise-free transmission techniques be employed to convey the signals to the computer.

Model Equipment Description

Commercially available electronics and sensors can be used for most measurement requirements. Statham P23De pressure transducers are interfaced with Hewlett-Packard 78205B electronics for processing of the intraarterial pressures. Atrial pressures are acquired with Statham P23BB transducers and processed by Hewlett-Packard 78205B electronics. Model 78214A modules accommodate Yellow Springs thermistors for measurement of surface and rectal temperatures. Disposable electrodes pretreated with electrode paste are attached to the patient in a monitoring configuration to obtain the electrocardiogram. The Hewlett-Packard 78203A ECG preamplifier has a band width of 0.05–100 Hz and a voltage gain that is adjustable between 200 and 4000. A cardiotachometer circuit continuously derives average heart rate and provides the computer with an analogue signal of 1 V per 100 beats/minute. Respiration rate is derived from the variations in thoracic impedance with each breath. The ECG electrodes provide the signal, which is processed by the Hewlett-Packard 78202B respiration module. Respiration rate is calculated and transmitted to the computer at a level of 2 V/100 respirations per minute. The intraarterial modules electronically extract systolic, diastolic, and mean pressures from the arterial waveforms and present these signals to the computer's analog input at 1 V/100 mm Hg. Small pressure variations in the right and left atrial pressures contributed by the cardiac cycle are electronically filtered from the signals; however, the wider fluctuations phasic with respiration remain. Computer programming is used to derive end expiratory values from the incoming signals. Voltage levels are 1 V/10 mm Hg for atrial pressures, and the signal range of 0–3 V represents rectal temperatures from 30°C to 41°C. Hewlett-Packard 78304A oscilloscopes provide continuous visual monitoring of the ECG, intraarterial pressures, right atrial pressures, and left atrial pressures for all patients.

A Mennen–Greatbatch digitally programmed pump is used for computer-controlled infusion of vasodilating agents to regulate arterial blood pressure in hypertensive patients. Rates of infusion range from 0 to 90 ml/hour. The pump can also be operated in the manual mode.

Commercial devices for three of the clinical functions did not exist, necessitating development of subsystems for measurement of chest-tube drainage and urine output and computer-controlled blood infusion.

Chest-tube measurements are derived from the output of a weighing system and expressed in ml by assuming a constant specific gravity. The signal from a Statham UC3 load cell, incorporated in a Wheatstone bridge network that is excited with direct current is amplified and transmitted to the computer's analogue input. The glass suction bottle normally used for collection of chest drainage is clamped firmly by a steel platform attached to and supported by a UL4-10 load cell adapter. Fluctuations in weight caused by the plastic tubes connected to the patient and the wall suction unit are prevented by anchoring them with specially designed clamps to the frame, which also serves as a protective enclosure. The constant weight contributed by the tubing and the bottle is measured when the patient first arrives in the coronary ICU by instructing the computer to acquire an empty weight reading, which is subtracted from subsequent measurements.

Incorporated within the same framelike enclosure is a UC3 load cell for the measurement of urine output. Suspended from the UL4-5 load cell adapter is an aluminum frame with hooks for attaching the plastic bag, which is used for urine collection. The plastic tubing connecting the patient's urinary catheter to the collection bag is anchored to the frame. Measurement techniques are as described for chest drainage.

The essential elements of the computer-controlled blood infusion pump are a power unit, a control unit, a stepping motor, a roller pump head, and a drip sensing assembly. The blood infusion subsystem is designed to deliver 20 ml of blood in 40 seconds. The pumping cycle is initiated by activating two time-delay relays (in series) from the computer's electronic contact. Switching in the control unit enables the translator to gate power to the stepping motor. An oscillator pulses this translator to advance the rotation of the motor at a fixed stepping frequency. Blood flow is monitored by sensing the drips with a multiple photodiode and light-source assembly affixed to the drip chamber. The pulses from this device reset an alarm circuit as each drop is detected. If a reset pulse does not occur within a prescribed time interval after the previous pulse, it is assumed that the unit of blood is spent or normal sequencing at the end of 40 seconds has occurred. This condition results in interruption of power to the motor and transmission of a signal to the computer's process interrupt signifying the no-flow condition. A status signal from the control unit enables the computer to determine whether the process interrupt occurred prematurely or was caused by normal time delay relay sequencing. The clinical personnel are alerted by way of the bedside display in the event of detection of a spent unit. Initial setup and replenishment are accomplished through the keyboard/

display terminal. A disposable intravenous infusion set is used for infusion by threading the plastic tubing between the rollers and the housing of the pump head.

Four of the beds in the coronary ICU are instrumented as described and connected to an IBM 1800 data acquisition and control system. Two additional beds, equipped with custom-engineered systems developed by Mennen-Greatbatch Electronics, are connected to the 1800. A stand-alone two-bed system with its own PDP 11/20 minicomputer was developed and installed by Roche Medical Electronics. The computer programs were written by Roche, utilizing those we developed for the 1800 based system as a model.

Model System ICU

Repetitive collection of the clinical measurements followed by presentation in the ICU is carried out automatically at 2-minute intervals. Keyboard entry of information is managed on a demand basis. Organization of the data and frequent logging to auxiliary storage such as disk establish the source data for subsequent computer processing. Data retrieval and display formating are executed quickly to allow structured review of the automated and manually entered measurements to assess the patient's current status and progress. Complex computations for derivation of information include calculation of base excess and oxygen saturation from blood-gas measurements, cardiac output from a thermodilution or dye dilution curve, body surface area from height and weight. Full exploitation of the computer's data management potential is realized through preparation of the hospital record by tabulating the patient's clinical data.

As patient management protocols are developed, the care of critically ill patients becomes more structured. This trend toward decision making on a logical basis from data analyzed according to rules has made it possible to enlist the computer's aid in the appraisal of patient condition and the choice of treatment.

Patient management programs for the cardiovascular subsystem have been computerized to assist in the detection of diminished cardiac performance, the decision to intervene, and the selection of the appropriate intervention. Reoperation rules for the analysis of chest-tube drainage measurements provide automatic evaluation of postoperative cardiac surgical patients for early detection of excessive bleeding.

Computerized ICU monitoring systems can relieve nurses of many of the time-consuming tasks such as routine measurement and charting, enabling them to devote a much higher percentage of their time to those aspects of patient care that can only be done manually by skilled personnel. Further support of the nurses can be provided by biomedical instrumentation technicians to clean and sterilize the transducers, set up and calibrate the clinical measurement subsystems, interconnect the newly arrived patient to the measurement devices, collect arterial blood samples and perform the blood gas analyses, and carry out the steps necessary for measurement of cardiac output by the dye dilution method. These paramedical personnel are essential to the smooth operation of the system, providing expert technical support and continuity for a staff that typically experiences very high turnover among the registered nurses.

The system has been designed to allow fall-back to manual procedures if a malfunction occurs. Each electronic module digitally displays the derived measurement transmitted to the computer. Chest-tube drainage and urine-output volumes can be observed visually since the collection containers are housed in an open frame. Even though system failures have a very low incidence, once or twice per year, these back-up features are essential in those rare instances, requiring the nurse to rely on manual data recording until full system function is restored.

However, achievement of clinical results depends on intensive operations analysis *before* the system is designed. A complete understanding of the problem is absolutely essential. The following principles must be strictly applied to produce a system in which technology has been utilized intelligently:

1. Identify the clinical needs
2. Define the problem
3. Completely analyze the manual or existing system
4. Establish realistic objectives
5. Devise relevant solutions
6. Implement with robust technology
7. Integrate the system into the operation of the unit and
8. Follow through with training, maintenance, evaluation revision, and updating

39

THE CLINICAL ENGINEER IN CORONARY CARE

W. Steawen

The CCU concept was developed and implemented in the early 1960s. It was considered that the prognosis for recovery of patients from the acute stage of a myocardial infarction could be greatly enhanced in a hospital unit dedicated to their care. The concept was based to some extent on the early detection and treatment of premature ventricular beats—a harbinger of sudden death during the early postinfarction phase.

The primary element of a CCU consists of close nursing surveillance supported by electronic monitoring of patient parameters; a patient setting remote from other patients suffering more severe physical trauma; personnel especially trained for this special-care function; and facilities, supplies, and equipment required to treat a cardiac emergency.

The majority of CCUs are probably in the range of 4 to 6 beds with extremes of from 2 to 30 beds. The physical layouts include miniwards, cubicles, and private rooms. Separate facilities may be available for the patients during the acute (3 to 5 days) and progressive (approximately 3 weeks) stages of recovery. Constant electronic monitoring of the patient in the acute area is usually done by connecting the patient directly with wires to the monitoring equipment. In the progressive coronary-care area, some patients are monitored by radio telemetry. These patients may be ambulatory. Some CCUs have incorporated computers into their monitoring systems.

Engineering technology is an essential ingredient of coronary care. In order to achieve maximum success in the CCU, the engineering facilities must be properly managed.

The clinical-engineering involvement in the CCU is multifunctional. Clinical engineers and BMETs can work directly with the nursing and medical staff in the care and treatment of patients. In such cases, they are responsible for the patient's life in addition to the equipment. Since the CCU is dependent on equipment, facilities, and patient-monitoring techniques, clinical engineering involvement must be broad based. The clinical engineer should thus be active in all of the following:

1. Planning
2. Facilities design
3. Monitoring equipment system design
4. Equipment installation
5. Scheduled and repair maintenance
6. Electrical safety
7. Updating and expansion of equipment and facilities
8. Equipment operation and utilization problems
9. Special procedures
10. Device development
11. Teaching and training

In many hospitals with existing CCUs, the clinical engineer will not have an opportunity to get involved in the planning, facilities design, monitoring system design, and installation. However, older units will be redesigned or moved, and the same principles apply as well as to other special-care units. Therefore, these clinical-engineering roles merit emphasis.

Planning

The responsibility for planning a special-care area such as a CCU is usually delegated to a hospital committee. The committee is generally comprised of administrators, physicians, nurses, hospital engineers, architects, and consulting engineers. Major decisions concerning location, number of beds, layout and room size, special facilities, staffing, protocol, logistics, and equipment needs are solved. All of these problems are relevant to the planning of equipment utilization in the unit.

The CCU should be designed so that the staff is able to treat the patient efficiently. This requires easy access to and around the patient. Consideration must be given to the plan so that the monitoring equipment and patient attachments do not hamper the staff. Supplies should be readily accessible. Patient comfort and safety cannot be compromised. Electrical wiring, lighting, medical gas systems, plumbing, waste disposal, furniture, nurse calls, emergency systems, ventilation, and temperature controls are factors that must be considered. The clinical engineer, understanding the disease state of CCU patients, their special needs, monitoring and safety facilities required, should be able to provide valuable input into the solution of these design problems.

Case Problem

The design of a 10-bed acute CCU with an accompanying 18-bed progressive-care unit included a central ECG monitoring console for the 10 acute-care patients.

It was decided by the planning committee to include extensive visual observation of the central monitors as a requirement of the operation of the unit. After reviewing the staffing situation, it was determined that it would not be possible to recruit enough nurses to include monitor watching in their duties. The clinical engineer on the committee was asked to propose a solution to the problem.

Solution

The clinical engineer recommended that BMETs be hired to perform the monitor-watching function. He rationalized that fewer BMETs than nurses would be required; they could be easily trained to interpret electrocardiograms; they would not be overwhelmed by equipment problems; it would allow the hospital to expand its clinical engineering services to 24 hours a day. The recommendation was accepted and has been operating successfully for 5 years.

Facilities Design

The design of the electrical distribution, medical gas (oxygen, vacuum, CO_2), lighting, and heating and ventilation systems are very important. This responsibility is usually left to the architects and consulting engineers. The clinical engineer should be active in the design of such systems. Basic guidelines and regulations in the form of standards and codes will greatly influence the final design, but they frequently require careful interpretation. In addition to cost, there are several important factors that must be considered for each of these systems.

1. Electrical distribution
   a. Patient safety (grounding, insulation, isolation)
   b. Ampacity
   c. Number and location of receptacles
   d. Emergency generator circuits
   e. Location of circuit-breaker panels
   f. Phasing
   g. Two systems (normal and X-ray)
2. Medical Gas
   a. Number and location of outlets
   b. Number and location of trap bottles
   c. Plumbing
   d. Maintenance
   e. Additions and changes to the system
3. Lighting
   a. Types (examining, reading, room)
   b. Location of fixtures
   c. Location of switches
   d. Light-intensity requirements

4. Heating and ventilation
   a. Central or individual room units (efficiency, patient comfort, etc.)
   b. Controls
   c. Noise
   d. Infection control

Other aspects of the facilities design include monitoring-equipment mounting, selection of beds, plumbing and waste disposal, and emergency nurse-call systems.

Case Problem

Members of the CCU committee wished to use electrically operated beds because of their overall convenience rather than hydraulic-type beds. However, the possibility of the metal frame becoming electrically energized or ungrounded because of an electrical malfunction had to be prevented.

Solution

Electrically operated beds were specified with insulated side rails. This prevents the patient or personnel from contacting any conductive surfaces on the bed. Beds with this feature were not available at the time. Existing models had to be modified for this design criteria. However, they are now standard items.

Monitoring Equipment System Design

Obviously, the clinical engineer should be responsible for the patient-monitoring-system design. However, he must work closely with the medical staff in designing a system that will meet their exact requirements, accept additional equipment as needed, but not be overdesigned. Cost is very important, but quality and patient safety cannot be compromised.

ECG waveforms and heart rate are the basic variables for CCU monitoring at each bedside. Arterial and venous blood pressure, temperature, respiration, and cardiac output are frequently monitored but may not be required for most patients. The larger units have a central monitoring console remote from the patient. The ECG and heart-rate information are repeated at the central console. Heart-rate alarms are incorporated into the bedside equipment. These alarms usually present both an audible and visual signal. If there is a central console, the audible alarm is detected there and silenced at the bedside. ECG recorders should be available for bedside use and at the central console where they will automatically record the ECG of a patient who triggered an alarm.

To assist in the detection of premature ventricular beats, an arrythmia monitor can be used at the central console. This is a small computer dedicated for that purpose alone. In recent years, larger computers have become available and are able to monitor at least 16 patients. They are useful in interpreting a variety of some arrhythmias. However, specific interpretation of complex rhythms is still left to the observer.

The unit must be equipped with cardiac pacemakers and defibrillators for emergency situations. Battery-operated pacemakers are preferred for electrical safety considerations. Pacemaker generator and catheter electrode terminals should be insulated to prevent accidental contact with conductive paths. Battery-operated defibrillators should also be considered. This will allow them to be used in an emergency if there is a facilities power failure.

Based on his knowledge of equipment and the particular requirements of the CCU, the clinical engineer can write detailed performance specifications. Consideration should be given in his design scheme relating to cost, safety, quality, reliability, maintenance, instruction manuals, service, versatility, ease of operation and warranty.

Case Problem

There was a need to add 4 beds with radio biotelemetry monitoring for progressive-care patients into an existing 10-bed acute CCU monitoring system. ECG waveform and heart-rate monitoring with high- and low-rate alarms were the essential characteristics.

Solution

The clinical engineer designed the radio telemetry system so that it could be incorporated into the central monitoring console in the acute area of the CCU. Four radio transmitters, receivers, and heart-rate modules with digital displays and alarms were designed to be packaged into the central console. Open ECG monitor display channels were already available, and some shifting around of the monitor modules was all that was necessary to accommodate the four new channels. The new heart-rate monitors were connected into the alarm display and patient identification system at the console and the direct writing recorders that recorded the patient's ECG automatically with the onset of an alarm.

The main feature of the clinical-engineering input into this system was that he designed the original system so that additions such as this could be added later on at minimum cost and would enhance rather than disrupt the design features of the system. Because of advances in the state of clinical and technological art, it is important to design initial patient monitoring systems for additions and changes in the future.

Equipment Installation

Equipment installation involves mounting the instruments, pulling cables from bedside to central console, interconnecting instruments, equipment checkout, and debugging. It is important for someone on the hospital staff to verify that the entire system is wired correctly and functioning as specified. The clinical engineer and BMET are the most competent to do this.

When monitoring or checking out the installation, the clinical engineer should make certain that nothing in the installation technique will compromise the safety of the patient or the reliability of the equipment. Careful inspection and performance evaluation of individual instruments should be conducted. Many instruments received directly from the factory have a major defect. Some of these defects could go undetected by the installer or hospital personnel who do not have engineering experience. This also gives the clinical engineer and BMET an opportunity to become familiar with the total system. This will be of considerable value when they assume full responsibility for maintenance of the system.

Case Problem

Upon delivery of a 10-bed CCU monitoring system and before installation, the clinical-engineering department tested each instrument for safety and performance. There were many problems detected, but the most significant was open ground connections in 10 of the instruments.

Solution

The instruments were repaired before installation in the CCU with better-quality power cords and plugs.

Scheduled and Repair Maintenance

As with any instrumentation system, a protocol must be established for routine scheduled maintenance and repairs. This can be done most efficiently by an in-house clinical engineering department. Studies have also been conducted to demonstrate that this method of maintenance can also be cost effective.

The scheduled maintenance is required to verify the calibration of the instruments and to detect problems that are not immediately apparent. Electrical safety checks of the equipment are also included in the schedule. The clinical engineer must develop a routine maintenance schedule based on equipment usage, failure-rate experience, and priorities. Occasionally, he will receive guidelines from the equipment manufacturer.

Repair maintenance is done as needed, and priorities must be considered. By performing the repairs in-house, minimum downtime of equipment is achieved. To further reduce equipment downtime, an analysis of the problem should be made at the location of the equipment. Frequently, the problem can be solved there without having to take the instrument to the shop for repair.

Case Problem

Routine testing of defibrillators in the CCU by a consulting clinical engineer revealed two units that were grossly defective. The maximum energy that either of these defibrillators could deliver was 120 J as measured on an energy meter. These problems were not detectable by nursing personnel because of inadequate test methods available to them.

Solution

The defibrillators were sent to the manufacturer for repair. A recommendation was submitted by the clinical engineer to the hospital that would allow the nursing personnel to more accurately assess the performance of the defibrillators.

Electrical Safety

Electrical safety for the hospital patient is a commanding issue. This is particularly true for an area like the CCU in which many patients have cardiac catheters. The clinical engineer must plan for optimal electrical safety in the design stages. He must then establish a procedure for continually monitoring the electrical integrity of the unit and be prepared to make changes when necessary. Knowledge of the principles of electrical safety, standards and codes, and safety techniques and devices are essential for the clinical engineer. He should be quick to respond to any problem that may affect the safety of the patient and personnel.

Equipotential grounding is a basic requirement for CCU patient rooms. Additional protection is achieved through the use of isolated patient connections in monitoring instruments and insulated patient settings. All of these safety methods preclude the need for an additional safety scheme—isolation transformers. There has been considerable controversy over this subject, and the hospital's clinical engineer can provide knowledgeable advice in this area.

Case Problem

Measurement of chassis leakage currents of ECG recorders in the CCU revealed a significant increase over a 1-year period. The typical original values were 15 μA, and they had increased to an average of 130 μA.

Solution

The clinical engineering group investigated the problem and determined that a screw bonding two separate chassis in the recorder had built up a resistive coating because of a dissimilar metal affect. This produced a significant resistance between the two chassis, effectively causing one chassis to become ungrounded. The manufacturer was notified of the problem and sent a new screw to bond the chassis that would not cause the same problem.

Updating and Expansion of Equipment and Facilities

After a CCU has been in operation for a period of time, it becomes necessary to update and add equipment or make some changes in the unit. This is caused by the need to offer new services, improvement in equipment because of advances in the state of the art, the need to replace obsolete instruments, and the need to improve existing services and techniques.

The clinical engineer must determine the present needs of the unit and make recommendations on how to improve services. It may be necessary to add additional beds to the unit, to expand monitoring capabilities into the progressive area, or to modernize the central monitoring console with computers and memory-type nonfade display monitors, to mention a few.

Any changes or additions that are made should be compatible with the existing system as much as possible. This will minimize costs and maintain the basic integrity of the unit. The significance of the changes should be understood and approved by the medical staff before the changes are implemented. It may frequently be necessary to allow the medical staff to conduct a clinical evaluation before reaching a final decision.

Case Problem

The central monitoring console of an existing CCU did not have a delay system that would permit "hindsight" recording of ECG events. The nursing personnel considered it important to document transient events such as single PVCs or short runs of ventricular tachycardia.

Solution

The clinical engineer considered three methods of providing delayed recordings of ECG signals, that is, magnetic tape delays; solid state delays; or memory nonfade display monitors. He concluded that a nonfade display would be the best solution. This would provide the needed delayed recording (both on alarm and by manual selection from an observer) and would permit replacing the existing "bouncing-ball type-displays" with a superior monitor.

Equipment Operation and Utilization Problems

Medical equipment (patient-monitoring instrumentation in particular) is not flawless in terms of human engineering. In addition to internal breakdowns, the equipment functioning is very susceptible to human error. The nature of the physiological variables that are being measured also make the operation of medical devices something considerably less than routine.

In addition to strict training needs for the user, this also presents the clinical engineer with frequent problem-analysis tasks—noisy ECG signals, malfunctioning pacemakers, and defibrillator burns—just to mention a few. The clinical engineer is familiar with the operating characteristics of the instruments and their clinical application. It is essential to have someone available to the CCU staff with these qualifications to solve problems that may affect the care and treatment of the patient.

Case Problem

It was observed by the medical staff that a patient's demand pacemaker was not sensing properly. The patient's ECG demonstrated that the pacemaker was not delivering a stimulus each time the patient required one. The clinical engineer was asked to investigate the problem.

Solution

The clinical engineer investigated the situation and learned that the patient had two catheter electrodes in the heart, that is, the permanent transvenous pacemaker catheter for the implanted unit and a temporary transvenous catheter that is routinely left in place for 24 hours in case the permanent pacer that was just implanted would fail.

The clinical engineer demonstrated (through intracardiac ECG recordings) that the two catheters would occasionally touch and produce an electrical signal that fooled the demand pacemaker. This signal had characteristics that were similar to a patient's R wave, and it was sensed as such by the pacemaker.

Special Procedures

The CCU staff is sometimes confronted with the problem of using complex equipment for special procedures. This may include devices such as intra-aortic balloon pumps and cardiac-output computers. Arterial and venous blood-pressure measures may also be required but not on a routine daily basis. When devices such as these are used, occasionally it may be difficult for the medical personnel to manage them. The clinical engineering personnel with their instrumentation training and experience can function well as the technical experts on this equipment. They can be depended on to set up the instrument, verify its performance, and solve problems that may develop during the course of the procedure. This eliminates the need to hire specially trained personnel to be responsible for equipment that is only used sparingly but for crucial situations.

The clinical engineer and the BMET can also provide assistance during emergency procedures. They can handle equipment problems during cardiac-resuscitation procedures, provide extension cords if needed, and reset circuit breakers if they tripped during an emergency. It is extremely important to have people available with technical competence during emergency situations. The medical staff, being preoccupied with the treatment of the patient, occasionally are confronted with simple equipment problems that can be disastrous in a critical situation.

Case Problem

A resident had just inserted a temporary transvenous pacemaker catheter during an emergency procedure at the patient's bedside. After attaching the catheter to the external demand pacemaker, the resident was attempting to adjust the rate and stimulus controls on the pacemaker. However, he noted that even though the patient had no intrinsic rhythm, the pacemaker was inhibited and appeared to be sensing a signal from the patient.

Solution

A BMET attending the procedure observed that the patient was lying in an ungrounded mechanical bed. The physician was touching the bed while he was holding the pacemaker. He was able to transmit enough 60 Hz interference from the bed to inhibit the pacemaker, a problem that had earlier been observed by the clinical engineering department during its routine testing of pacemakers.

The BMET grounded the bed, and the pacemaker functioned correctly. *Note:* It is not necessary for someone to touch an ungrounded object directly to cause this problem. If the person touching the pacemaker is in close proximity to the interference source, it may be enough to produce a signal that the pacemaker will sense.

Device Development

As in most areas that provide medical treatment, there is often a need for a device that is not commercially available. There may also be a need to modify an existing device or to fabricate something that would improve or add to the function of an instrument. The hospital's clinical engineer will be able to evaluate the problem and determine if he can design the necessary option. He must base his design on good engineering and clinical practice. The device or modification must do the job reliably and effectively. The need must be real and not simply a whimsical gadget project. Frequently, the clinical engineer will take the initiative in determining the need for a new instrument, circuit, device, or a modification, a very important area of responsibility for the clinical engineer. By being an active observer in the CCU and communicating with the CCU staff, he can develop an awareness for needed changes and improvements.

Case Problem

A paraplegic patient was admitted to the CCU, which has private rooms for its patients. The patient was not able to use the normal nurse-call system, which required pressing a button. The clinical engineer was asked to devise a device that would allow the patient to activate the nurse-call system.

Solution

The clinical engineer determined that the patient was only able to move her lips, tongue, and eyelids. He devised a sensitive switch that the patient was able to control with her tongue.

Teaching and Training

One of the most important functions of the clinical engineer is training. This is particularly true in the CCU in which complex electromedical equipment is used extensively. It is extremely important that the CCU medical and nursing staff is well trained in the principles of the operation of their equipment, electrical safety, and the clinical application of specific instruments. The clinical engineer should establish training and retraining programs. He should become aware of specific operational problems and hold training sessions so that the staff is properly informed on the correct procedures. It is difficult to rely on the hospital's nursing staff to conduct instrumentation training. The equipment manufacturer cannot be expected to supply continuing education of the hospital staff. There are very few nurses who should be expected to fully understand enough about instrumentation to have a teaching command of the subject. Further, there may be a high turnover of nursing personnel in the CCU. Provisions must also be made for doctors who rotate in and out of the unit.

Case Problem

There was a need to establish a training program for new CCU nurses to teach them the principles of electrical safety and the operation of monitors, defibrillators, and cardiac pacemakers.

Solution

That the clinical engineer establish training sessions that would be included in the new CCU nurses 6-week training program.

40

A MODEL IN IMPLEMENTATION OF CORONARY CARE

D. Lubin

In 1968, detailed planning started for a hospital's CCU. From the outset, the hospital's clinical engineers participated in all phases of planning and provided liaison with the architect and design engineers in the development of the unit's design. The 28-bed CCU consists of "acute and progressive" areas. The rooms were designed for intensive supervision, monitoring, and resuscitation. Monitoring equipment is silent, out of the view of the patient, and has isolated input connections. Specially designed electric beds have completely insulated safety sides. The wiring distribution system is designed to provide an equipotential environment. The individual rooms are attractively decorated, provided with large outside windows and speakers for soft background music that can be controlled from the nursing station. The oscilloscope monitors at the central station have nonfade display and are provided with a tape-loop delay.

The criteria for admission to the unit include definite myocardial infarction, suspected myocardial infarction, and any cardiac condition requiring intensive electrocardiographic monitoring, with no restrictions regarding age of the patient or severity of the disease.

By virtue of continuous clinical engineering participation in the operation of the unit, there is continuous inspection, maintenance, and repair capability. In addition, the clinical engineering technicians are always available for technical assistance.

Recent experience in the treatment of myocardial infarction in this CCU has been documented during a five-year period and details 1246 cases of diagnosed myocardial infarction in a unit population of 2636 admissions.

The seriousness of possible shock hazard from a nonequipotential environment has not been satisfactorily documented. It was decided, nevertheless, to construct an equipotential system in the new unit.

Documentation and observation indicated primary hazards could be caused by:

1. Poor-quality wiring devices, particularly receptacles, attachment plugs, and power cords and their strain reliefs
2. Difficult and time-consuming access to the patient for resuscitation and routine medical and nursing care. Architectural and equipment placement obstructions were prime offenders
3. Insufficient electrical and medical-gas outlets
4. A conventional environment that could cause apprehension because of equipment noise and deprivation of normal sights and sounds

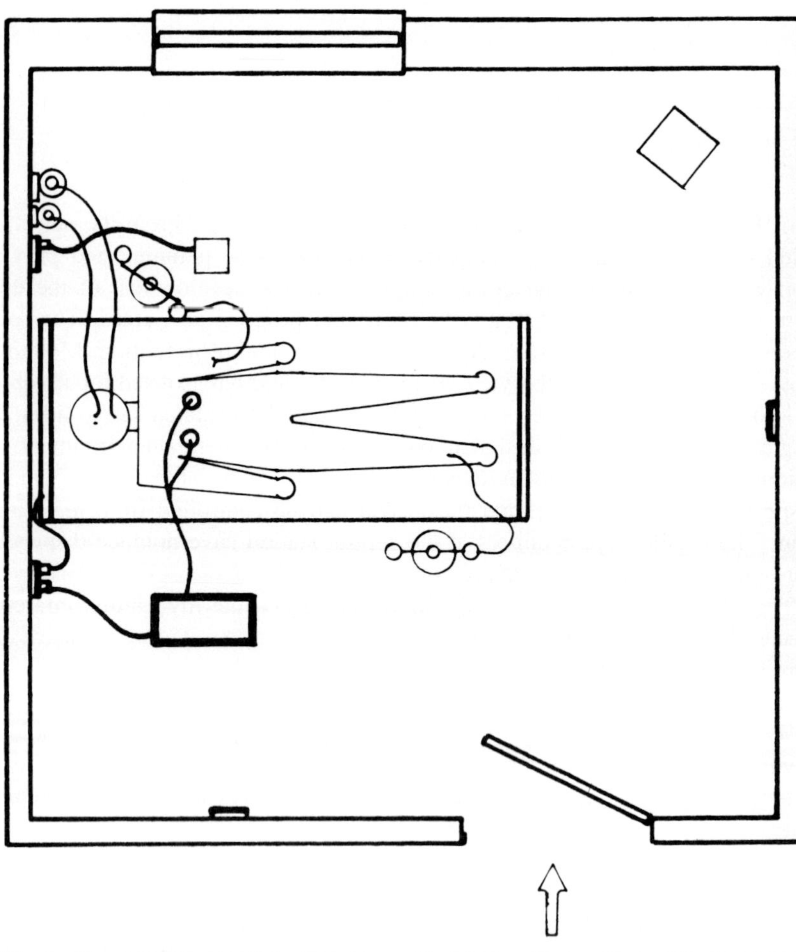

Fig. 1. The general layout of the intensive-care bed in the old area. During the planning stages, clinical engineers were involved in study of the various areas of possible improvement. Many of these are related to safety in its broadest aspect.

Features included:

1. An equipotential environment with exposed metal that could not be insulated bonded to a central ground point—now called the room or patient reference ground
2. A grounded electric bed with fully insulated safety sides
3. Ensuring rapid access by placing the bed diagonally with the headboard removed and the head of the bed always away from the wall
4. Full instrumentation for each bed; all power connections made to dedicated receptacles having full mechanical protection against damage
5. Redundant medical-gas outlets placed to shorten patient connection tubing

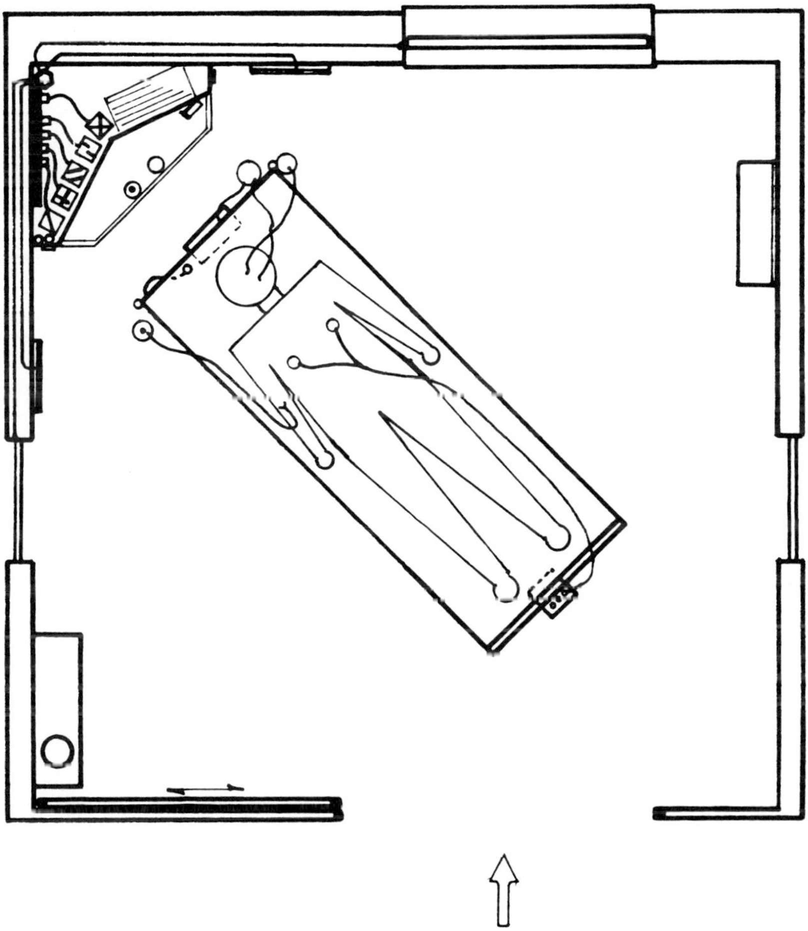

Fig. 2. Basic changes in design resulting from clinical engineers working with the medical and nursing staffs and the architect.

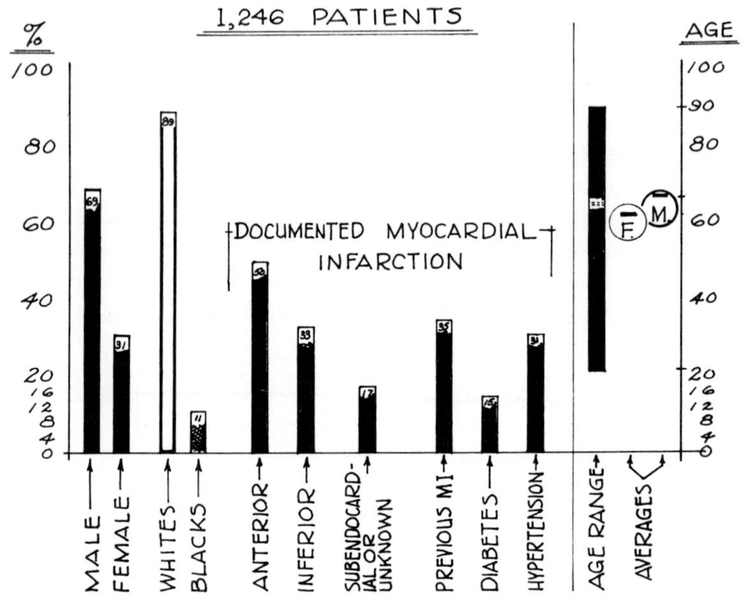

Fig. 3. Profile of the 1246 cases of myocardial infarction documented in this study.

6. All tubing, monitor lead, and power-cord connections to floor pedestals to eliminate any obstructions between the bed and the walls
7. Use of ''hospital duty'' wiring devices which was before the advent of the ULs ''hospital grade'' classification
8. Attenuation of apprehension-generating factors by eliminating monitor noise, providing attractive décor, good visibility for the patient and the staff, and optional background music
9. Twenty-four-hour presence of clinical engineering technicians manning the central monitoring console, and continuous clinical engineering supervision

The very low incidence of primary ventricular fibrillation, fibrillation that could be attributed to the design of the unit, indicates the high quality of engineering design and maintenance.

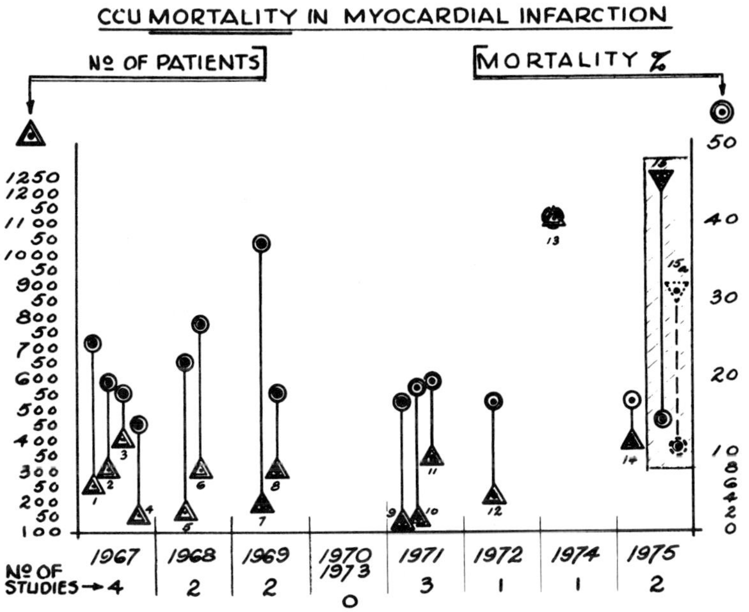

Fig. 4. A comparison with somewhat similar studies in 14 other CCUs reported in the literature between 1967 and 1975. It shows the largest case load in 15 studies and the lowest mortality rate.

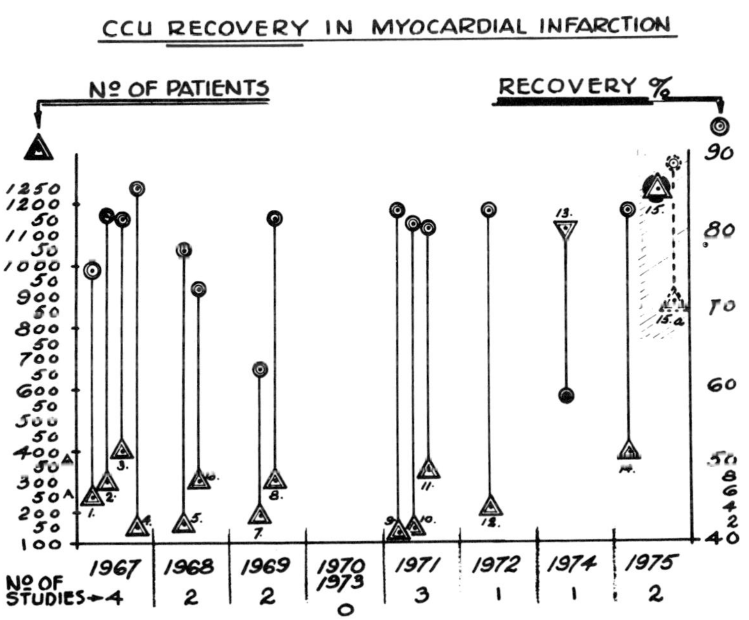

Fig. 5. The same comparison as in Figure 4, only graphing recovery rather than mortality.

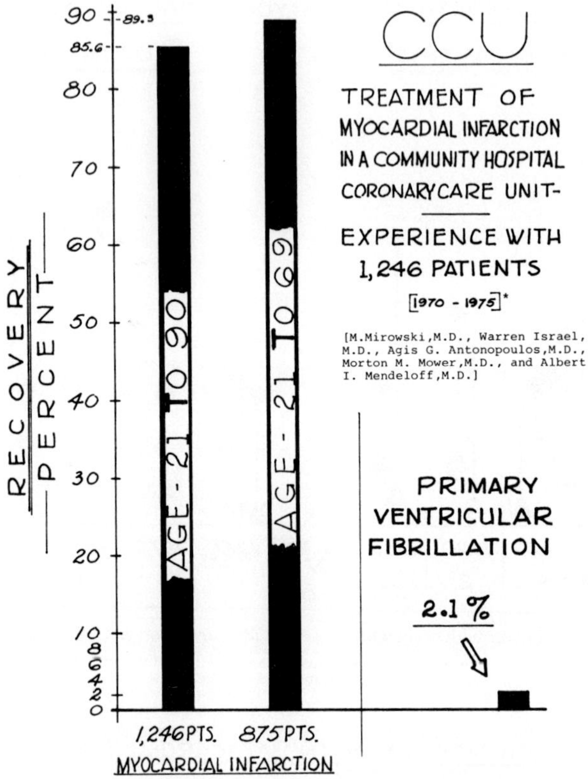

Fig. 6. An index of the success of the CCU. The recovery rate of 85.6% provides an indicator of medical and nursing excellence and the influence of clinical engineering participation in the daily operation of the unit.

41

QUALITY CONTROL IN AUTOMATED LABORATORIES

G. R. Cooper

Need and General Problems

Quality performance in automated laboratories demands quality control. The need for quality control is intimately connected with the need for valid data. A great concern is that the clinical laboratory, responding to the stimulation to install large-volume analytical and computer systems, may produce massive but incorrect and insignificant data. When we think, we realize that regardless of the quantity, incorrect data lead to worthless conclusions and are worse than no data.

Automation helps the laboratory accomplish the daily workload but has presented huge problems of its own that must be controlled for quality performance. Each type of automation has its own specific problems, and one only changes from one set of problems to another set of problems by changing from one type of automation to another. Because of the remarkable accomplishments in building automated systems and in the extensive applications of these, there is the widespread and unjustified tendency to conclude that the problems in the use of automation have been essentially solved. Automated analytical systems are often also a composite of rapid and fairly nonspecific methods susceptible to many physical and chemical interferences. Automation thus has not reached the stage at which the major problems are to acquire the funds for a "black box" and employ any personnel who can be trained to punch buttons in the correct sequence.

Variability and error are associated with the use of automated equipment as with any other laboratory equipment. Because of the potentially high productivity, it is possible to produce large quantities of results before excessive errors become obvious. Major elements necessary for quality performance that must be monitored in order to be able to detect these errors and make corrections quickly are: (*a*) knowledgeable, trained, and careful personnel with adequate motivation; (*b*) regular use of primary standards, bench controls, and external reference materials; (*c*) regular checks and calibration of all parts of the automated equipment; (*d*) proper collection, handling, shipping, and storage of samples; (*e*) stable and uncontaminated reagents; (*f*) proper care and calibration of auxiliary pipetting, weighing, drying, or other instruments and glassware; (*g*) adequate working facilities and control of personnel problems in the laboratory; (*h*) record of all significant changes made in the laboratory; (*i*) explicit written instructions outlining all steps of the methods, calibration, and preventive measures. The first step in quality control is to accept the fact that errors will occur and prepare oneself to be able to detect and correct these quickly.

Special Problems

Major problems in the application of quality control to automation reside in all parts of the clinical laboratory, but clinical chemistry only will be used as an example. In clinical chemistry, major obstacles exist even in the tests that have been widely used for years. For the determinations of glucose, urea, and uric acid, there exists indecision about the preferred reference method, question about stability and correctly labeled values of serum and blood reference materials, suspicion that collection, handling, and preservation techniques may cause deterioration in the sample or add interferences to the sample, and realization that results from different methods differ. Contamination with microorganisms essentially has some type of effect on all determinations in clinical chemistry, particularly the determination of glucose. The neocuproine method for the determination of glucose yields values significantly higher than those for ''true'' glucose, while the ortho-toluidine method may vary considerably in specimens with elevated values. In the case of the determination of urea, questions have been raised about excessive sensitivity to ammonia contamination, consistency of urease reactions, uncontrolled errors in automation from deterioration in stream lines, and lack of similar reaction on standard solutions, reference materials, and unknown samples. With the determination of uric acid, concern has been expressed repeatedly about the purity and stability of available primary standards of uric acid, the specificity of colorimetric methods, and the suitability and stability of serum pools of uric acid for use as reference materials. In all of these determinations, intake of drugs may influence either the level of the determined constituent in serum or the chemical reaction utilized in the test.

Many practical standardization problems still exist with the determinations of calcium, electrolytes, bilirubin, and serum proteins. For instance, in the case of the determination of serum proteins, different laboratories use (*a*) different conversion factors to calculate protein content from nitrogen data; (*b*) various methods based on different physical or chemical properties; and (*c*) reagents sometimes unstable with respect to sensitivity and specificity. A decision is needed whether to base calculation of protein content on calibration with a pure compound such as ammonium sulfate, on a highly purified preparation of animal or human albumin, or on a known human serum of defined "normal" characteristics.

Many difficulties in methodology and standardization exist in the automated laboratory for the determinations of diagnostic enzymes and lipids. Tests for diagnostic enzymes cannot be calibrated with pure standards because enzyme preparations are not absolutely pure. Points of reference for the determinations of enzymes must be based on functional activity, and control must be attempted through checks on instruments, reagents, conditions of assay, carefully described procedure for calculation of results, and well-defined units. Each of the lipid determinations, cholesterol, triglyceride, and lipoproteins, possesses unique problems. Multiple relatively nonspecific methods for the determination of cholesterol exist where each may be sensitive to different interferences, may not be properly referenced to available cholesterol standards, and may not be calibrated against multiple reference serums covering both the "normal" and abnormal ranges of values. The determination of triglyceride currently is quite variable because the procedure involves steps that are difficult to reproduce, and the calculation of results suffers from lack of one accepted standard and use of multiple units to express results.

Approach of Quality Control to Automation

The approach of quality control in automated laboratories utilizes the same principles applied in laboratories employing manual procedures. Tools are needed for calibration and both internal and external surveillance. Essential to the success of a quality-control system is that these tools are available and are used properly, and corrective actions are taken immediately when a problem exists. Needed tools and information are: stable and correctly labeled primary standards and serum reference materials; stable bench serum or urine controls of both known and unknown values; reference methods to furnish reference points; and "normal" values for method, place, and time of interpretation. A plan must be devised to use these tools systematically and regularly to attain appropriate surveillance and maintenance of the same level of values. Institution of an effective quality-control system is a prerequisite for standardization and consistent success in proficiency testing.

Quality control can be divided into five essential phases:

1. Planning and achievement
2. Measurement of variability
3. Evaluation of stability of performance
4. Correction and control of sources of excessive variation
5. Documentation of quality of performance

Quality performance must be achieved before it can be monitored by measurement and evaluated with respect to the functions of the laboratory. Stability of performances must also be achieved before documentation can be gained about quality of performance. Each phase of the quality-control system, in order to be highly effective, must include all steps in the processing of specimens and results. Particular attention must be paid to mixup of samples, transcription errors, and handling of data in an automated laboratory. To gain maximum benefit of a quality-control system, it seems reasonable that the essentials of the system must be incorporated into the entire operation before routine analyses are performed.

Quality-Control System of CDC High-Volume Automated Laboratory

The CDC (Center for Disease Control) Automated Analytical Services Laboratory utilizes the following in the quality-control system: (*a*) bench controls; (*b*) commercial reference materials; (*c*) duplicate analyses; (*d*) blind controls; (*e*) interlaboratory comparisons; (*f*) low-temperature stored samples; (*g*) comparison of results with reference manual methods; and (*h*) data review.

Bench Controls. Serum and urine bench control aliquots are prepared from pools and placed in small vials and frozen. After each lot is analyzed on 18 different days, the mean concentration and standard deviation of the analyses are calculated. Two concentration levels, usually samples of a "normal" and a high concentration, are introduced at random into each run. Deviations for the daily pool value that are greater than 2 S.D. from its previously established mean are reported to the supervisor. Both pools are inserted immediately after the primary standards at the beginning of the run, and this permits the run to be stopped immediately if excessive deviation is noted in the value of either pool. The readings of the primary standards at the beginning of the run and the pools immediately after them must give acceptable values before the remaining unknown specimens are analyzed.

Commercial Reference Materials. These are used primarily as a further check on serum pools. These are used also to help check on new reagents, new manifolds, or any other significant changes in apparatus or conditions.

Duplicate Analyses. Forty specimens are arranged in two groups of 20 each, one a duplicate of the other. Both groups are analyzed in sequence within the same run. Analysts compare the results of the duplicate analyses and determine that the duplicates agree within preestablished limits. If the difference between duplicates exceeds these limits, and the run is considered in control, another set of duplicate analyses is performed.

Duplicate analyses are utilized mainly to decrease the likelihood of clerical error. In our experience, clerical errors exceed any other type of laboratory error in an automated laboratory. Mixups in specimens, mistakes in sequences on turntables, misreading of recorder charts, and transposition of digits in a result or of two patients' results may occur quite often under continuous working conditions in an automated laboratory. An error in sequence can make almost an entire run invalid. Duplicate analyses also can detect an unknown source of error that can cause an obviously excessive difference in duplicates in about 3% of the patients.

Blind Controls. Previously analyzed specimens, with fictitious names and identification numbers, blindly inserted into runs, can give unbiased evidence of the between-run and between-day variability.

Interlaboratory Comparisons. Participation in national and international standardization programs can determine the relationship of results to reference data of standardization groups.

Low-temperature Stored Samples. Vials are stored at −80°C to test long-term storage and to make comparisons of results of analyses over long periods.

Comparison of Results with Reference Manual Methods. Manual methods selected as points of reference were established for certain determinations to detect possible long-range drift and change in automated analytical conditions and to help control potential interferences.

Data Review. The review is performed not only to examine the results as a laboratory director but also to evaluate the results as related to clinical findings. The data review is comprised of four parts: (*a*) daily reviews of computer printout evaluation of standards and controls and check by analysts and data clerks for clerical errors in input of data; (*b*) monthly reviews of monthly summaries of daily controls, such as standards and two serum controls; (*c*) monthly reviews of distribution of all patient data to detect trends; and (*d*) monthly review of individual patient data to detect obvious inconsistencies in the data of the same patient.

The focal point for the quality-control operation is at the bench, where the trained analyst can exert control at the most effective time and place. Also essential is the laboratory supervisor, who must examine summaries to detect trends and obvious changes in data and to assess quality of total data.

Quality Guidelines for Laboratory Multitesting

"Quality guidelines" is a highly comprehensive term. It connotes concern about how to build quality into every aspect of an endeavor. In automated laboratory multitesting, this term becomes even more expanded to include the attitude, planning, design, operation, reporting, and follow-up of each of the multiple procedures.

Since quality has to be achieved before it can be monitored, the essential factors for quality performance in all aspects must be selected and instituted and tested for suitability during the preoperation stage. Guidelines therefore should not be considered relevant only after the program is initiated but should be applicable as well in the planning stage. Maintenance of quality can be accomplished by appropriate monitoring and by setting up a requirement that certain corrective actions must be taken when out-of-control values or other problems arise in the operation. Quality assurance of an operation depends greatly on strict attention to the quality guidelines.

The following questions should probably be asked about quality guidelines for laboratory multitesting:

1. Are the essentials for quality operation covered in the guidelines?
2. Are the laboratory procedures now known to be useful to medical practice included?
3. Will the data be satisfactory for the objectives of laboratory multitesting and valid for use during the lifetime of the participant and for other potential users of the data?
4. Is the quality of the operation such that the results are used confidently by the physician, are suitable for educational purposes, and are acceptable for individual and community characterization?

These suggested questions, along with discussions about the quality of assumptions, approaches, technical points, and organization, probably can best be discussed from a general point of view. The remainder of the guidelines will be presented, therefore, under the headings: (*a*) Most Common Problems; (*b*) Controversial General Ideas; and (*c*) Comments on Specific Technical Points.

Most Common Problems

Quality guidelines should make recommendations about the most common problems involved in procedures, equipment, and data handling:

1. Procedures
   a. Unsuitable specimens
   b. Nonspecific and nonprecise procedures
   c. Inadequate quality-control procedures
   d. Overestimation and underestimation of machine capability
   e. Inadequate scheduling for cleaning, maintenance, and repairs
   f. Poor understanding of scientific principles
   g. Inability to read, translate, or properly phase measurements
   h. Inability to utilize results as planned
2. Equipment
   a. General design uses simplest chemical reactions
   b. Sample identification is complex
   c. Reagents are not thoroughly mixed
   d. Colorimeter cannot be kept cleaned or easily calibrated
   e. Conditions are not well controlled

3. Data handling
   a. Humans can cause errors at any point
   b. All ''abnormal'' values should be checked for validity

Controversial General Ideas

Certain concepts probably used as a basis for planning, making choices, and instructions for operations are not accepted universally, such as:

1. Technological automation developments have increased precision and accuracy. Automation can increase precision, but use of a more specific method or more reliable standards for calibration is the only way to increase accuracy. Automation can actually decrease accuracy by using a relatively nonspecific method or an inadequate calibration procedure. Automation, though, may show decreased precision from day to day without effective internal and external controls.

2. Automation is the answer to inadequate application of known useful techniques. Many specific chemical and physiological methods are not suitable for existing automation. At the present time, therefore, automation will not solve the needs for certain highly specific methods. Also, it is debated whether effective laboratory services can be rendered to the medical profession more by multiphasic analyses than by efficient and intelligent use of conventional laboratory support.

3. The primary objective of laboratory multitesting is to detect high-risk individuals and groups. Many believe that of equal importance is characterization of the individual and providing educational opportunities for medical profession and populace.

4. Quality guidelines should cover all feasible types and needed supporting services, including such things as special batteries of tests for mental, genetic, and metabolic diseases for special situations. Selection of tests should be directed at major problems in the examined area. Single automation units might be needed to handle special objectives. Eventually, the mass of data produced will require computer assistance for correlating medical and laboratory results.

5. Quality performance can be accomplished simply by installing a standard operating procedure. There is no controversy about the desirability of having guidelines for developing and using a standard operating procedure, but it is not necessarily true that this will lead by itself to quality performance. Standardization, continuous surveillance, and the competence to respond to technical problems are needed for quality operation of the equipment and methods. When different types of automated equipment are used in the facilities, the approach using standardization of results is advised.

Personnel factors are extremely important in the use of standard operating procedures. Personnel must be motivated to implement, maintain, and not to change standard operating procedures.

6. Tests that show a high degree of variability in some individuals from time to time have no diagnostic value. Varying of values within the same individual is not

always caused by diet or difficulties in sampling. This variability also can indicate existence of stress or risk factor.

7. Automated equipment can be operated by any person. This is far from the truth. Automated equipment requires considerable expertise to make it work and to maintain it. We must not provide just a machine but in-depth support in competent personnel and suitable controls. The handling of massive amounts of data will require well-organized and careful personnel and exploitation of computer systems for data handling, storage, and retrieval. Good management practice is the key to success.

8. Attitude is relatively unimportant in laboratory multitesting. It is not true that automation removes the personal factors. Experience has shown that quality depends too much on attitude and interest of the personnel. It is difficult to develop quality guidelines to describe a dedicated, interested, competent, and knowledgeable staff.

9. Laboratory multitesting is an essential part of a true health service. Obvious minimum service objectives should include the hopes of the physician that multiphasic testing will help him control long-term chronic illness and the hopes of the populace to get the best care at the least cost. The types of examinations that can be expected to benefit the patient and justify the expenditure of any large-scale funds should be discussed in depth during the planning stage. Incomplete programs, such as a battery of chemical tests, could have little value unless supported by in-depth health examinations and indicated follow-up.

Quality guidelines, in addition, should provide for continuing evaluation of relative merits and benefits of the various multiphasic procedures. Adequate clinical examinations and sufficiently long follow-up of each participant are necessary to gain the data for this evaluation.

Laboratory multitesting is a true health service only if we make it one by using it as a component of total medical health services.

Comments on Specific Technical Points

Certain technical points are worthy of mention in quality-control guidelines:

1. Choice and use of equipment. The quality guidelines should be applicable to and encourage the use of all types of automated equipment. It is important that a decision be made about quality guidelines for equipment since this can stimulate commercial efforts toward more dependability, durability, and reasonable flexibility. Plans should include acquisition of critical parts, systems for rapid repair on a preventive basis, and recalibration after each repair or change in equipment.

Utilization of instrumentation and automation should be on a scale to justify the investment, operating costs, and supporting efforts. Highly automated operations can easily be under-utilized and their real costs readily underestimated—causing lack of quality in productivity and economy. Work output can easily be overestimated;

quality performance demands realistic allowances for maintenance, scheduling for suitable calibration and controls, recovery from machine failures (including recalibrations and repeat analyses), and sufficient time to do quality work.

The statement that minimum requirements for automated equipment performance is 95% reliability will cause considerable concern among laboratorians. The feeling exists now that we are too complacent about accepting poorly developed, underdesigned, and underengineered equipment. It seems more reasonable to plan for rapid repair and recovery for about 99% reliability of operation time, or 1% "down" time.

Quality guidelines should assume that considerable time will be needed initially to make automated equipment work. Most automated systems have relatively fixed designs and are limited in how much change can be made to fit the needs. Specialized automated equipment sometimes must be selected that can be applied to definitely needed specific chemical and physiological tests.

2. Staffing pattern. Knowledgeable and experienced analysts, supervisors, and professional directors and consultants are essential for quality performance. It is not true that less trained and less educated and less expensive personnel are required. A high-quality staff is needed on a sustaining basis and intermittently for problem solving. The inference that laboratory multitesting can get along with unsupervised, inexperienced operators let loose on a monster analyzer is the attitude that will surely lead to poor-quality results.

3. Calibration of clinical chemistry procedures. One of the more controversial and more difficult concepts to accept by the clinical chemists is the use of serum reference materials for calibration. The current opinion, though, is that this is the only feasible approach. Quality guidelines must therefore be instituted to prevent misuse. Serum reference materials must be checked against accepted reference points, evaluated for interferences by other constituents and additives, and followed for stability against environmental insults. We must find a way to get dependable serum reference materials and checks to know what values mean.

One shudders at the thought of utilizing commercial serum reference materials from multiple sources as a basis of quality calibration. It seems more reasonable to make certain one set of serum reference materials in the concentration range of the values being measured is accurate and stable by checking these with aqueous standards, other methods, serums with known interfering substances, and any other available points of reference. Quality guidelines should therefore present suggestions about how to correct the variation caused by the use of different commercial serum reference materials by the same laboratory over a period of time and by different laboratories at multiple locations.

4. Choice and use of procedures. Quality guidelines are difficult to prepare for determining priority of choice of procedures. Not only must the capability of analytical technique be considered, but also the clinical usefulness and educational value should be assessed. For instance, one hesitates to accept the statement that the determination of uric acid should be given a lower priority. The recently recognized greater range of values in the population without clinical signs and the suspicion

that interreactions with unknown constituents affect clinical symptoms could be interpreted to mean that the value of uric-acid determination indicates proneness not only to gout but possibly to other metabolic derangements. Uric acid is a constituent that can change slowly in serum concentration over an extended time period, just like cholesterol and certain other constituents of significance in chronic diseases.

Quality guidelines for analytical competency should include demands for specificity, sensitivity, and reproducibility of chosen technique. Important, also, are recommendations for valid ways to control sampling, preservation, storage, and interference factors.

On some occasions, it might be useful to get a qualitative result, but in general it is advised to seek a quantitative measurement because (*a*) precise data are less likely to mislead physicians; and (*b*) a precise and accurate method, once automated, can produce a result just as economically as an automated nonspecific or qualitative method.

Mention of possible use of organ, body, and system tests in clinical chemistry assumes capability of enzyme, hormone, and metabolic product testing that does not currently exist. As an objective of the future, this should be given high priority.

The detection and measurement of bacteriuria is discussed with reservations. Automation is not an impossibility. Applied research on new ideas about application of known scientific facts can accomplish automation of a test for bacteriuria.

5. Allowable limits of performance. Acceptability of the results of a procedure is based on the ability (*a*) to discriminate between "normal" and "abnormal" ranges; (*b*) to determine any clinically significant unique relationship between the results of two or more procedures; and (*c*) to follow any excessive variation within the individual. Quality guidelines should plan for periodic review of all allowable limits to ascertain that results are valid for the objectives and that laxity has not occurred in maintaining the allowable limits of errors for each procedure.

The range of "normal" values selected for use as part of the basis for determining allowable limits of performance for each procedure should be reviewed to see if corrections for variables such as sex, age, and location can be made in order to increase the discriminatory power. Computer handling of the data should help increase discrimination by more easily making corrections for these variables.

6. Reference and substitute procedures. Quality guidelines should provide that procedures selected for the operation be related to standard reference procedures either within the unit or in a referee laboratory. Comparability of results over time and with other installations can be helped by use of common reference materials and methods.

Substitute methods should not provide less valid results. One should not substitute a qualitative method for a quantitative method as mentioned for the determination of glucose. It seems more desirable to spend the time to correct a problem rapidly rather than to substitute a less useful method.

7. Verification, validation, and integrity of data and reported results. A patient-identification system must be satisfactory to follow the patient through the different parts of laboratory multitesting and to maintain identification from collec-

tion of samples through analysis, reporting, and interpretation of results. All suspect and "abnormal" results must be verified and validated. Experience in automation now suggests that automated analyses can be controlled more easily than human errors. The two main components in erroneous reports are improperly calculated or transcribed results and mixups of patient identity. In one survey, these amounted to an apparent 11% rate of undetected laboratory-data errors.

Heavy reliance must be placed on a valid system of quality control in order to recognize less than optimal or unsatisfactory performance without overt failure. These types of errors are difficult to detect and cause large expenditures in time and effort to correct.

Quality control can operate effectively in an automated laboratory. Insistence by the entire staff on high-quality results, institution of essential factors of quality control before beginning routine operation, and maintenance of these essentials of quality performance on a stable basis are necessary for effectively and successfully conducting a quality-control program. Sampling, analytical, and data-handling areas, as well as human sources of error at every stage, need continuing surveillance. Availability of checks and controls for each stage of the operation is not sufficient in itself to ensure a successful operation; also needed are continuing supervision by competent personnel and continuous rethinking about ways to handle changing equipment, procedures, and rising problems.

42

CLINICAL ENGINEERING AND HOSPITAL SAFETY

K. S. Kagey

To many, juxtaposition of the terms clinical engineering and hospital safety means protection from microshock electrical problems. In actuality, this is only one facet of safety for hospitalized patients in relation to medical instrumentation. This facet drew considerable attention to the clinical engineering field in the mid- to late-1960s and still retains a significant effect on the field in many ways.

Microshock

In 1964, a paper reported 1200 deaths per year. The paper reported ventricular fibrillation threshold studies for canines and also reported on thresholds studied on a few humans undergoing open heart surgery with fibrillatory arrest and gave clear documentation that both humans and dogs can be fibrillated at very low current levels when the current is applied directly to the heart. Scattered additional reports on humans have appeared. Although fibrillation is commonly used during open-heart surgery, the equipment is extremely simple, providing only gross control over dose level since no further refinements have appeared clinically necessary. Thus, a careful study requires more sophistocated equipment and enough time to evaluate threshold.

At about the same time, a few reports of instrumentation-related fibrillation episodes in patients appeared and also reports that many then-existing pieces of equipment could, under certain conditions, produce currents at least in theory of fibrillatory magnitude. As far as the real world goes, what is the magnitude of this problem? The first question is what are "dangerous" and "safe" levels for current potentially applied to the heart? Several factors influence threshold: First, it is clear that low levels of current are life-threatening only when applied to one of the ventricles. The atria are far less vulnerable, and should atrial fibrillation occur, it is rarely a life-threatening situation. When the current source is in one of the great vessels—vena cavae, aorta, pulmonary artery—far greater current levels are required to cause arrhythmias. Thus, concern should be restricted to ventricular application. Epicardial application requires higher currents than endocardial application, but since the vast majority of clinical situations encompass transvenous catheters with endocardial stimulation, we should reasonably look at the lower measured thresholds. These have been found as low as 80 μA and as high as over 2 mA. Canine work has shown fibrillation to occur in a few cases with currents of 20 μA, in the majority at somewhat higher levels, and in some cases over 1 mA.

A number of people have recommended setting safety limits at 10 or 20 μA on the basis that this provides severalfold safety margin below reported thresholds. Undoubtedly, this will be far lower than most patients need; theoretically, it could be lethal to one patient. Obviously, zero would be ideal but impractical.

The early recommendations for microshock protection were leveled at any and every electrically operated device in the patient vicinity. They also tended to consider any patient with an externalized cardiac catheter to be critically ill, tethered to bed, and surrounded by sophistocated and well-delineated devices. Unfortunately, the patients are more often rather well. Many patients are out of bed a lot, may take care of their own personal needs, and stroll down the corridor at will. The concept of someone running after them with a cage (nonconductive, of course) to keep evil spirits away is ludicrous. Even in the situation in which the so-called susceptible patient is truly critically ill, a wide variety of devices may surround him, including TV and the housecleaning devices necessary to prevent serious infectious complications.

It is now better recognized that the primary protection from microshock lay in protecting the externalized heart (catheter) from unwanted contacts with possibly hazardous surfaces and in care as to what was connected deliberately to the catheter. It is also becoming more widely accepted that somewhat "imperfect" devices, priced so they are affordable, are usually of more clinical benefit than "perfect" devices beyond the reach of most institutions.

The present generally accepted current limits are 10 μA for circuits likely to be connected directly to the heart (20 μA sink current limit with normally used cables), 50 to 100 μA for patient-connected circuits not likely to be connected to cardiac leads, and 100 to 250 μA chassis leakage current.

It is extremely important to remember that regardless of the leakage current available from an instrument chassis, it cannot reach the patient's heart until two separate faults occur: (*a*) loss of grounding; and (*b*) contact with the externalized catheter. Given careful attention to protecting the externalized contacts, this double fault should have essentially no chance of happening.

How is this achieved? By realistic protocols for cardiac-lead care in each hospital (simple and very cheap), by emphasis on new pacer and pacing-catheter designs having built-in protection, and by special design of those few types of circuits that are apt to be connected directly to ventricular muscle. The latter two technical aspects are being implemented. The first is less clearly being implemented. After availability of a pacemaker use protocol from the Peter Bent Brigham Hospital was reported, during the first year, over 80 requests for copies were received, but only one protocol has been received in return from another hospital. Almost half the requests were from the engineering side, with many of the remaining from nurses. As a group, physicians would seem to have only minimal concern in this area, while engineers are very concerned.

Perhaps the following hypothesis can explain this dichotomy. Engineers have read the reports and see what seems to be a major hazard. Physicians who have handled externalized cardiac leads since the technique became clinically accepted have seen countless situations in which theory would shudder but the patients remained healthy.

Actually, one does not see many cases of induced ventricular fibrillation. Such cases of fibrillation are relatively few since most of the patients required pacers, and those who died, had bradyarrhythmias eventuating in standstill as the terminal event, not fibrillation. They became irresponsive to the pacer. One particular case of fibrillation occurred a few hours after open-heart surgery. A patient with prophylactically placed epicardial leads appeared to be doing fine and then fibrillated. He reverted immediately with countershock. Out of interest, possible sources of fibrillatory current were checked around him without finding any. This patient was being monitored by computer, with pressure readings recorded at minute intervals to test a new program. On reviewing these, a slow but clear downward trend was evident, suggesting he needed more blood transfusions, although this had not been evident at first glance. Clinical judgment over the next hour bore this out. However, had the fibrillation not been reversed, had the computer trends not been available, and had some small problems been found in the equipment later, it could have been made to read like an "obvious electrocution."

To summarize the microshock story:

1. Implement good catheter practice protocols among all the personnel who care for such patients, including but not limited to insulating the externalized conductive parts with plastic carafe or other bags, or rubber. (Gloves do insulate but are very awkward.) This will give microshock protection; protect against static if that becomes documented as possible hazard; satisfy those who feel that stringent equipment/facility regulations are needed because "no one" is protecting the patient; and provide protection against more common hazards of disconnected leads (alligator clip connections) and shorting between wires. This last is especially a problem with temporary transthoracic wires and can lead to cessation of pacing unless care is taken to coil the uninsulated wire around the terminal and secure it with tape.

2. When purchasing new ECG equipment and anything else that may be connected to cardiac leads, opt for isolated patient input circuits. They are readily available.

3. If you must use older equipment with nonisolated leads for direct cardiac monitoring, know what, if any, hazards exist. Whenever possible, this equipment

should perhaps be used in intensive-care units in which the staff knows what to do, not for the ward emergency in which these procedures are uncommon.

4. When purchasing new equipment, look for chassis leakage currents under 100 μA if possible, or under 250; it should definitely be below 500 μA, which is the recommended limit for general-use equipment. However, remember that this simply makes the equipment relatively safe under open-ground fault conditions and gives it a margin in which to fail before becoming very hot; so long as the grounding wire in the cord connects to a reasonable facility equipment grounding (green) wire, almost any equipment is safe.

There have been several dialysis machines with leakage currents in the milliampere range (up to 90 mA), but there never was a problem because the heavy line cords and heavy caps maintained grounding integrity at all times. The reason the extremely high leakage current was discovered was that the equipment began to be used in a unit with isolated power and a line-isolation monitor. The hospital electrician who was familiar with the equipment pointed the problem out, but it took some convincing to persuade the company that the heaters and thermostats were not suited for use in hot saline solutions.

Perceptible Shocks

What are some other safety aspects that should concern the clinical engineer? Perceptible shocks are not unheard of and usually are associated with open grounds; two-wire cords; removal of grounding pins; cheaters; open ground in facility wiring. Elimination of these hazards requires close working arrangements, including floor personnel, clinical engineers, and physical plant engineering personnel. All the rigorous safety routines practiced on monitors and similar equipment will be sorely limited in effectiveness if there is no one worrying about the ubiquitous bedside lamp, housekeeping equipment, food carts, TVs, and where allowed, patient-owned equipment.

One of the most important aspects of an electrical safety program is to impress on all employees that ungrounded equipment and damaged equipment are not to be used and at the same time to provide a sensitive and responsive system so that a complaint is easily made to the right party and corrective action taken at once. The employee who reports an apparent hazard but sees no action taken rapidly loses impetus to report subsequent observations.

Emergency Power

The above situations deal with too much electricity in the wrong place; what about ensuring power when and where it is needed?

One aspect is that of emergency power. What is available, what is the available capacity, how is it distributed, and do the people who need to use it know about it.

The clinical engineer should be knowledgeable about what emergency power is available in the house and where there is none. Are there situations in which portable battery-inverter power might be needed? What is the branch circuit distribution in each area? In a dialysis unit, there was a duplex marked EMERGENCY at each bed, but review of the circuits revealed that two or three beds were on each branch circuit, thus making it important that heaters not be used to avoid an outage since each machine draws about 5 A plus 10 A for the heater. Since heaters cycle, it could be possible for two machines to run without causing the breaker to open if the cycles did not coincide, but Russian roulette in patient care leaves much to be desired. By knowing the limitations of the power system, the staff could intelligently plan their activities to maintain optimum patient care.

This particular unit also impresses the need to have clear, precise, information made known to the staff. For example, a major power failure occurred in the hospital, and after getting areas secured, the dialysis unit was checked to see if there were any problems. It had been 5 minutes or so before someone remembered having seen some outlets that said EMERGENCY. They were placed in an awkward position, but the equipment was now connected and operational. However, the staff was concerned about "how long the batteries" would last. They were much relieved to learn that the DC power running the motor generator set was from the power house rather than from batteries. The clinical engineer should be in a good position to obtain and understand the technical information from the plant engineering department and then distill the clinically significant material needed by the staff.

Another constraint to power availability, locally, is matching branch circuit distribution and equipment load. The monitors, ECG recorders, even most DC defibrillators, do not represent a serious power demand. However, dialysis machines, hypothermia machines, some line-operated respirators, heaters for burn patients, and similar items need from 5 to 15 A running (exclusive of start-up surges). Understanding of branch circuit distribution in a given area will make it possible to recognize the limitations that may exist.

Hypothermia machines are often requested for use in general-care hospital areas. Beyond the question of medical desirability is the question of whether the circuits can handle the load. In some areas, it is possible to use a machine by blocking off use of other outlets on a particular circuit; in others, there is no reasonable way that the equipment can be used safely (it can be used, certainly, but not safely), and the optimum patient-care consideration is to move the patient to a more suitable area.

Decision making on the basis of branch circuit distribution presupposes knowledge of the distribution. This is frequently not known with certainty, and there is relatively little concern shown by administrators for the support needed to obtain the information, then keep it updated. Another spinoff is that when circuit distribution is well known, it should be possible to open the breaker when a switch or receptacle is to be repaired rather than working the circuit hot. An example occurred at a time when the intensive-care area was full, had several respirators going, and had in addition a patient on the membrane oxygenator—essentially long-term partial cardiopulmonary bypass. A simple switch change was being done, and a short circuit occurred as the switch was returned to the box. In this case, it was not the involved branch circuit breaker that opened, rather the breaker feeding the *panel* containing the breaker in question that resulted in power loss to about one-third of the unit. Since the panels were all in the unit and readily accessible, the problem was quickly resolved, and no harm was done. However, had the panels been remotely located, serious problems could have ensued. The whole situation could have been avoided had the electrician known that the circuit distribution in that unit was well described and had turned off the breaker involving the switch.

Safety

One must realize that clinical areas are not always ''shipshape,'' that spills of various conductive and sometimes flammable materials do occur. When selecting equipment for purchase or when simply reviewing existing equipment for safety, one must be concerned with how easily foreign materials can enter. This requires consideration both of the physical aspects of the device and the anticipated use. As an example, there are a number of portable monitors that have completely solid top surfaces but openings on the sides for ventilation. It is hard to imagine how anything could drip into the instrument, but indeed coffee with sugar did. It was learned from talking with the hospital electronics man who serviced these monitors that this was not unusual.

The company was then asked to make some sort of shield. They had originally designed the equipment for wall mounting and assumed there would be no problem. Actually, there could be, as IV fluids under pressure infusion can pop and splash far and wide, and cleaning agents can enter. Another case involved equipment from a different manufacturer that could be either rack mounted or mounted on a cart. For rack mounting, the equipment came with perforated side panels for ventilation. This was safe since the rack sides prevented spills from reaching the equipment. However, some units were surface mounted with the same perforated side panels, and failures did occur due to entry of spilled or splashed material.

This last example brings in the responsibility for ensuring that clinical instruments are properly matched to the job they will be expected to perform. This does not mean simply that an ECG monitor will pick up ECGs or that pumps will pump but how each actually fits the specific and individual purpose for which it is purchased. For the clinical engineer involved in purchasing decisions, this means first of all truly understanding what the physicians, nurses, and other involved personnel need. This means talking with them and over time developing an understanding of how each patient-care floor and each ICU functions. Clinical staff frequently are not familiar with options and appreciate information. While perhaps not strictly safety, cost must be considered as one variable. Where little money is available, care in selecting suitable but moderate cost equipment may be crucial in whether services are to be available. Selection of a modular device that can be added to as needs dictate may be invaluable. Even where the immediate goal may seem simple, a little forethought may provide much later benefit.

Accuracy

Patient safety in relation to pressure monitoring includes accuracy of information obtained with the equipment. One aspect is accuracy of the readout device; if 100 mmHg is applied, what does the monitor say? However, the degree of accuracy demanded should be based on what is actually needed. Arterial pressure fluctuates slightly with respiration, perhaps more with the length of the nurse's skirt. There are also no absolutes; each patient is very much an individual. Therefore, an error of one or 2 mmHg at the 100 mmHg level is less than normal physiological variation. Efforts at maintaining extreme accuracy, if they tie up a great deal of effort, may mean that the patient gets shortchanged elsewhere. Of more immediate benefit to the patient is having a simple, properly set up mercury manometer to allow the nurse to check the system if questions arise.

More "errors" in readings reflect the numbers being different from expected rather than being system errors. Use of the mercury manometer checks the system from gauge to readout and, being a rather basic, familiar standard, is accepted by most nurses and physicians. All the calibration work in the world aimed at the electronics of the system will never replace the need for this quick bedside check.

While a properly designed manometer system and proper technique render the calibration procedure quite safe for the patient, there are always possibilities for line contamination and air embolism, so there is a definite advantage to electronic calibration for routine checks so long as the primary standard is available and its use familiar to the staff.

Another technical aspect to pressure accuracy is frequency response. While it is of importance in high-fidelity ventricular and central aortic pressures for special analysis, it is not a serious problem in routine clinical monitoring. A variety of connecting tubings has been used over the years of different diameters and wall type, with lengths ranging from 40 to 120 in. (this range sometimes spanned on a single patient) without appreciable effect on the waveforms. Excessive concern over system frequency response, if it has negligible effect on patient care in a given setting, can be expected to lead to reduction in other attentions to safety in patient care.

Digital and meter displays are good but only if the information entering is without artifact. Systemic arterial pressure presents the fewest problems since the waveform is well defined and respiratory fluctuations are normally minor. On the low-pressure side, however, well-defined waveforms are absent in the atria and may be absent from the pulmonary artery. Respiratory variations may be 5–20 mmHg with quiet breathing, 50 mmHg or more with struggling. Mean pressure processing circuits integrate all pressure variations; they cannot evaluate which are cardiac and which respiratory artifact. Therefore, it is possible to have a reading of, say, 18 mmHg for right atrial pressure when the meaningful end-expiratory pressure is 10 mmHg. Clinically, this can be the difference between high and normal pressure, thus dictating a wrong mode of therapy. Reflected V waves from the ventricle or catheter advancement from an atrium to its ventricle can totally invalidate presented data. Cure? Careful training of the staff in what the scope pattern means (every pressure channel must be observable for waveform) and use of end-expiratory readings from the scope when the respiratory pattern renders "computed" readings invalid.

It is important to have adequate-sized waveform display for the low-pressure systems, a combination of adequate gain and adequate scope channel size. It is desirable to be able to modify gain, especially for pulmonary artery monitoring in which systolic pressure may range from 10 to 100, though more commonly ranging from 10 to 50 mmHg. Passage of a Swan-Ganz flow-directed catheter depends in part on accurate recognition of the changes in pressure as the catheter advances to right atrium, right ventricle, pulmonary artery, and on to the pulmonary capillary wedge position. Once the catheter is in place, there is need to see the systolic peaks to watch for damping and to accurately recognize migration out to the pulmonary capillary position.

Another point is to ensure that ECG cables cannot be connected to a pressure circuit through use of common connector types. If needle electrodes are used, the excitation current can produce burns. With surface electrodes, burns are unlikely, but patient complaints are heard.

Design

Safety in instrumentation also includes optimizing the array of equipment. CCUs designed as arrhythmia monitoring units frequently have just ECG at the bedside. When pressure monitoring is needed, another device is brought in. When cardioversion is needed, another unit is brought in.

When it is necessary to bring in an extra monitor, it may be desirable to have the capacity for connecting both pressure transducers and ECG to the portable monitor and slave the ECG from that to the bedside unit to maintain central station monitoring. Safety also dictates extension ECG and transducer cables, where needed, to prevent serious trip hazards to personnel.

When separate cardioversion units are used, it is not uncommon to have the patient connected both to the cardioverter and to the bedside monitor. This may subject the patient to some degree of risk and usually produces an added number of wires for the staff to step over. An alternative solution used in two ICUs has been to utilize a defibrillator with 1 mV ECG sensing capability and synchronization circuit, with the bedside monitor as the readout. The cardioverter can be equipped with a long cable with male and female connectors common to all the unit ECG monitors. One simply disconnects the ECG cable from the monitor, plugs it into one connector of the cardioverter cable, and connects the other to the monitor. Since the cardioverter has no oscilloscope, it does not get tied up on one patient for monitoring, can readily be slipped in and out of a room, and has maximum work space and drawers for storage of pacing and other cardiac devices. In an ICU in which any patient potentially needing cardioversion is on a monitor, anyway, adding duplication of equipment on the cardioverter seems to be a waste of time, money, and ever-insufficient space. The specific unit is also chosen for an essentially fail-safe characteristic, whereby it is always set for unsynchronized defibillation unless deliberate adjustments are made for synchronizing. Thus, it is a simple device for anyone to use for treating ventricular fibrillation, a versatile device for use by knowledgeable personnel for special purposes.

The foregoing is not meant as an indictment of full capability units, including scopes for emergency areas, portable use, etc.; rather, it is a matter of tailoring equipment to specific needs.

Surveillance

Safety in equipment use includes constant surveillance for equipment problems and function problems. One must circulate with the user to run across unmet needs. As an example, efforts to curtail use of electrical ''cheaters'' in the OR uncovered a sigmoidoscope light source that had a three-prong connector potted with the step-down transformer. Not only did the plug not fit the OR receptacles; the cheater was also used to provide extra length to the cord. Several exchanges of correspondence with the company established that they would not supply a cord with an OR-type connector, but that they did have an extra-long cord that was not in the catalogue. One of those cords was purchased, and a permanent connection to an OR plug devised for it. This seemed an excellent solution. The sigmoidoscope was often used in the sterile field, and the short length of cord on the instrument that connected to the new power cord made it difficult to keep the unsterile power cord off the field. Another letter brought the news that longer instrument cords could be purchased, and they solved the problem. What started as an apparently simple electrical safety problem ended up in resolving both that problem and a potential source of sepsis for the patient. Without open lines of communication, the first might not have been solved; the second certainly would have been unanswered.

In another situation, evaluation of electrical safety for various fiber-optic light sources revealed a problem in that various types seemed to be needed to fit different diagnostic and therapeutic devices. The reason was that varying connectors were used to connect light cable and light source. Several manufacturers were consulted who had partial solutions at best. In an effort to learn more about basic principles, someone in the field for whom clinical instrumentation testing had been done in the past was also contacted. He was helpful in this regard; he also determined that he could make a half-inch bundle for the preferred light source that would fit several end-use devices. This is now available ''off the shelf'' for the same price as other half-inch bundles and has done much to minimize the need for additional light sources while ensuring that special procedures will not be canceled because a unique light source failed.

Specifications

Ensuring hospital safety is a multifaceted communication challenge within the institution, including active dialogue with manufacturers and suppliers. Specific problems may often be solved as some of the previously mentioned situations illustrate, but is it not better to avoid problems if possible?

A well-designed prepurchase evaluation can do much to ensure safety in equipment and in safe usage techniques. However, this does not necessarily refer to having equipment brought in to be taken apart by experts. This method has been used and should continue to occur in certain leading institutions, but at the risk of offending some people, it is suggested that these techniques have in some ways made life much harder for many since no demands for data were made on the manufacturers. The first step for most, once needs are defined, should be to obtain factual data from manufacturers. A written statement of data requested should be developed to avoid confusion. Direct contact with manufacturers may be needed if suppliers are slow to respond. Even with this, it can be difficult.

What kind of data should be sought?

1. Power requirements: amperes and/or watts; "power" information appearing in terms of volts and Hertz is surprisingly frequent and says nothing about whether special wiring may be needed to handle the equipment. Such special wiring may include a new circuit for a 5-A device if the existing circuit already carries its maximum rated load.

2. Line voltage needs for stable operation; knowledge of one's institution's commonly encountered voltage ranges is needed to properly assess the suitability of equipment under consideration. If one is likely to have long periods of voltages of 135 V or 110 V, one should be certain that the equipment is capable of operating in this range.

3. Frequency range tolerable, especially if frequency control of emergency power is not very closely regulated.

4. Battery information: rechargeable or not; number and type; special purchase or available at any hardware store. If rechargeable batteries are used, how long will they last under specified running conditions, how long do they take for recharging, and will the instrument operate from line if the batteries are completely discharged?

5. Line cord size and type: While one may reasonably well assume that the size will be adequate for the power requirements, there is neither current assurance that physical durability will be considered by the manufacturer nor special code requirements such as may be found in OR standards. Use of #16 or larger sizes of extra-hard usage type (ref. National Electrical Code) will help to maintain integrity

for cords of portable devices. While it would seem that this information would be readily available from a manufacturer's purchasing agent, two separate situations have been encountered with medical instrumentation companies that *could not* provide information on cord type. One gave as a reason that his cardiac output computer was expected to be operated on battery, so the line cord would not be used in a patient area. The possibility that the device would be set up in a corner and left connected (if it were really a major clinical help in patient care) was never considered.

6. Line cord length: What is normally provided; what provision will the manufacturer make to give a different length if needed? The normal 8–10-ft cord is outright dangerous when the device is used free-standing at the foot of a bed. Fifteen feet is necessary, or extension cords and/or trip hazards predominate. In a large OR, 25 feet may be a must. Lack of input to manufacturers and to listing groups compounds this problem. It is nice to say that short cords reduce leakage current, but if that is at the risk of physical injury to personnel/patient/equipment or fosters wide use of extension cords, no benefit is obtained.

7. Type of cord cap normally provided: Is it a light-duty molded cap, rugged molded cap, good or bad replacable cap? If the device is to be used in an operating room, provision with proper cap is desirable. In this instance, compromises may be required, especially if the device is not ordinarily used in operating rooms or areas with special receptacles. However, strong insistence on proper plugs for equipment, the use of which is restricted to anesthetizing areas, and for provision of adequately heavy duty and proper-length line cords should be made.

The clinical engineer must be familiar with pertinent codes and standards if he is to (*a*) communicate with manufacturers effectively; and (*b*) aid in fostering changes in codes and standards when they do not meet current clinical needs. A few months ago, a prominent clinical engineer stated that companies could not provide equipment with needed 15-foot cords because "United Laboratories" wouldn't let them. The reference actually was to Underwriters' Laboratories and Subject 544 (Medical and Dental Equipment)! (Not being familiar with the document he did not know the limit is actually 15 ft.) Even this is too short for some applications.

8. Provision of manuals and schematics should be insisted upon *before* a device is brought into the hospital, whether for trial or purchase. The manuals and schematics could be demo copies, just as there are demo units of equipment. By careful screening of prospects on paper, an intelligent decision is more readily reached, and if equipment is brought in on trial, one will know better what to look for. A device "on trial" is costing the manufacturer money, and the costs eventually get back to the consumer. A company that has reasonable manuals and data should have no qualms about releasing this to prospective customers. The customer also knows what quality documentation he will purchase with the equipment. If the manufacturer cannot be bothered with providing this information, one may wonder whether he really knows his equipment.

9. Information on nominal leakage current data is needed to ensure the device will fit the institution's requirements and also to make more relevant incoming-

inspection testing. If the observed leakage current (ungrounded) is 95 μA and the limit 100, it would seem acceptable. However, if the nominal value is 20, that value of 95 should be examined very closely. Conversely, if the nominal is 95 and the observed 105, it may reasonably be elected to accept this as one knew it would be right around the limit before it was purchased.

When new equipment is brought into the hospital, whether for trial or permanent use, it is very important that pertinent instructions for use within that institution be drawn up, including correlation of basic principles with similar devices of other manufacturer or model. Reliance totally on manufacturer's instructions can lead to staff considering every ECG or pressure monitor as a different entity from other ones rather than recognizing the common principles and adapting to different control knobs. Another factor is that certain procedures may be off limits to nurses by local rules, and a decision may be needed about who will undertake such procedures. Such local tailoring is not something that manufacturers can do; it must occur within the institution.

When equipment comes in on trial, the above comments hold, and also the need for a carefully planned trial protocol. The tendency for equipment to come in for informal "trials" that generate only individual anecdotal comments does no one any good. Designation of one individual to bird-dog the trial, having specific comment sheets, and similar controls will help both the hospital, the patient, and the manufacturer. Information gained in such trials must be maintained in some central information center, too, so that the information thus gained is available for future use.

To summarize, safe use of clinical instrumentation involves the clinical engineer's being familiar with all aspects of its function, use, and the environment within which it is to operate. It is also important that clear information is available as to what equipment is available, where replacable parts are obtained, instructions written for the user in that institution, and where to call for help.

The clinical engineer will not perform all of these tasks, but he seems the most likely coordinator to *think* of the needs and nudge in the right places to get the needs met.

PART VII

MAINTENANCE

43

JUSTIFICATION FOR THE TECHNOLOGIST

J. K. Kerekes

The medical profession today faces a dilemma. In conformity with its ethics, practiced custom, and indeed the law, the profession has conscientiously sought to provide the highest quality of patient care consistent with known methods and the technological achievement of better diagnostic equipment. The art of healing has cooperated with the science of engineering to construct a vast amount of electronic diagnostic devices. This instrumentation is so flexible in its ability to monitor body functions and so precisely accurate as to make its use mandatory to those hospitals and clinics exceeding minimally acceptable medical care. Unfortunately, a critical shortage exists in the number of technologists and technicians properly trained to evaluate, maintain, and operate this highly sophisticated equipment.

The problem is complicated. The educational institutions, which have traditionally trained nurses and technicians, suffer a technological lag. Knowledge in the field has vastly increased in the past few years. Limited budgets prohibit the acquisition of either the many types or current models of such expensive equipment. Even universities, which are dependent on endowments from their alumni for their financing, have their operations stretched to provide educations sufficiently comprehensive for their medical-degree students. They cannot afford the duplication occasioned by special programs at the technician or technologist level. The result is that doctors and other members of the health team all too frequently enter the field with less than complete skill in the use of the new biomedical electronic instrumentation.

Nor do the hospitals or clinics provide the type of instruction needed to fill the gap in training. They have fallen into the error of relying on the instrumentation industry itself to perform this vital educational responsibility, completely forgetting the inescapable fact that operation of such equipment itself depends on a considerable amount of technical know-how.

What is the manufacturer's responsibility and its limits? The manufacturer does have a marketing organization, but its duties are very circumspect. The vendor's salesmen may promise the customer that the company will provide training for an operator of the equipment. Once sold, the company representative will drop off an operator's manual and spend an afternoon with the person designated as the operator. The manual is prepared by engineers, and it takes an engineer to understand it. To believe that the person given the task of operating this equipment might have a substantial engineering background is an unwarranted assumption. If the customer is fortunate, his contract includes clauses respecting the duty of the company to train personnel to a competency level. Usually, such courses are conducted at the distributor's classrooms in order to cut training costs. In the event of labor turnover, the customer would then have no recourse whatsoever, the manufacturer having performed according to his contract. Companies decline to train a second set of operators on the basis, justifiably, that the expense of education would exceed the profit on the sale of the equipment. The courses, moreover, are rather superficial. When a man buys a car, the manufacturer does not undertake a full driver's education program, which would qualify him for a driver's license.

Many otherwise competent administrators fall into the trap of not fully digesting the actual impact of the contractual duties assumed by the equipment manufacturer It is true that such companies have a qualified guarantee of biomedical electronic equipment, but what are the conditions limiting that promise? Any damage arising from mishandling or negligent use is specifically excluded from the guaranty clause. As a practical matter, the hospital operates on a 24-hour schedule. It is next to impossible to prevent access to the equipment; it must be immediately available for emergency use. Most vendor's contracts also include the requirement that the equipment be periodically checked and serviced by the seller, and failure to comply absolutely voids the guaranty. If service personnel are then needed, all parts and labor associated with the repairs must be paid. All of these things considerably increase the costs of using this indispensable equipment. It must be concluded that the residual responsibility for training biomedical technologists and technicians will ultimately fall on the hospitals and clinics utilizing their services.

To assist in alleviating this technological dilemma, an indispensable partner in the modern health care team is the biomedical electronics instrumentation technician. For the first time, technicians are being trained to operate all medical electronic equipment likely to be used by even the most progressive hospitals and doctors and to continue this competency through rapidly successive technological advances. Ambitious? Yes, but not before its time. A lot of money is spent on this type of equipment, and few people know how to operate more than one machine. A versatile and competent technician can considerably broaden the potential of any health-care institution to serve better more people in its community.

Open-heart surgery, heart catheterization, ICUs, kidney dialysis, and total automation and computerization of the electrocardiographic field provide proof that two professions, medicine and engineering, can effectively work together.

The advance of medical science has placed a great demand on industry and technology to develop not only advanced machinery but also qualified men and women to monitor, operate, trouble-shoot, and possibly repair the vast amount of new equipment manufactured each year. So far, however, most educational programs have concentrated basically on electronics. Biomedical engineering and other technological programs have proliferated in colleges, universities, and private institutions. There have been recognized deficiencies in past training programs for biomedical engineering technicians. Training must include basic electronics, related physiology, shop mechanics, and intensive physiological laboratory training to perform related biomedical functions in hospitals, clinics, and other medical enterprises.

The development of new equipment has proceeded rapidly with broadened knowledge on the part of doctors and the engineering and technological supporting teams. The earlier attitudes of freezing a technician into a single-function classification is anachronistic. Today, as a result of engineering's significant advances in sophisticated medical equipment, newer and better equipment and new diagnostic capabilities have been created for the practicing physician. The full recognition of his potential hinges, in part, on the versatile and well-educated technician who is enthusiastic about increasing his expertise, welcomes new equipment, and assists actively with the capability of his sponsoring institution.

The continuing influx of sophisticated electronic equipment in hospitals and institutions has resulted in unfavorable expenditures for maintaining, repairing, and utilizing the instrumentation. Formerly, most instrumentation repair was conducted by an outside company or distributor. This service may have been performed in an inadequate, partial, and costly manner. Recently, government-imposed electronic safety requirements and periodic checking of medical instrumentation have increased the overall cost of operation. Therefore, some hospitals have initiated biomedical technologist programs to reduce costs and improve the technical service within the hospital. Technicians are available who possess many years of experience in the biomedical instrumentation field; however, they are very few in number, and there are simply not enough available at a reasonable salary for small institutions. Programs must be directed particularly at small institutions that attempt to operate on an acceptable professional and academic level. The biomedical technologist can help the clinical engineering profession establish high standards for small institutions, which they could not afford otherwise.

44

QUALITY IN PREVENTIVE MAINTENANCE AND EQUIPMENT CONTROL

L. Goodman

An NAE study reported

> (*a*) . . . hospitals generally lack the in-house capability for servicing medical electronic instruments; (*b*) . . . industry feels that, ideally, hospitals should have their own facilities for the maintenance of biomedical equipment. However, the general feeling is that within hospitals there is little awareness of how equipment is operating and a lack of personnel with the capability to determine whether or not equipment is in calibration; (*c*) Hospital and clinical personnel are inadequately trained in the use, operation, and maintenance requirements of technological products and services, and administrators do not appreciate the existence or impact of this inadequacy.

Excerpt (*a*) is well documented in the professional, trade, and popular press; and (*b*) suggests that industry might well reevaluate the relative emphasis they place on market sales versus customer service. Regarding (*c*), it may be agreed that hospital personnel are inadequately trained in the given context. It is not clear, however, how much technical expertise should be expected from nurses, orderlies, interns, and medical practitioners. Furthermore, in fact, probably no one appreciates the existence and critical impact of this inadequacy more thoroughly than the hospital administrator himself. Some of his keenest frustrations derive from the difficulties he faces in obtaining the skills and services he desperately needs. Hospital directors and senior medical staff members have every right to expect that all equipment function reliably, safely, and effectively. Theirs is a critical responsibility, taken very seriously. Small wonder that they may feel impatient and seem somewhat unreasonable about the lack of competent personnel, funds, facilities, and rational guides for action.

The planner's first task is to select the most important problems faced by those concerned with technology and health. The biomedical equipment maintenance service program is one of them. Such medical-equipment maintenance-service programs must be intended to be of significant value to governments, hospitals, clinicians, researchers, bioengineers, educators, and allied biomedical workers and provide comprehensive information on staff, facilities, financing, safety, standards, and related issues pertinent to a variety of technological, social, and economic settings.

The number of conferences and symposia placing emphasis on the practical aspects of equipment management is growing steadily. New technical journals featuring authoritative, useful guidelines for dealing with medical instrumentation are well received.

Innovative university-based programs have emerged that feature direct involvement of engineers in the clinical setting and emphasize the practical aspects of health-care instrumentation. A myriad of relevant summer training courses and special-purpose workshops are regularly conducted by academic institutions, professional organizations, and private enterprise. Substantial resources are being allocated to biomedical-equipment technician training; at least 25 formal BMET training programs are now operational in the United States, with approximately 60 more in the planning stages.

Private entrepreneurs are finding it profitable to offer comprehensive technical services, including equipment maintenance, to health-care institutions. The VA has established a Central Research Instrument Program at their hospital in Little Rock, Arkansas, that devotes considerable energy to devising effective instrumentation management programs for the entire VA system. The Air Force Medical Material Field Office at Phoenixville, Pennsylvania, has innovated methods that provide excellent examples for others to follow and demonstrates the imagination and deep commitment of our armed forces. Individual hospitals and biomedical research institutions are operating comprehensive programs for equipment maintenance, using modern computerized techniques and automatic data processing.

The systems maintenance section (SMS) of the biomedical engineering and instrumentation branch of the NIH maintains and repairs a substantial segment of the scientific apparatus used at NIH in Bethesda, Maryland. SMS is concerned with an equipment inventory valued at approximately $36 million. This represents 60% of the current total NIH scientific equipment complement. The types of instruments it deals with are numerous and may be compared to a typical equipment inventory for a medium-sized research hospital. This suggests the magnitude of the task faced by equipment technicians and biomedical engineers.

In the fiscal year 1972, SMS completed 10,000 "jobs." An average "job" required 4.86 man hours of technician time, with replacement parts and material amounting to 22% of labor costs. These figures might be useful as guides to one who would estimate potential costs for a particular institution. Citation of the actual dollar costs for the SMS operation, although potentially informative, would not be useful here because of the unique circumstances of the federal system.

A task analysis was conducted on a random sample of 2400 from the 10,000 jobs performed in 1 year (Table I). Two particular observations from the study merit

TABLE I
Task Analysis

Man hours	Remove and replace		Performance check		Trouble-shoot and repair		Preventive maintenance		Minor modification		Major modification		Fabrication		Total	
	Jobs	(%)	Jobs	(%)	Jobs	(%)	Jobs	(%)	Jobs	(%)	Jobs	(%)	Jobs	(%)	Jobs	Avg.
0 ≤ 1	30	12.1	43	16.3	79	5.4	8	2.4	4	7.7	2	15.4	2	8.7	168	7.0
1 ≤ 4	163	66.0	151	57.4	720	49.0	119	35.7	17	32.7	3	23.1	4	17.4	1,177	49.0
4 ≤ 8	44	17.8	56	21.3	384	26.1	81	24.3	16	30.8	2	15.4	5	21.7	588	24.5
8 ≤ 40	10	4.0	13	4.9	286	19.5	125	37.5	15	28.8	6	46.2	12	52.2	467	19.5
Total	247	10.3	263	11.0	1,469	61.2	333	13.9	52	2.2	13	0.5	23	1.0	2,400	100

comment. Of the 2400 jobs analyzed, 1469, or 61.2%, were classified as primarily trouble-shooting and repair, and 333 or 13.9% were classified as preventive maintenance.

The significance of the first observation lies in the recognition that trouble-shooting, which constitutes the major fraction of jobs performed, is by far the most challenging task faced by the equipment technician. Very high levels of knowledge and skill in technical fundamentals are required, as well as an intimate awareness of the context of application, be it laboratory, clinic, or surgery. Quality performance in this key function may be expected from well-trained, experienced people who, necessarily, command salaries commensurate with their qualifications. Further, to be effective, they should be regular members of the institution's health-care team. One cannot expect the level of quality required from an odd-job mechanic or part-time television repairman. Although certain private technical services companies might provide adequately skilled technicians, they suffer from being limited to vicarious participation in the everyday work of the institution, its people, and its problems. We are all advised, therefore, to guarantee that the very best technicians are attracted, motivated, trained, and rewarded; to do otherwise is clearly shortsighted and economically false.

The second observation worthy of mention relates to the 13.9% of jobs devoted to preventive maintenance. This perhaps surprisingly low figure is not a result of deliberate design; it derives from the fact that necessary budget constraints forced the section to operate with less than adequate staff over the year of experience described. As a result, priorities had to be given to emergency demands, and scheduled preventive routines had to be delayed. It is felt that a more effective distribution would find twice or more the 13.9% devoted to preventive care. It is certain, given more attention to this area, that the costly and difficult tasks of trouble-shooting and repair would be far less in number than the majority reported.

It is generally agreed and amply demonstrated by experience that a well-designed preventive maintenance program can substantially enhance equipment life and performance while markedly reducing expenses. Explicit quantitative documentation of the economic and operational effects of preventive maintenance is not available for the general category of health-care instrumentation. Certain normative benefits have been claimed, but this author is aware of no thorough controlled study of relevance.

It is agreed that the costs are substantial and may loom enormous when contemplated by the hospital fiscal officer and the board of trustees. The real question, however, is not how much it costs to provide for adequate technical support and preventive maintenance but how much it costs *not* to do so.

One example illustrating this case is the heart-lung bypass machine now used during open-heart surgery on an almost routine basis. It is usually taken for granted that it will work as intended. If, however, it should fail to perform as expected during an operation, a life could be lost. A typical heart-lung machine contains a large number of components, including:

4 peristaltic blood pumps
4 pump speed indicators
2 arterial and venous pressure gauges
1 blood-flow rate meter
1 oxygen-flow-rate meter
2 blood-temperature indicators
1 blood-oxygen sensor
2 oxygenator blood level and tilt indicators
1 oxygenator disk drive indicator
1 blood "debubbler"
1 blood heater
1 multichannel oscillograph
8 variable control circuits
8 manual and automatic fluid valves
6 electric motors
6 override circuits and clutches
24 electrical and mechanical switches
Scores of electrical and fluid connectors, vacuum tubes, transistors, and passive components
Over 500 feet of wires, tubes, and pipes

Normally, nine man hours of cleaning, calibrating, and preventive maintenance are required for a 3-hour duty period in surgery. Standby heart-lung bypass machines, in case of emergency, are not feasible because the time lost during a switchover could be fatal to the patient. (An occasional equipment technician, who feels unappreciated, might comment that standby surgical teams are feasible.)

Several pertinent aspects of preventive maintenance can be revealed by reviewing the experience of one rather substantial ongoing activity. NIH conducts a preventive maintenance program (PM) on light microscopes. The following comments are taken from a discussion with a senior technician who is regularly involved with microscope maintenance and repair.

At present, there are roughly 4000 microscopes on the NIH reservation. Approximately 800 of these are incorporated within the PM program, with about 35% scheduled for semiannual or annual PM depending on usage.

A typical PM routine requires eight man hours and costs, including parts, approximately $135. Many scopes are so old that standard parts are not available; these parts must be specially fabricated in the shop.

In SMS there are two technicians who spend about 60% of their time and one man who spends 35% of his time on microscope maintenance. A supervisor is available for consultation when needed.

Outside firms usually charge about $20 per hour, portal to portal, for labor;

many investigators complain about delays in obtaining service from outside firms and large bills for unproductive time.

Investigators complain about the quality of service provided by many outside firms; the comment is often heard that only the particular item that is broken is repaired and little or no effort is made to check optical alignments, mechanical movements, etc.

Because of continuous and intensive use, the microscopes of the blood bank are routined every 6 months. One area would like to have their scopes serviced every 3 months. At present, this is not feasible because there are not enough people.

Routine PM service reduces emergency calls that might prevent professional researchers from finishing their projects. PM is scheduled between research projects when possible so as to prevent loss of experiments that are in process. If the microscopes break down once a project is ready for microscopic or photographic study, any delay could nullify the results completely.

On routine PM, problems are discovered and corrected while they are minor and are not permitted to develop to a point at which a major overhaul is necessary to place the scope back in operation.

On many occasions, electrical shorts in microscopes have been discovered and corrected on routines. This was computed *before* it became a safety hazard to personnel using scopes. In many labs, personnel are working in wet areas; a 110-V shock could cause an electrocution.

The routine checking of all mechanical movements as to dovetails, rack and pinion, backlash, ease of operation, and other areas for wear and stiffness makes the use of scopes easier on the researchers, who need their attention on their own problems and not on minor irritations of a poor microscope.

On routines, prisms and lenses are heated and corrected that are in the stage of deteriorating, becoming uncemented and cutting down on light transmission, not permitting the scope to be used to its maximum benefit.

Lubrication dries out because of conditions in many labs, such as temperature changes, ultraviolet lighting, ventilation problems, and other reasons. If not serviced routinely, this deterioration will cause damage to the mechanical parts of the scope.

Occasionally, a routine service detects that a lens has been replaced backward by a lab technician. This could have been the cause of severe eye damage to the operators had the situation not been corrected. There are many times that this and similar problems are discovered and corrected on routines. Prior to the present PM program, it took a month for personnel to get action on a trouble call and possibly another month to repair the scope. Researchers cannot tolerate this type of delay in their projects. Thus, every effort is made to keep the delays at a minimum. If a routine is required or desired, it is completed in 2 to 3 days.

On one occasion, an individual had contacted the scope company and was advised that her scope could not be repaired. They could, however, sell her a new one. She was aware that certain particular types of cell formation were present in her slides but could not verify the facts. SMS was called on, and after cleaning, realignment, and a complete overhaul of her microscope, she was able to complete her project satisfactorily with no undue delay and no bill for a new scope.

These same sorts of comments are typical of those made by all who work on preventive maintenance for other types of equipment, such as balances, centrifuges, oscilloscopes, physiological monitors, and X-ray apparatus.

45

MEDICAL EQUIPMENT MAINTENANCE

J. A. Hopps, J. Busser, N. Anderson, A. Colombo, D. Djordjevic, C. Laszlo, J. Lenihan, J. Matauschek, J. McCormick, M. Meyers, M. Milosevic, F. Norman, P. Paraskevopoulos, B. Pendic, S. Pocock, A. Remond, R. Thorner, R. Tomovic, B. Van Eijnsbergen, J. Weinman, M. White, T. Williams, and T. Zeren

Modern health-care delivery depends in an ever-increasing manner on the technology of physical science. The introduction into hospitals of X-ray equipment for patient diagnosis and later for therapy paved the way for a number of diagnostic and therapeutic instruments. Today, there is not a hospital department that does not use electrical, electronic, or mechanical instrumentation in its daily routine. The development of such equipment represents a considerable contribution in research and development by engineers, physicists, and medical investigators and is the more remarkable because, by and large, it has come about without an adequate interface between the scientist or engineer and the medical practitioner.

Thirty years ago, the amount of medical instrumentation was such that a community hospital could manage with a small staff of X-ray technicians and perhaps one or two technically trained people to look after such items as electrocardiographs. The impetus of wartime innovation subsequently led to a new generation of sophisticated equipment that required more maintenance and technical expertise. This advancing technology supported medical developments and, in turn, created a demand for further instrumentation.

The consequence of this trend was an increasing complexity of equipment and dependence on a technology in which few hospital personnel had knowledge or training. Ironically, the design of equipment that simplified its operation by non-technical staff required a complex technology that, in turn, added to maintenance demands.

The repair and maintenance of biomedical instrumentation has become a major concern of health-care institutions. Various procedures for maintenance and repair will be reviewed and criteria recommended for policy determination by a health-care authority, and recommendations will be presented for the structure and operation of a maintenance and repair service.

What Is Biomedical Instrumentation?

Biomedical instrumentation is comprised of any apparatus used to gather or present information about biological systems involved in the science and practice of medicine. It includes equipment designed to monitor a physiological state, diagnose the state of the patient, or effect therapeutic treatment. In a broader sense, it sometimes includes specialized apparatus required to assure the safe and effective care of the ill. In this latter category, data-handling equipment, patient environment control apparatus, and even ''hotel'' items such as beds may be added, for they often involve technical considerations in hospital use. A variety of instrumentation has evolved that generally fits into one of the following categories: diagnostic, therapeutic, monitoring, or housekeeping.

Comprising the diagnostic group are all instruments used for detecting and displaying body potentials (electrocardiograph, electroencephalograph, electromyograph, etc.), equipment for direct or indirect measurement of physiological parameters (electromanometers, blood-flow meters, oximeters, etc.), and apparatus for laboratory analysis of specimens (electrophoresis, spectroscopy, automated chemical analysis, etc.).

Therapeutic equipment includes apparatus for applying radiant energy to the body (X-ray, microwave, diathermy, ultrasonic), equipment for resuscitation (pulmonary respirators, cardiac defibrillators, etc.), prosthetic and orthotic devices (including cardiac pacemakers), physical therapy devices, muscle/nerve stimulators, and surgical support equipment (electrosurgery, pump oxygenators, dialysers, etc.).

Monitoring devices are essentially diagnostic devices used for continuous indication of body parameters (in the OR, ICU or CCU, etc.) or for the patient/staff environment (radiation monitors, ground current detectors, etc.).

Housekeeping items that may be considered as bioinstrumentation in this context include electric beds, signal systems, certain sterilizing apparatus, and, in some instances, data-handling equipment.

The significant factor that differentiates bioinstrumentation from other hospital equipment is that it is *patient oriented* and usually involves a higher level of technology in its design. Hospital authorities sometimes fail to see the difference between the two categories and combine their maintenance services. For any but the simplest of bioinstrumentation, a qualified technical staff is required for routine maintenance and repair.

Maintenance and Repair Service Policies

The introduction of biomedical instrumentation has been a gradual process, although accelerated in recent years. Most medical-care institutions first encounter the maintenance and repair problem in their X-ray departments. It became accepted that technical staff was required for radiological operations. Later, other departments added technologists and technicians to their staffs to handle their individual requirements. Eventually, however, the sheer volume of instrumentation, much of which involved complex technology, required servicing facilities beyond the scope of any individual department. For maintenance and repair of the growing amount of biomedical equipment, a more effective solution was needed.

Several approaches to the maintenance and repair problem have been explored. In some instances, manufacturers' representatives or commercial agencies provide consultation and servicing. Small health-care institutions may depend on the facilities of other medical centers. Health-care institutions may also have to look to government or university sources for technical advice, maintenance, and repair.

For some hospitals, the practical solution has been to establish a medical engineering department responsible for the routine maintenance and repair of all instrumentation. Recent concern about patient safety during investigative or treatment procedures has given impetus to the appointment of technical staff to scrutinize the operation of such equipment. The hiring of biomedical engineers or technicians has added a new dimension to patient care. Several environmental circumstances determine whether or not an in-house biomedical facility will affect the economy of operation, but it will certainly improve the quality of medical care. These are the common modes of managing instrumentation maintenance; however, in addition, there are hybrid combinations.

Economic Considerations

From an economic point of view, maintenance and repair of equipment should be regarded as an integral part of the investment made at the time of instrumentation purchase. Without proper maintenance, instrumentation cannot perform its assigned functions or yield a reasonable lifetime of operation. The cost/benefit considerations applicable to capital investments are equally valid for equipment maintenance. Furthermore, complex considerations involving systems of multiple instrumentation must be resolved in many instances before deciding what combination will give the best performance at the best price with the least outlay for maintenance over a number of years.

Maintenance planning must therefore include the economic aspects. It must reflect operating and maintenance costs, outlays for new equipment, updating of existing items, replacement costs, servicing equipment and instrument expenditures, the availability of funds for quick purchase when necessary, and the economic significance of equipment breakdown.

The economic aspects of maintenance are closely related to the managerial factors at the various levels of health care, a fact rarely considered in developing countries. The acquisition of new equipment is assumed to represent the total financial expenditure for its operation; little thought is given to the costs of maintenance. Inadequate maintenance inevitably degrades the quality and quantity of medical service, and such losses may seriously affect the economy.

A review of the statistics on expenditures for biomedical equipment will provide some idea of the magnitude of the maintenance problem. In short, the biomedical equipment market value averages 3.4% of the total electronic equipment market.

In 1971, the annual market for medical electronic equipment in the United States was approximately $411.5 million. The expenditure per capita in the same year totaled $2.0 million. The annual market for medical electronic equipment by category was (*a*) X-ray, $208 million; (*b*) other diagnostic equipment, $65.6 million; (*c*) therapeutic equipment, $39.8 million; (*d*) patient monitoring equipment, $27.4 million; and (*e*) unspecified equipment, $70.7 million. Thus, it is seen that X-ray apparatus costs account for more than half of the total expenditures.

While these statistics give the overall magnitude of expenditures on biomedical equipment, it is important to note that the actual cost to health-care institutions is considerably higher. For this reason, before the decision is made to purchase a new piece of equipment, the following costs should be considered.

1. Purchase price, including accessories
2. Costs of expendable supplies, plus a minimum stock of supplies for 6–12 months
3. Installation and building costs, if applicable
4. Costs of special tools and equipment for repair and maintenance
5. Cost of special training for operating and maintenance staff
6. Operational costs for maintenance services, power, etc.
7. Funds to cover eventual replacement.

The average life-expectancy figures vary widely depending on the type of equipment, extent of use, and replacement policies; the average value being 8–10 years.

The technical personnel in charge of these instruments should be in a position to provide factual data on the stock of parts and special tools, costs of operation, installation, and maintenance as a routine part of their normal work.

Frequently, hospitals accept gifts of equipment without realizing the full financial, administrative, and technical implications of commissioning operations and subsequent maintenance. There must be a continuing commitment of costs throughout the life span of the equipment. It is important that this concept be emphasized.

Other Factors

There are other considerations beyond economic ones involved in the determination of a hospital policy for the selection and maintenance of biomedical instrumentation. Dependability is of prime importance. How will a breakdown affect the routine of patient diagnosis or treatment? Will equipment failure endanger the patient? Will the selected instrument offer optimal service for the medical workload of the institution? Will it be compatible with other equipment?

The present concern for the safety of a patient undergoing diagnosis or treatment arises from the multiplicity of instrumentation that may be used simultaneously. Each item of equipment may be inherently safe but may interact with other equipment via common connection to the patient. Protection against such hazards requires a systems approach requiring technical expertise in both selection and operation of the components of the system. Such expertise may also be necessary for the calibration of complex equipment to ensure that safe limits of dosage are applied or that measured values are within the desired level of accuracy.

It is apparent that the level of instrumentation in a hospital must be influenced by the quality of its technical service. The corollary is also true: the determination of a maintenance and repair policy must be influenced by the level of instrumentation. It should be noted that instruments that are designed for safe and effective use by nontechnical personnel often involve complex technology and require special expertise in maintenance and repair, whether provided by an in-house service or obtained whole or in part from outside sources.

In order to best utilize the tremendous potential of technology that is available to the health-care system, medical institutions at all levels should consider the establishment of suitable services for their needs. Within the framework of these services, operational mechanisms must be provided to satisfy clinical demands, optimize the cost/benefit ratio within existing economic and technical restraints, allow for professional freedom, and provide opportunity for training, research, and education in the medical-technical area.

The implementation of technological services within a medical institution must begin with an assessment of the required technology. On the basis of such analysis, objectives for technological services can then be defined and a policy delineated for employing technical personnel. The policy should provide incentive, professional recognition of qualified staff, and opportunity for career development.

The Present Role of Bioengineering in Health Care

Until its recent proliferation, the invasion of technology into the hospital had been a progressive one and for many years did not require any particular reorientation of medical practice. The new advances were assimilated, one by one, in the various areas of patient care, and discrete accommodation was made for staff and facilities. However, as this practice continued, it became no longer economical to maintain separate islands of technical expertise. Indeed, the interplay of these services forced an integration of both procedures and personnel.

There is no hospital department that is not dependent on some instrumentation, whether simple or complex. The sum total of their investment in technology grows constantly, and the multiplicity of available equipment presents them with a problem of evaluation that, when added to that of maintaining instrumentation after purchase, requires expertise not often possessed by hospital personnel. Even routine equipment operation requires scrutiny by qualified technical staff to ensure effective and safe use.

Extensive diagnostic or treatment services offered in a hospital involve complex systems of equipment, interconnected by the patient's body. Each component can be used with relative impunity, for it is, or should be, designed with intrinsic safety. When several are used concurrently, there are subtle patient hazards. Many large medical institutions employ professional bioengineers or clinical engineers to consult on the selection and use of equipment and to supervise its maintenance and repair.

Bioengineering techniques serve the modern hospital in several ways. Used in conjunction with medical expertise, they offer diagnostic accuracy and information not attained by other means. In presentation, data storage, or speed of operation, they affect an economy in which labor costs are a significant factor. Bed-occupancy time may be reduced by the use of equipment that gives prompt analysis or diagnostic record.

Modern technology has introduced new noninvasive measuring techniques. Ultrasonic devices delineate internal structures. Infrared scanning detects skin tumors. New electrocardiographic techniques add to the cardiologist's diagnostic information. Skin transducers detect variations of pressure, temperature, and volume. Implanted or ingested radiosondes measure similar parameters within the body. Blood oxygen can be measured with fair accuracy on the ear lobe or finger.

Numerous biomedical devices are used routinely for respiratory control; cardiac resuscitation; pacing; extracorporeal blood circulation; blood dialysis; critical patient monitoring; protein analysis by electrophoresis and other analytical processes; ultrasonic, radio frequency, or microwave heat therapy; electro- and laser surgery; neuromuscular therapy; and a score of other procedures. Electronic devices control patient dosage, program angiography procedures, and intensify X-ray images with low levels of radiation. Powered prostheses use myoelectric and other complex controls.

Computer-based data processing is utilized in hospitals for patient diagnosis, medical-record storage and retrieval, and for many housekeeping operations.

Projected Trends in Biomedical Instrumentation and Services

There are many indicators that suggest the future course of bioinstrumentation. Miniaturization of electronic components and integrated circuits now permits the design of smaller, more compact instruments for medical diagnosis, monitoring, or treatment. Such equipment generally has a low electrical power requirement and can operate from self-contained battery units. The trend to battery-powered instruments will reduce the risk of electric shock that is derived from leakage of electrical service power through equipment.

Miniaturization will also offer new techniques for monitoring or treatment within the body. Small sensing transducers coupled to encapsulated transmitters will provide continuous data on physiological parameters. Similarly, passive implanted units can be commanded from outside the body to stimulate or inhibit muscular excitation. Such devices will find increasing application in techniques and equipment for the handicapped.

The implanted device that has already had great impact is the heart pacer. If lower energy thresholds become possible, one can visualize a pacemaker stimulator of very small proportions implanted on or within the heart without the need for vulnerable leads to the stimulating electrodes.

Clinical measurements require high-technology instruments, and these will increase in number and variety. As more complex instrumentation appears, the need for specialized services for maintenance and repair will become more critical. It is unlikely that the training of hospital staff will provide more technical competence than now exists. Clinical tests based on microscopy, visual cell counting, or blood chemistry analysis will become increasingly more automated. The trend is less apparent in other assessment procedures, and greater effort will be required in such areas.

It is inevitable that the application of computer techniques will increase. Small computers are already in evidence as component parts of medical instrumentation. There will be an expanding role for computer-aided diagnosis. In large institutions, medical computation departments are already appearing. They bring with them a requirement for engineering staff at both professional and technical levels.

At the present time, some of the supposedly immutable analytical techniques are being displaced or challenged, and new concepts will be inevitable in the future. Clinical tests will probably require smaller samples for evaluation. It is probable that the future will bring relatively fewer manufacturers of biomedical instrumentation, thus enhancing the possibility for improved standardization.

Future Delivery of Health Care

The increasing complexity of health care will inevitably prompt more effective planning and control of available resources. The present trend of diminishing general medical practice will continue, with more specialization of medically qualified staff. The rising costs of medical diagnosis and treatment will result in fewer but larger hospitals, supplemented by more health centers and polyclinics offering concentrated facilities for maximum utilization.

Mass screening will play an important role in preventive medicine, an area that offers the optimum economic return for health expenditures. Increasing government support of health care will accelerate this trend. As chemical assessment procedures grow in number and complexity, clinical chemistry "factories" will develop to serve large areas.

Hospital services will become more and more dependent on technological procedures, and nonmedically qualified staff will find greater acceptance. They will handle most of the maintenance of electrical and electronic equipment, with more adequate training and detailed information provided by the manufacturers. In-house staff will probably do most of the first-line maintenance of instruments in clinical or research laboratories. Policies for repair or replacement of equipment, as outlined in this report, will replace the present hit-or-miss procedures.

The present-day concentration on improved reliability of hospital services should be reflected by a trend toward more reliable instrumentation, perhaps with built-in redundancy of power supplies and other subassemblies to reduce breakdown outages. Although the workload will increase, its percentage of the total health-care effort will remain about the same.

In the area of maintaining biomedical instrumentation, this workload will have to be undertaken by staff not involved in plant operations. Past experience has shown that combining these operations seldom produces satisfactory results. Equipment interfacing with the doctor or patient must be the exclusive responsibility of the bioengineering staff. The organization of bioengineering services will vary according to the needs of individual institutions, available technical services and facilities, and considerations of cost effectiveness. The rationale for such determinations is presented in subsequent sections of this report.

Guidelines for the Selection of Instrumentation and Determining a Policy for Its Maintenance and Repair

The Interrelationship Between Instruments and Service

The boundary conditions that apply to the selection of medical instrumentation and to the maintenance and repair service for that instrumentation overlap and interlock. It is, therefore, desirable to consider the two topics together if at all possible.

The types of instrumentation in any given medical care facility are determined primarily by the demands of the medical-care service and second by the kind of maintenance and repair service that is available to keep the instrumentation calibrated and in running order at all times.

In turn, the maintenance and repair service is determined by the types of instrumentation, their design for use in the particular environment of the particular medical-care facility (which are interrelated), the organization of the maintenance facility, and the people who are available to staff the facility (which are also interrelated).

Instrument Selection Guidelines

The needs of the medical-care service will dictate the particular kinds of equipment and instrumentation that will be needed in the performance of that medical care. Thus, in the normal course of events, one will find a certain group of equipment and instruments in use in pediatrics and another, perhaps similar but certainly different in significant degrees, in orthopedics. As the needs of medicine change and become more sophisticated or complex in response to social pressures or advances in medical knowledge, so the instrumentation and equipment that is used will change.

In the selection of particular pieces of equipment or instrumentation to satisfy the needs of the medical service, there are two readily identifiable extremes of choice. Assuming that both extremes will perform the needed function or measurement equally well, one may be extremely simple to operate, have automatic adjustments and calibration functions built in, and indicate to the user when it is in need of maintenance or repair. The other may have many manual adjustments, require calibration with each use, and require some sophistication in the user to tell when it is in need of servicing.

The choice seems obvious and in favor of the automatic device. The choice is not so obvious when one examines the demands placed on the maintenance and repair service by the two kinds of equipment or instrumentation.

The automatic system, which has taken many burdens away from the user/operator, probably required sophistication and/or complexity in its design and the use of a higher level of technology in its construction and functioning. This, in turn, will place a much heavier burden on the maintenance and repair service that must keep it in running order. Building into a device the capability of "knowing" when a given control setting should be changed is much more complex than providing the control and relying on the user or operator to readjust that control. That this kind of design is probably reflected in the selling price of the device is not germane to this discussion. What is important here is the demand placed on a maintenance serviceman or his organization. It is this hidden requirement, which is often not known to the purchaser of the device if he has not had the advice of a bioengineer, that can suddenly place such equipment in the class of undesirables in a particular hospital or medical care facility.

Biomedical Engineering Staff in Hospitals

Levels of Staff

Four levels of biomedical technical staff are commonly found in medical institutions. They are the junior technician, the senior technician, the biomedical engineer, and the physical scientist. Many small hospitals employ an electronics technician to maintain and repair equipment. When the workload requires three junior technicians, a senior technician may supervise their activities. The addition of a biomedical engineer provides the nucleus of a biomedical engineering department. Such a unit would probably require an administrative assistant. Two teams, comprised of three junior and one senior technician and a bioengineer in each, constitute a department that may profit from the addition of a physical scientist. The combined unit can then be classified as an applied science or a biophysics department. Large teaching hospitals may require additional personnel for teaching assignments, inventory control, clerical duties, etc.

It is not enough for a hospital administration to decide on its required number of technical and scientific personnel in a biomedical unit. There is need for careful consideration of the scope of operation; the financial and facility resources for its function; the hierarchy of its administration; its status in the hospital family; in-house training of and by its staff; salary scales and opportunities for career advancement; required staff qualifications; and probable interface with other hospital departments or health-care organizations, the industrial sector, and, where applicable, government.

The Junior Technician

This individual carries out minor repairs and assists with the maintenance of relatively simple equipment. His qualifications can range from high school education with some technical training to more extensive technical experience without formal training. In a small institution, he may be responsible to a specific medical department head. In a larger organization, he will probably be supervised by a senior technician or bioengineer. A specific budget and simple tools and test equipment must be provided for his needs. His salary scale and advancement prospects must be comparable to those of medical technicians in the institution. Although a relatively junior employee, he may be the only person who can give intelligent advice on equipment operation, and he should have reasonable opportunity to do so.

The Senior Technician

The need for such a person arises with the purchase of sophisticated equipment that requires preventive maintenance, repair, and calibration. The senior technician should have a high school diploma plus 2 or 3 years of technical training or the equivalent education through experience, trade schools, and/or special courses. It is desirable that he be well qualified in electronics or medical instrumentation principles.

His responsibility is the maintenance and repair of complicated apparatus, and he should understand the physiological rationale of its application. He should also have competence to recognize problems in measurement and calibration and to solve the more basic ones. He must be able to specify replacement of spare parts, install equipment, and direct junior technicians. In a small organization, he may be the individual on whose technical opinion the medical practitioner must depend. He must, therefore, have the capability to carry out his task without technical guidance.

The senior technician should have an appropriate shop or small laboratory equipped with test equipment, tools, and commonly used components. His responsibility should be to either the hospital administrator or a senior medical official. There should be an explicit budget to improve his facilities as the workload changes or expands. It has been suggested that his salary and career prospects be at least comparable to those of a registered nurse in a progressive health-care institution.

A qualified senior technician is an expert in his field and should have recognition as such. Every effort should be made to provide easy communication between him and the medical personnel so that mutual education is possible. He should keep himself informed about industrial developments and keep up with the state of the instrumentation art so he can advise on the selection and purchase of new equipment.

The Biomedical Engineer

In a larger facility, the bioengineer administers the department, supervises the technical personnel, coordinates the technological activities of the institution, analyzes data, and advises the administrative and medical staff on technological matters. His academic background should be at the university graduate level, preferably with biomedical engineering training with emphasis on systems engineering, data processing, electronics, and clinical procedures.

The major task of the bioengineer is to organize his department in all the functions of instrumentation selection, installation, maintenance, and repair; be responsible for the teaching and training of medical staff who will operate the equipment; modify and occasionally design apparatus for specific needs; consult; and participate in technological planning.

The bioengineer should report to the hospital administrator for administrative and financial matters. He should have the rank of head of department and represent it at meetings with other department heads. It is essential that he be given status in the hierarchy of the hospital, with a salary scale and career potential equal to those of an engineer with equivalent responsibilities in industry or government. He must be provided with the opportunity to advance or update his education.

The hospital administration should recognize the biomedical engineer as its spokesman in technological discussions. The biomedical engineer should provide interface with colleagues in related fields (statisticians, physicists, etc.) and develop cooperation and constructive interaction with medical and paramedical personnel. Above all, he must be aware of his moral and ethical responsibility to the doctor and the patient.

The Scientist

The scientist enters the health-care environment when the interaction of technology and medicine is required at a high level, as in a teaching hospital. He must be a scientific generalist, with such multidisciplinary backgrounds as biology, medicine, and technology. His academic training must be at the master's or doctorate level.

In the context of this report, it is assumed that the scientist will head the technical services department, which will generally include medical physics in its title. With this assumption, the scientist must have the responsibilities listed for the biomedical engineer. However, the facilities provided must include an up-to-date research laboratory with the backing of specialists, as he will have additional responsibility for research, whether independently or as part of a clinical program. In the teaching hospital environment, the design and development of instruments may become an important function of the scientist's organization.

It is customary for a hospital scientist to have a university appointment at the professorial level. He may direct or administer in-house or external research programs. Several budgets may be required to satisfy the operational, research, development, and teaching programs under his control.

Not all health-care institutions require extensive technical services. They may draw their help from regional centers or larger units of the health service. However, somewhere in the system, technical personnel must cope with the maintenance and repair of biomedical instrumentation. The staff categories listed herein are those most commonly encountered where in-house service is provided, with the exception of the scientist, whose function is unique to a specific type of institution. This last position is included merely to complete the classification, not to suggest that maintenance and repair services require a staff scientist. Subsequent sections will give guidelines for determination of the specific needs of various types and sizes of health-care units.

In the context of this article, the term technician refers to the instrumentation technician with training in physical science, not to a laboratory technician with a biological background. It has become practice to make this differentiation clear by use of the term *biomedical equipment technician* (BMET) and to classify the staff members who use the equipment for patient diagnosis or laboratory analysis as technologists. The emphasis on their training and function is different and it is important that we recognize the distinction.

Hospital patient care depends more and more on the technology of science, and it is essential that the decision to employ technical personnel be made with cognizance of the need for their integration into the health-care family. The medical practitioner must realize that technology will play an increasing role in his profession and that he must make an adjustment to both technology and technically oriented staff. On the other hand, the technical staff must recognize that the doctor has the final responsibility for the care of his patient. Both must work together for the good of the patient.

It must also be observed that the structure of a biomedical engineering department or equipment service facility as presented here is not necessarily the best solution for all hospitals. Every health-care institution has its unique and individual needs, and the technological support organization must be tailored to these needs. Health-care systems and structures vary widely throughout the world and even within a region. Health-care demands are dictated by the local environment and the services by many restraints. An attempt has been made only to touch on the broad aspects of biomedical equipment maintenance and to stress the essential human and social aspects of technological services in a hospital.

What Equipment Should a Hospital Accept?

The choice of the proper equipment to satisfy a specific clinical need affects the speed and efficiency of the desired medical service. Its proper selection is the first step toward an effective equipment maintenance program and should be made with great care. Too often, the hospital administration is dependent on the literature or promotion offered by manufacturers or their agents. Technical guidance invariably leads to a more intelligent determination. This function is in fact one of the more important contributions that can be provided by a medical engineering service, whether in-house or external to the institution. The medical engineer can and should evaluate the design quality of the instrumentation, its mode of operation and performance, and, above all, its probable maintenance demands.

Commitment to a maintenance and repair policy begins from the moment of purchase. The initial investment in equipment may be much smaller than the cost of its maintenance. Thus, a relatively small savings in the purchase of a less expensive instrument may result in increased maintenance costs. This is true in other areas of endeavor, but in the delivery of health care, the consequence of failure makes it a mandatory concept.

If quality is the first consideration in purchase of equipment, availability of parts or service must come second. The most sophisticated equipment is of little use if it cannot be maintained or repaired without delay. The wise purchaser will examine the service policy of the seller, the advisability of buying reasonable spares, the accessibility of the instrument for servicing, the maintenance data provided by the manufacturer, and the local availability of parts, service facilities, and expertise. Since all these desirable features are seldom available, the buyer should seek to optimize his choice.

Standardization is an important concept in the selection of instrumentation. Whether it be within an institution or a widespread system, the consistent use of proven models of equipment reduces the volume of spares that must be stocked and the number of maintenance and repair procedures that must be undertaken. It also strengthens the bargaining power of the health-care system in dealing with the manufacturer in purchase or repair contracts.

Compatibility of new items with existing equipment is essential. In modern clinical practice, instruments are often integrated into a diagnostic or therapeutic system. The buyer who attempts to purchase without technical guidance may well end up with an "orphan" that will not fit into the system.

Compatibility of power sources will become of greater importance in the developing trend toward battery-powered instruments. Not only will it be necessary to standardize the types of batteries used in order to reduce inventory, but the investment for recharging facilities may be decreased. Standardization of power connectors and other hardware will also affect economy and contribute to safety.

Closely associated with compatibility is versatility. A patient-monitoring instrument with provision for external display or interchangeable functional modules is more useful than single-purpose equipment. Additional channels may be added as the need arises. The module concept also facilitates replacement or repair.

The next consideration must be the suitability of equipment for its intended use, environment, and local custom. Thus, equipment that automates many functions that can be done safely and in an acceptable time manually may not be advantageous in an economy in which labor is plentiful and inexpensive. Similarly, an instrument designed for laboratory research may not be appropriate for clinical use, and equipment designed for a temperate climate may break down when subjected to the high temperature and humidity of tropical regions.

On the other hand, there are occasions when the buyer may seek equipment that reduces the decision-making demands by the user in order to obtain the maximum utilization with the minimum expertise. In such instances, he must accept the more complex technology inherent in the design of such instruments. In a sense, he must trade off medical for technical expertise and must weigh the cost of this when he makes the purchase.

Operational costs may be a significant factor in selecting equipment. Does the instrument consume excessive power? Does it require expensive chart paper? Does it need conditioning of the environment for dependable operation? Will it require extensive staff training for operation or maintenance?

The probable period of use before obsolescence of either the equipment or the clinical need should be considered. Solid-state electronics (transistors, printed and integrated circuits) revolutionized the design of most electromedical instruments in a few short years. In many instances, its improved performance, reduced size and power demands, and longer operational life rendered the previous generation of equipment obsolete. Many complex systems have been developed for automated chemical analysis at a great savings of time and effort. However, some of the routine tests are now being replaced, as diagnostic needs change. A complete generation of this equipment may be obsolete within the next 5 years. Obsolescence cannot be predicted with certainty, but there are indicators in technology and clinical practice that need to be read in determining instrumentation requirements.

Concern must be focused on safety in medical instrumentation. Most instruments are intrinsically safe when their interface with the patient is at the body surface. However, we are becoming committed to more and more diagnostic or therapeutic procedures that invade the inner tissues of the body. In that milieu, the threshold of electric shock hazard is much more critical. Many safety standards now call for classification of electromedical instrumentation into categories according to the hazard associated with its use. These standards specify safe design features and designate acceptable limits for fault currents. Compliance with such specifications should be an invariable condition of purchase.

These are the cardinal guidelines for the selection of medical instrumentation. They should be applied, where possible, to the acceptance of donated equipment. Gifts of equipment and instruments pose very special problems in a health-care system. They may create operational and maintenance expenditures far in excess of their initial cost and in every case will require some continued outlay by the recipient. The embarrassment involved in specifying requirements for donated instrumentation may be far less than the embarrassment incurred later in explaining why it is out of service.

The selection of equipment must be followed up by inspection on arrival. Failure to do so may invalidate any claim against the supplier and will invariably increase the maintenance and repair burden. If this seems to be an unlikely occurrence, consider what happens when equipment is ordered at the time of construction of a new facility. It usually remains in a packing case until the facility is completed. It is later discovered that the patient applicators are missing, there is no maintenance manual or parts list, rodents seem to have eaten the insulation off wires, and the shipment has been dropped in transit. If the warranty is located, it will probably have expired. The work and expense of repair commences before the equipment ever sees service. It is essential that inspection be linked to selection as the first step in an equipment maintenance repair program.

What Are the Bioengineering Demands?

Before attempting to determine a policy for the maintenance and repair of instrumentation, the health-care authority should look at the demands of the institution or system for bioengineering services. These will be dependent on many factors and may differ widely between hospitals or regions.

Maintenance requirements are dictated by the amount of instrumentation and equipment, its use (and abuse), complexity, and environmental conditions that may accelerate degradation or failure. The amount and type of instrumentation is determined in turn by the size of the health-care establishment, the nature of patient treatment, indigenous health problems, the extent of dependence on other regional facilities, and economic limitations.

Other bioengineering service demands are conditional on the sophistication of diagnostic or therapeutic procedures; safety considerations; the extent of clinical research, development or hospital planning; and the need for technological consultation in the procurement or installation of equipment. The complexity and amount of instrumentation are good indices of service requirements.

Some instruments are relatively insensitive to damage from extended use. X-ray equipment is not. The manufacturer usually gives guidance on the recommended duty cycle. If it is ignored, the life of the X-ray tube and perhaps the high-voltage supply will be foreshortened. The X-ray transformer oil cooling system demands rigorous attention in hot climates. Since radiography equipment constitutes a large proportion of hospital instrumentation, its extent and use offers a useful index to the probable service needs of the institution.

Climatic extremes influence service demands. Electrical components are vulnerable to damage from high humidity. Solid-state circuitry is sensitive to excessive heat. Exposure to cold may destroy components of diagnostic instruments or defibrillators. Sand or other airborne pollution has a most deleterious effect on equipment.

A large health-care center has unique demands for maintenance expertise, depending on the services it offers. Neurosurgery and cardiac surgery involve complex support equipment and diagnostic instruments. The postoperative monitoring array alone may well equal the total volume of instrumentation of a small institution. Automated analysis and other laboratory equipment have diverse maintenance and servicing needs.

In large hospitals, there are many complex diagnostic systems in which technical expertise is mandatory to effect compatible and safe application to the patient. If computer data-handling services are provided, they will require maintenance staff in addition to the technically trained personnel who process the data.

The consequence of equipment failure must be considered in the assessment of technical service requirements. Will a delay in restoring it to service endanger life-support systems or even slow up treatment procedures and extend the bed-care period to an overload condition? If so, in-house technical staff or quick access to external help must be itemized as a bioengineering service demand.

The quality of public utilities and other services will affect maintenance needs. If the line voltage of the power system varies beyond normal limits, it will degrade the performance of instrumentation and perhaps lead to its failure. Failures or impurities in the water supply will increase the incidence of equipment breakdown.

There are a number of bioengineering services usually associated with various types of health-care institutions. Some of these services include number of beds, purchase evaluation, incoming inspection, safety inspection, instrument calibration, etc. In all cases, there is a need for some sort of preventive maintenance and basic technical instruction on the use of instrumentation.

The mass screening unit or clinic is primarily a diagnostic center and has an additional demand for instrument calibration service. The consequence of failure generally does not require a staff allocation for emergency repair unless the unit is large.

On the other hand, to a rural hospital, some sort of emergency repair facility is much more vital than instrument calibration. Neither type of institution is likely to need in-house staff specifically for maintenance and repair or safety inspection. This should not suggest that these areas are totally neglected. In small hospitals, the medical, paramedical, and nursing staff traditionally accept some responsibility for the maintenance and safe use of their instrumentation. Many urban hospitals have some sort of inspection service for new equipment or instruments, and the large university teaching hospitals usually draw on bioengineering services for the purchase of medical equipment.

What Is the Best Maintenance Service Policy

The dependence of modern health care on technology in diagnosis of diseases, therapeutic procedures, and monitoring of the critically ill makes the maintenance and repair of medical instrumentation a vital necessity. Inevitably, equipment will need maintenance or repair, and medical institutions at all levels must consider the establishment of a service structure for this purpose. It may be an "endoskeleton" or an "exoskeleton," but if it is not provided, effective patient care will collapse.

The determination of a maintenance service policy must take into account the restraints imposed by socioeconomic factors, geographical limitations, the environment, the level of medical practice, and the available technology.

As previously stated, health-care authorities often fail to recognize that the economic aspects of hospital equipment maintenance are linked to essential managerial concepts. There is frequently no acceptance of the fact that it may cost more to maintain equipment than to buy it and that such continuing expenditures must be considered as part of the total investment. The additional costs incurred at breakdown because of disruption of normal procedures and possible damage to other facilities must also be considered. In economic terms, poor maintenance will lead eventually and inevitably to a waste of the health system's assets.

Any effective program for management of medical instrumentation must be based on a realistic appraisal of instrumentation costs and available financial resources. The program will be limited by its financial support and must therefore, eliminate areas of endeavor that are out of economic reach.

If a health-care authority chooses to establish its own service agency, it should examine the cost of staff, training, testing, repair facilities, spare-parts inventory, and the maintenance plant itself. It should then compare these costs with those incurred in hiring commercial service plus dispatching defective equipment for repair. It may be practical to utilize the maintenance services of government departments, research laboratories, or universities; however, the consequence of inadequate repair or excessive delay must be considered in deciding on such an alternative.

The effectiveness of maintenance and repair may be influenced by accessibility, assessed in terms of time rather than distance. It may be quite feasible to provide effective service at a remote location if transportation is fast and available. In today's world, distance no longer imposes an insurmountable barrier, while speed of execution becomes increasingly more important. This concept goes beyond national boundaries. It may be more satisfactory, in some instances, to ship equipment abroad than to attempt to provide home facilities for its repair. This is particularly true for developing countries in which priorities must be assigned to domestic development. The administration, however, must ensure that provision is made for prompt dispatch to minimize the out-of-service period.

A comprehensive maintenance and repair policy may include both in-house and contracted services. It is realistic to use the latter where available and concentrate the in-house facilities on services that are less accessible.

In some areas, commercial or other outside facilities are more limited. The greatest likelihood of such help is in X-ray technology. Manufacturers' representatives offer maintenance and repair services and will usually cooperate with a health-care system in planning a program to serve its needs. Other major suppliers of biomedical equipment may not have regional agents, but generally are sympathetic to the maintenance and repair problems of the user and can give constructive advice on routine servicing and maintenance manuals and offer recommendations on the quantity and number of spare parts required in normal repair procedures. The recommendation simply expressed is "do not compete with outside services, collaborate with them."

It is an almost inevitable conclusion that some in-house technical maintenance and repair staff will be required. This staff should not be associated with the routine plant maintenance services. Such an association has been attempted by many hospitals and has proved unsuccessful. If the institution or system is large, a bioengineering service should be organized as an autonomous department. It is best located at a large medical center so that it maintains contact with clinical programs. If it serves a system of other institutions, the autonomous structure is essential to ensure equitable service to all.

The central service agency concept works very well if provision is made for prompt response to the needs of the more remote parts of the system. It may be supplemented by institutional or regional representatives whose function is to provide routine preventive maintenance and minor repairs. A hospital of 100 beds will have a minimum of 80 items of biomedical equipment. The average time required for service of each item is about 10 hours per year. Thus, this activity will occupy about half of one technician's time. The balance can be profitably spent in assistance to or training of equipment operators, maintenance of spares, institution of safety measures, updating of his own training, and other activities. By comparison, if each piece of equipment were sent to the manufacturer or an agent for service, the cost at current rates would be about $20,000 per year. Even if available, such services would not cover all the activities essential to the effective operation of a biomedical maintenance and repair program.

Consideration should be given to establishing a pilot-plant prototype at a large medical center, which could become the nucleus of a bioengineering service or a model for further development. Thus, a focal point would be established for the development of technical and professional bioengineering expertise.

The development of a maintenance and repair facility should be linked with the planning of new health-care centers. The role of a central medical engineering agency in technical training should not be overlooked. In an area in which there is little or no research or industrial activity in bioengineering, there is no other base from which to draw expertise.

The health-care authority, in planning the facility best suited to its institutional needs, should consider possible adjuncts to a maintenance and repair operation. The bioengineering center might provide an instrument pool to serve transient hospital needs and allocate the disposal of older equipment for staff training, research use, rebuilding, or dismantling. A pool of laboratory services could answer the needs of many institutions.

Finally, it must be repeated that no biomedical equipment maintenance service program will be effective if the need for funds, staff, facilities, and transport is not fulfilled; if the program is tied to general maintenance services; or if the organization is not given sufficient autonomy to implement the program.

46

IN-HOSPITAL MEDICAL EQUIPMENT MAINTENANCE: BIOMEDICAL INSTRUMENTATION DEPARTMENT

G. R. Goodman

In-hospital equipment maintenance has assumed a wealth of organizational structures and names. This and the following chapter are examples of two model systems: (1) the Biomedical Instrumentation Department of three hospitals functioning as a joint facility for St. Luke's Espiscopal Hospital, Texas Children's Hospital, and the Texas Heart Institute. These institutions are located in the Texas Medical Center in Houston, Texas, and (2) a Division of Electronics and Biological Engineering, which covers one facility, the Sinai Hospital of Baltimore. We begin with this chapter on the Biomedical Instrumentation Department.

The department strives to accomplish four basic goals: (*a*) documentation; (*b*) evaluation; (*c*) repair and preventive maintenance; and (*d*) training. Table I gives statistics showing the needs.

The organizational chart in Figure 1 shows the operation of a hospital-based maintenance group. The department director answers directly to administration, with no direct medical staff involvement in managing the department. It is a more difficult set-up to establish; however, it does give all medical services an opportunity to influence their own equipment needs. Also, it allows greater freedom to handle problems and needs by what is right technically and by what the medical service most directly involved desires. There are five levels of technicians and an attempt made to provide for both the 2-year technical school graduate and the 4-year technologists. All technicians answer directly to the department director as emphasis on the concern for a successful repair and preventive maintenance (PM) program. All junior-level technicians are on a 4-month rotation program through the equipment groups.

TABLE I
Relevant Statistics[a]

1.	1066 PATIENT BEDS.
2.	2600 FULL-TIME EMPLOYEES.
3.	100 PERMANENTLY MONITORED INTENSIVE CARE BEDS.
4.	80 PORTABLE EKG MONITORS FOR ADDITIONAL ICU NEEDS.
5.	31 PERMANENTLY MONITORED OR ROOMS.
	a. 8 CARDIOVASCULAR ROOMS.
	b. 1 NEUROSURGERY ROOMS.
	c. 5 CYSTO ROOMS.
6.	MONTHLY AVERAGE FOR 1974 OF *1760* SURGERY CASES.
7.	MONTHLY AVERAGE FOR 1974 OF *389* CARDIOVASCULAR SURGERY CASES.
8.	7 CATH LABS.
9.	31 ROOMS OF X-RAY.
10.	APPROXIMATELY 4000 INDIVIDUAL PIECES OF PATIENT-RELATED BIOMEDICAL EQUIPMENT.

[a]These statistics reflect the more than ample opportunity and motivation to establish engineering groups in many of the medical departments in the hospital.

Documentation

The first goal of the department, the documentation system, is the basis for all efforts. The records are required by both the Joint Commission on the Accreditation of Hospitals and the State of Texas' Department of Public Health. The documents are a modification of the system proposed by the Emergency Care Research Institute in 1971.

The basic record is the control card. The first part of the control card shows all necessary purchasing and identification information. The second half of the card shows the repair and PM information for the device. Each service report is reviewed, and a brief entry is posted on the card. The Kardex, of which there are three to hold 4800 individual cards, makes reference extremely easy. The top card is the general-information card, while the bottom card shows the maintenance history. The repair forms (Equipment Service Report [ESR]) are standard repair forms. They are four-part forms and are sequentially numbered for filing and reference. The PM form (Equipment Inspection Report [EIR]) is also sequentially numbered for easy filing and reference. All PM forms have a standard format.

Evaluation

The second goal of the department is the prepurchase evaluation of equipment. A condition of sale form is employed. These conditions are added to the purchase order prior to being sent to the purchasing department. The engineering specifi-

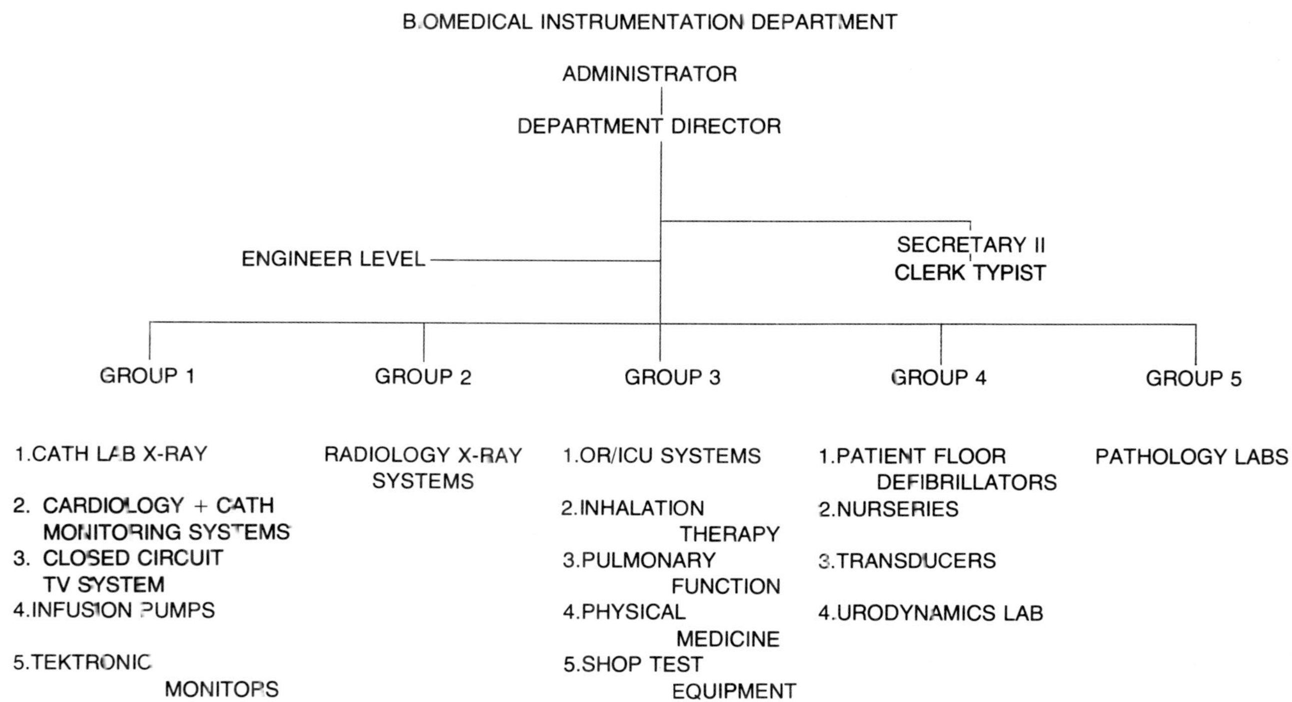
BIOMEDICAL INSTRUMENTATION DEPARTMENT
ADMINISTRATOR
DEPARTMENT DIRECTOR
ENGINEER LEVEL
SECRETARY II
CLERK TYPIST
GROUP 1
GROUP 2
GROUP 3
GROUP 4
GROUP 5
1.CATH LAB X-RAY
2. CARDIOLOGY + CATH MONITORING SYSTEMS
3. CLOSED CIRCUIT TV SYSTEM
4.INFUSION PUMPS
5.TEKTRONIC MONITORS
RADIOLOGY X-RAY SYSTEMS
1.OR/ICU SYSTEMS
2.INHALATION THERAPY
3.PULMONARY FUNCTION
4.PHYSICAL MEDICINE
5.SHOP TEST EQUIPMENT
1.PATIENT FLOOR DEFIBRILLATORS
2.NURSERIES
3.TRANSDUCERS
4.URODYNAMICS LAB
PATHOLOGY LABS

Fig. 1.

cations are evaluated as well as the actual performance of the device. It is possible for a device to meet design specifications but not perform clinically because the specifications are unrealistic.

There are, naturally, some problems. One problem arises from members of the medical staff who insist on a particular manufacturer. An attempt is made to abide by this desire unless there is a definite quality difference or if it varies from the brand of other equipment satisfactorily performing the same function in the hospital. Purchases made with private funds available to the physician were a problem until the hospital began to stress its ultimate liability for patient safety and diagnostic accuracy.

Repair and Preventive Maintenance

The third goal, repair and preventive maintenance, is the most active area. Nothing will decrease the support for a program faster than defective equipment and equipment endlessly delayed in repair. As mentioned, a sequentially numbered ESR for documentation is used. It is a four-part form with distribution to the owner department, accounting, and any outside service representative. The charge is by the hour for all work and billed once a month through accounting to the owner department.

The charge-back does two things. It first shows the exact cost to maintain a piece of equipment versus the inflated patient charge for the equipment usage. Second, it insulates the department from time-consuming and/or irrelevant tasks.

For the PM program, a form is used having a format showing a sequence of inspection results. This makes posting of old inspection data and filing much easier. Data such as leakage currents from previous inspections as well as any comments from the previous inspection are readily available. The forms are sequentially numbered for filing and reference.

A standard format is used for the EIR. This format reserves the first five items of all inspections to the same series of visual inspections and reserves the first two items of the operational checks to the leakage current from the chassis and leads, respectively.

The standard format gives a degree of organization to the forms and has made them appear more uniform and logical to the inspectors. The standard format is also necessary to simplify documentation of what the inspection involves. For this documentation, inspection notes are used that describe in detail the type of device inspected, the equipment needed, repair frequency, an item by item description of the test to be performed and the acceptable results, and a bibliography giving the source of the information used for the inspection procedure, even if it is only the manufacturer's service manual.

It is estimated that there are 5500 hours of preventive maintenance work (inspection, calibration, and cleaning) per year to cover the equipment. By comparison, an individual has available per year 1924 working hours if he is 100% efficient.

Training

The fourth and final goal of the department, training, has been the most difficult to achieve. Here, size of the institution does serve as a negative factor. The most effective technique seems to have the technicians make frequent rounds of their assigned areas looking for problems and instructing as they encounter problems or questions. In conjunction with the nursing in-service department, in-house-produced videotapes and slide presentations are being used because of the need to continually retrain and also to account for the traditionally high turnover rate of nurses.

For the technicians in the department, there is easy access to the nursing in-service program. For each technician on the rotation program, there is a response protocol. This document gives the technicians a written description of the dos and don'ts of the area to which they are assigned and also gives them a list of all supervisors in the area. It also serves as documentation that a technician has been given the proper basic information he needs to function successfully.

Conclusions

A series of efficiency reports have been developed to allow examination of proper direction of effort for the department. These efficiency reports give a weekly and monthly composite of how well each of the equipment areas performed in relation to actual hours worked. They show in what areas the time was spent, that is, repair, preventive maintenance, long-term projects, and supplemental activities. The same information is shown for the department as a whole. Supplemental activities, special procedure monitoring, such as Swan-Gantz and intracranial pressure, intraaortic balloon pumping, and the many service calls that are set-up problems or operator problems and do not involve an actual repair account for as much time as equipment repairs. The supplemental activities are extremely difficult to document. A great deal of success was found using a daily supplemental activity card.

The department has an average weekly efficiency of 64% broken down into the following categories:

1. Emergency repairs—28%
2. Preventive maintenance—12%
3. Long-range repairs—6%
4. Supplemental activities—18%
5. Total—64%

The department places the greatest emphasis on the establishment and continuance of an effective repair and PM program. The efficiency reports show that this is being accomplished. With this done, it is then and only then appropriate to begin the balance of a program and in particular the much sought after equipment modification and design phase.

Appendix

A number of the forms that have been successfully used can be used as models. They are reproduced in this appendix.

EQUIPMENT CONTROL RECORD — CONTROL NO.__________

ITEM			
MANUFACTURER			MODEL
SERIAL NUMBER	ACQUISITION COST	DATE PLACED IN SERVICE	WARRANTY EXPIRES
VENDOR			PURCHASE ORDER NO.
OWNER OR DEPARTMENT		NORMAL LOCATION(S)	
CALIBRATION FREQUENCY		PREVENTIVE MAINTENANCE FREQUENCY	

882 - RRNT-36038A

Fig. 1. The first part of the control card shows all necessary purchasing and identification information.

FINAL DISPOSITION OF EQUIPMENT	DATE

INSPECTION AND MAINTENANCE SUMMARY

882 - RRNT-36038 B

DATE	TIME OUT OF SERVICE	WORK PERFORMED	E S R NUMBER	E I R NUMBER	PARTS AND LABOR COST

CHECK HERE IF CONTINUED ON REVERSE SIDE__________ CARD NO.__________

TAG NUMBER	EQUIPMENT DESCRIPTION	MONTHLY SCHEDULING											
		JAN.	FEB.	MAR.	APR.	MAY	JUN.	JUL.	AUG.	SEP.	OCT.	NOV.	DEC.

Fig. 2. The second part of the control card shows the repair and PM information for the device.

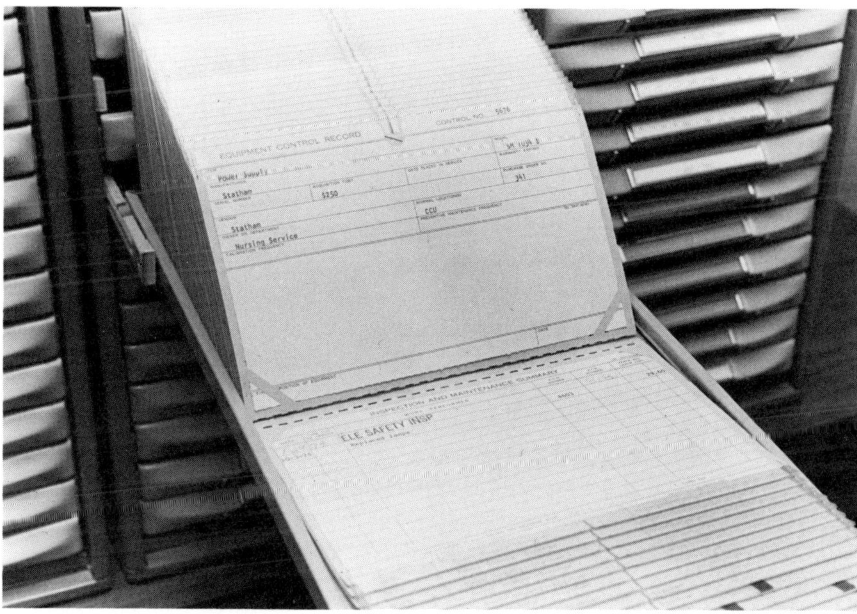

Fig. 3. The Kardex showing the general information card for one device (top card) and the maintenance history for this device (bottom card).

BIOMEDICAL INSTRUMENTATION DEPARTMENT
SERVING
St. Luke's Episcopal Hospital
Texas Children's Hospital
Texas Heart Institute
Extension 4277 or 3633

EQUIPMENT INSPECTION REPORT

NO. I-

CONTROL NO.

TYPE OF DEVICE ______

LOCATION ______ SERIAL NO. ______

MODEL ______ MANUFACTURER ______

VISUAL INSPECTION

	O.K.	ACTION NEEDED	ACTION TAKEN (Date & Initials)
1. ATTACHMENT PLUG ______			
2. LINE CORD & STRAIN RELIEFS ______			
3. PHYSICAL CONDITION:			
A. General condition of instrument ______			
B. Paddles, Cables, & Connectors ______			
C. Condition of Controls, Indicators & Meter ______			
4. GROUNDING RESISTANCE: ______ Ohms ______			
5. FUSE ______			
6. ELECTRODE PASTE OR SALINE PADS ______			
7. POSITION OF CONTROLS ______			
8. ______			

OPERATION

9. D.C. & A.C. LEAKAGE CURRENT TO CHASSIS (Circle unacceptable values):

	OFF		OPERATING (List Modes) ______		______				
PROPERLY GROUNDED	____	____ uA	____	____ uA	____	____ uA			
UNGROUNDED, Correct Polarity	____	____	____	____	____	____			
UNGROUNDED, Reversed Polarity	____	____	____	____	____	____			
	D.C.	A.C.	D.C.	A.C.	D.C.	A.C.			

10. D.C. & A.C. LEAKAGE CURRENT TO PADDLES OR CABLES (Circle unacceptable values):

	OFF		OPERATING (List Modes) ______		______				
PROPERLY GROUNDED	____	____ uA	____	____ uA	____	____ uA			
UNGROUNDED, Correct Polarity	____	____	____	____	____	____			
UNGROUNDED, Reversed Polarity	____	____	____	____	____	____			
	D.C.	A.C.	D.C.	A.C.	D.C.	A.C.			

SLTC-THI O-50 5/72

	O.K.	ACTION NEEDED	ACTION TAKEN (Date & Initials)
11. CHARGING TIME TO MAXIMUM ENERGY SETTING: ____ Sec. to ____ W-sec. Previous Value: ____ Sec.			
12. INTERNAL DISCHARGE OF STORED ENERGY ____			

13. OUTPUT ENERGY (watt-seconds):

CONTROL SETTING	INDICATED ENERGY	DELIVERED ENERGY	PREVIOUS VALUE	CHANGE

14. ENERGY DELIVERED AFTER 1 MINUTE, MAXIMUM SETTING: ____ W-Sec.

15. OUTPUT OF TENTH REPEATED DISCHARGE, MAX. SETTING: ____ W-Sec.

16. SYNCHRONIZER OPERATION ____

COMMENTS & DESCRIPTION OF DEFICIENCIES (Refer to item numbers) ____

☐ TYPE A INSPECTION TAG AFFIXED
☐ TYPE B INSPECTION TAG AFFIXED
☐ GROUND WARNING TAG AFFIXED
☐ EQUIPMENT SERVICE REQUEST FORM COMPLETED

ESR No. ____

INSPECTED BY ____

DATE ____

Fig. 4. Equipment inspection report (EIR). Space is adequate for one inspection only.

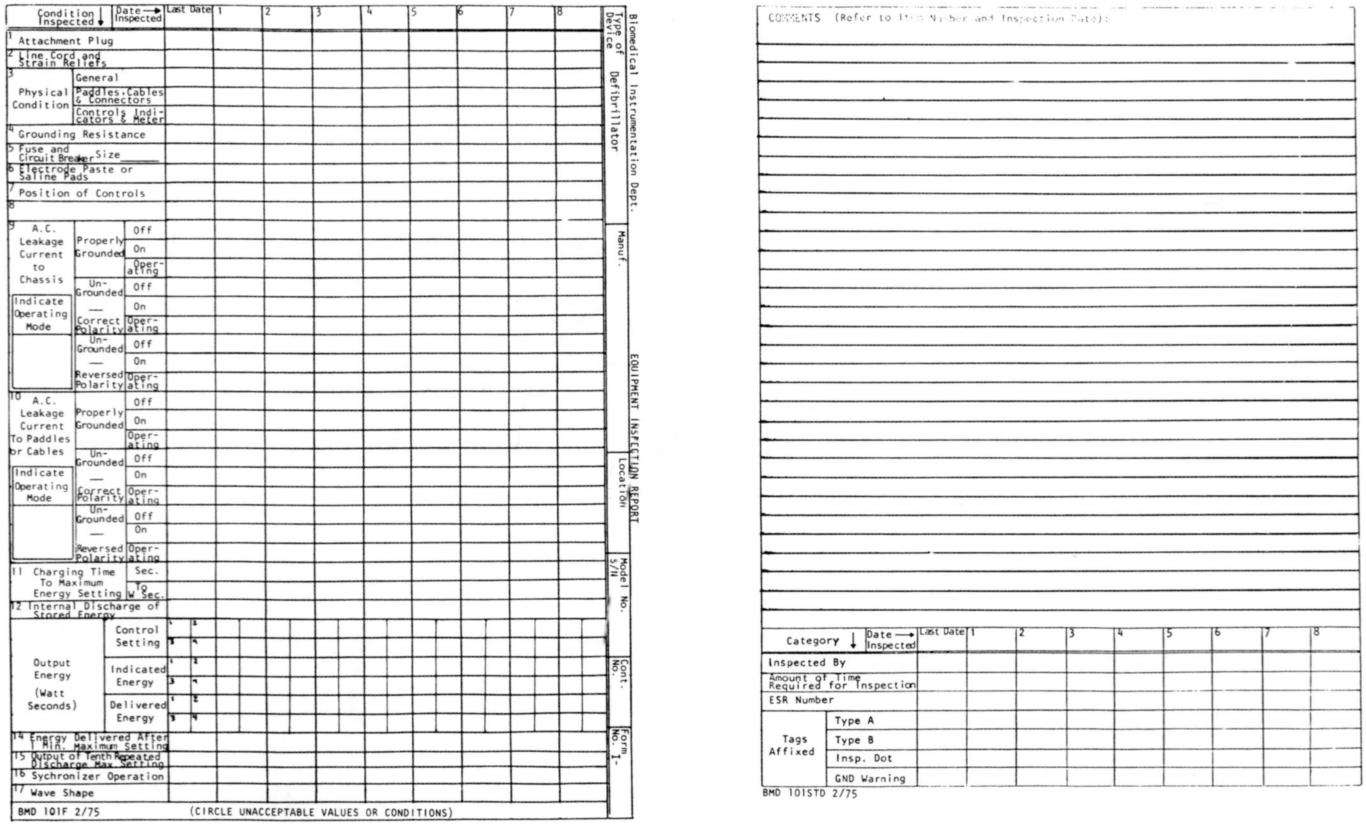
Biomedical Instrumentation Dept.
EQUIPMENT INSPECTION REPORT
Type of Device: Defibrillator | Manuf. | Location | Model No. S/N | Cont. No. | Form No. I-

Condition Inspected ↓			Date → Inspected	Last Date	1	2	3	4	5	6	7	8
1 Attachment Plug												
2 Line Cord and Strain Reliefs												
3 Physical Condition	General											
	Paddles, Cables & Connectors											
	Controls Indicators & Meter											
4 Grounding Resistance												
5 Fuse and Circuit Breaker	Size ____											
6 Electrode Paste or Saline Pads												
7 Position of Controls												
8												
9 A.C. Leakage Current to Chassis	Properly Grounded		Off									
			On									
			Operating									
	Un-Grounded		Off									
Indicate Operating Mode	—		On									
	Correct Polarity		Operating									
	Un-Grounded		Off									
	—		On									
	Reversed Polarity		Operating									
10 A.C. Leakage Current To Paddles or Cables	Properly Grounded		Off									
			On									
			Operating									
	Un-Grounded		Off									
Indicate Operating Mode	—		On									
	Correct Polarity		Operating									
	Un-Grounded		Off									
	—		On									
	Reversed Polarity		Operating									
11 Charging Time To Maximum Energy Setting			Sec.									
			To W Sec.									
12 Internal Discharge of Stored Energy												
Output Energy (Watt Seconds)	Control Setting											
	Indicated Energy											
	Delivered Energy											
14 Energy Delivered After 1 Min. Maximum Setting												
15 Output of Tenth Repeated Discharge Max Setting												
16 Sychronizer Operation												
17 Wave Shape												

BMD 101F 2/75 (CIRCLE UNACCEPTABLE VALUES OR CONDITIONS)

COMMENTS (Refer to Item Number and Inspection Date):

Category ↓		Date → Inspected	Last Date	1	2	3	4	5	6	7	8
Inspected By											
Amount of Time Required for Inspection											
ESR Number											
Tags Affixed	Type A										
	Type B										
	Insp. Dot										
	GND Warning										

BMD 101STD 2/75

Fig. 5. Front and back of a defibrillator inspection form. Space is adequate for a series of eight inspections, covering 2 yeras. The standard format reserves items 1–5 and 9 and 10 for the same series of inspections, regardless of the type of device being inspected.

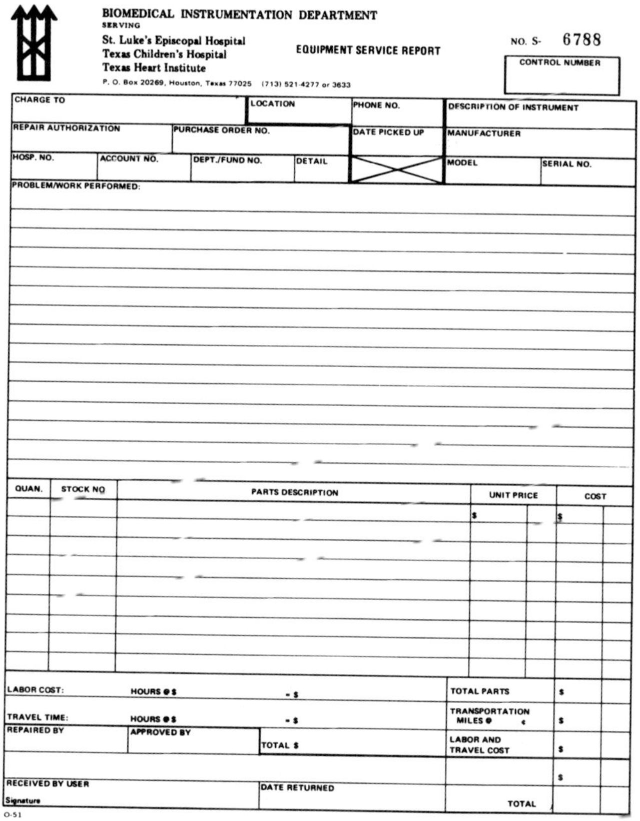

BIOMEDICAL INSTRUMENTATION DEPARTMENT
SERVING
St. Luke's Episcopal Hospital
Texas Children's Hospital
Texas Heart Institute
P. O. Box 20269, Houston, Texas 77025 (713) 521-4277 or 3633

EQUIPMENT SERVICE REPORT

NO. S- 6788

CONTROL NUMBER

CHARGE TO | LOCATION | PHONE NO. | DESCRIPTION OF INSTRUMENT

REPAIR AUTHORIZATION | PURCHASE ORDER NO. | DATE PICKED UP | MANUFACTURER

HOSP. NO. | ACCOUNT NO. | DEPT./FUND NO. | DETAIL | MODEL | SERIAL NO.

PROBLEM/WORK PERFORMED:

QUAN.	STOCK NO	PARTS DESCRIPTION	UNIT PRICE	COST
			$	$

LABOR COST: HOURS @ $ = $

TRAVEL TIME: HOURS @ $ = $

TOTAL PARTS $

TRANSPORTATION MILES @ ¢ $

REPAIRED BY | APPROVED BY | TOTAL $ | LABOR AND TRAVEL COST $

$

RECEIVED BY USER Signature | DATE RETURNED | TOTAL

O-51

Fig. 6. Equipment service report (ESR). This is a four-part form and is sequentially numbered for filing and reference. Distribution includes the biomedical instrumentation department file, the owner department, Accounting department, and any outside service representative.

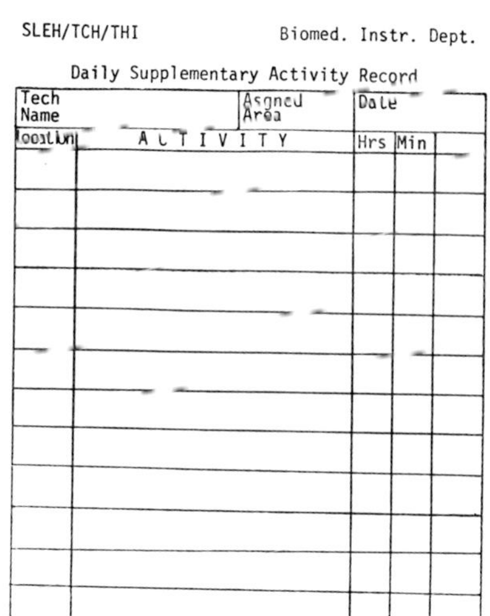

SLEH/TCH/THI Biomed. Instr. Dept.

Daily Supplementary Activity Record

Tech Name		Asgned Area	Date	
Location	ACTIVITY		Hrs	Min

Fig. 7. Daily supplemental activity card. Difficult to document minor repairs are noted on these cards, which are on pocket-sized red card stock.

St. Luke's Episc./Texas Children's Hospitals
Houston, Texas

Biomedical Instrumentation Dept.

COMPOSITE TOTAL DEPARTMENTAL & SECTION REPORT

Period

Week Ending Date	Payroll Hours					Total Dept. % Hours Used				Tot. Dept. Rep. & Maint.			Individual Sections - Hours/Job & % Hours Worked									
	Worked			Paid		Emer. Repair	Prev. Maint.	Long Range	Supplementary	No. Jobs	Hrs/ Job	% Hrs Worked	Radiology		Cath. Lab		Cardiology		OR-ICU		Inhal. Ther.	
	Reg	O.T.	E.P.	V&H	Ill								Hr/Job	% Hrs	Hr/Job	% Hrs	Hr/Job	% Hrs	Hr/Job	% Hrs	Hr/Job	% Hrs
Wkly Ave Prev Qtr																						

St. Luke's Episcopal Hospital
Texas Children's Hospital
Houston, Texas

Biomedical Instrumentation Dept.

WEEKLY BIOMEDICAL INSTRUMENTATION REPORT

SECTION:

PERIOD ENDING:

Week Ending Date	Hours Worked			Paid Hours		Emergency Repair			Preventive Maint.			Long Range Repair			Supplementary Activ			Total Repair & Maint			Amount Billed
	Reg	O.T.	EP	V&H	Ill	No. Jobs	Hours Used	% of Hrs Wkd	No. Jobs	Hours Used	% of Hrs Wkd	No. Jobs	Hours Used	% of Hrs Wkd	No. Jobs	Hours Used	% of Hrs Wkd	No. Jobs	Hours Used	% of Hrs Wkd	
Wkly Ave Prev Qtr																					
Totals This Qtr																					
Wkly Ave This Qtr																					

Mo.	Wks	WEEKLY AVERAGE BY MONTH																				

Fig. 8. Weekly and monthly composite report. The forms show how well each equipment area performed in relation to actual hours worked. The information is shown for each individual equipment group and the department as a whole.

St. Luke's Episcopal Hospital
Texas Children's Hospital
Texas Heart Institute
P.O. Box 20269
Houston, Texas 77025

BIOMEDICAL INSTRUMENTATION DEPARTMENT
(713) 521-4277 or 521-3633

CONDITIONS OF SALE

ITEM	P.O. NO.	DATE

VENDOR	MANUFACTURER

Part I - RADIOLOGY EQUIPMENT

In accepting this purchase order, the manufacturer or his licensed representative shall assume the responsibility of complying with the "Regulations for the Administration and Enforcement of Radiation Control for Health and Safety Act of 1968". In the event of noncompatibility, the manufacturer or his licensed representative shall petition for a variance to the Bureau of Radiological Health and make available to this institution a copy of this variance, whether the variance is accepted or not.

Part II - GENERAL PATIENT-RELATED DIAGNOSTIC AND THERAPEUTIC ELECTRICAL EQUIPMENT

The electrical equipment in this purchase order must meet the standards set forth by the Biomedical Instrumentation Department. No payment shall be made to the manufacturer or his licensed representative unless the following standards are met:

Applicable	Not Applicable	See Comments		
			1.	Equipment shall pass the appropriate electrical leakage current tests at 115 volts, 60 cycle power in the grounded, and ungrounded correct and reverse polarities. All measurements are referenced to ground:
			a	**Patient Contact Equipment** - 50 ua from leads and 100 ua from chassis.
			b	**Patient Contact Equipment, Isolated Patient Connection** - 10 ua from the leads and 100 ua from the chassis.
			c	**Nonpatient Equipment** - 500 ua from the chassis.
			2.	Equipment will be supplied with a 3-wire power cord & plug, both UL approved for hospital use. Molded plugs of any type are unacceptable.
			3.	Equipment shall pass an initial inspection of all the performance specifications advertised by the manufacturer of the equipment. All tests will be performed at this institution by the manufacturer, his licensed representative, or the Biomedical Instrumentation Department. Test results documentation will be filed with the Biomedical Instrumentation Department.
			4.	Upon successful completion of the initial inspection, a 30-day operational trial period will be required. If at the end of the 30-day evaluation period the equipment does not perform as advertised, the equipment will be returned at the manufacturer's expense.
			5.	Upon being placed in operation, ________ hours of in-service training will be provided to the hospital staff free of charge by the manufacturer or his licensed representative.
			6.	Two complete sets of operating instructions, schematics, and maintenance manuals for each separate identifiable item of equipment shall be provided.
			7.	The manufacturer will guarantee the direct sale to this institution of test fixtures and spare parts that are needed to maintain the equipment in proper operating condition.

COMMENTS:

CONDITIONS OF SALE ISSUED BY:	DIRECTOR, BIOMEDICAL INSTRU. DEPT.	DATE

CONDITIONS OF SALE MET - APPROVED FOR PAYMENT

PURCHASE ORDER NO.		DIRECTOR, BIOMEDICAL INSTRU. DEPT.	DATE

BIOMED COPY

Fig. 9. Conditions of sale form. This form is included in all purchase orders for biomedical equipment.

47

IN-HOSPITAL MEDICAL EQUIPMENT MAINTENANCE: DIVISION OF ELECTRONICS AND BIOLOGICAL ENGINEERING

W. Staewen

The Division of Electronics and Biological Engineering is a clinical engineering group at the Sinai Hospital of Baltimore. Its primary purpose is to ensure the optimal and safe use of electromedical devices on patients. Additional benefits derived from this group include extended life of the equipment, minimal downtime for repairs, occasional cost savings by providing engineering advice in the selection of equipment and procurement of the most suitable equipment because of engineering guidance. The division is presently organized as illustrated on the flow chart in Figure 1.

The chief clinical engineer has the following duties and responsibilities.

1. Administrative responsibilities related to personnel, equipment, budgets, job priorities, and physical facilities. The chief of the division must be responsible for personnel administration. He must interview and select new employees, determine the manpower requirements, and deal with personnel problems. He is responsible for determining the equipment and general operating budget needs of the division. When conflicts occur in the work schedule he must establish job priorities. He must establish suitable working facilities so that equipment, tools, and bench space are adequately maintained. He must also decide when instruments are beyond in-house repair and advise administration when equipment needs to be replaced.

2. Supervise the maintenance and repair facilities required to service the hospital's electromedical instrumentation. The chief of the division must direct, train, and assist the technicians. He must maintain an inventory of spare parts and accessories and also ensure that replacement parts are ordered for defective equipment. In addition, he must check maintenance and repair records and spot-check instruments and systems.

DIVISION OF ELECTRONICS AND BIOLOGICAL ENGINEERING

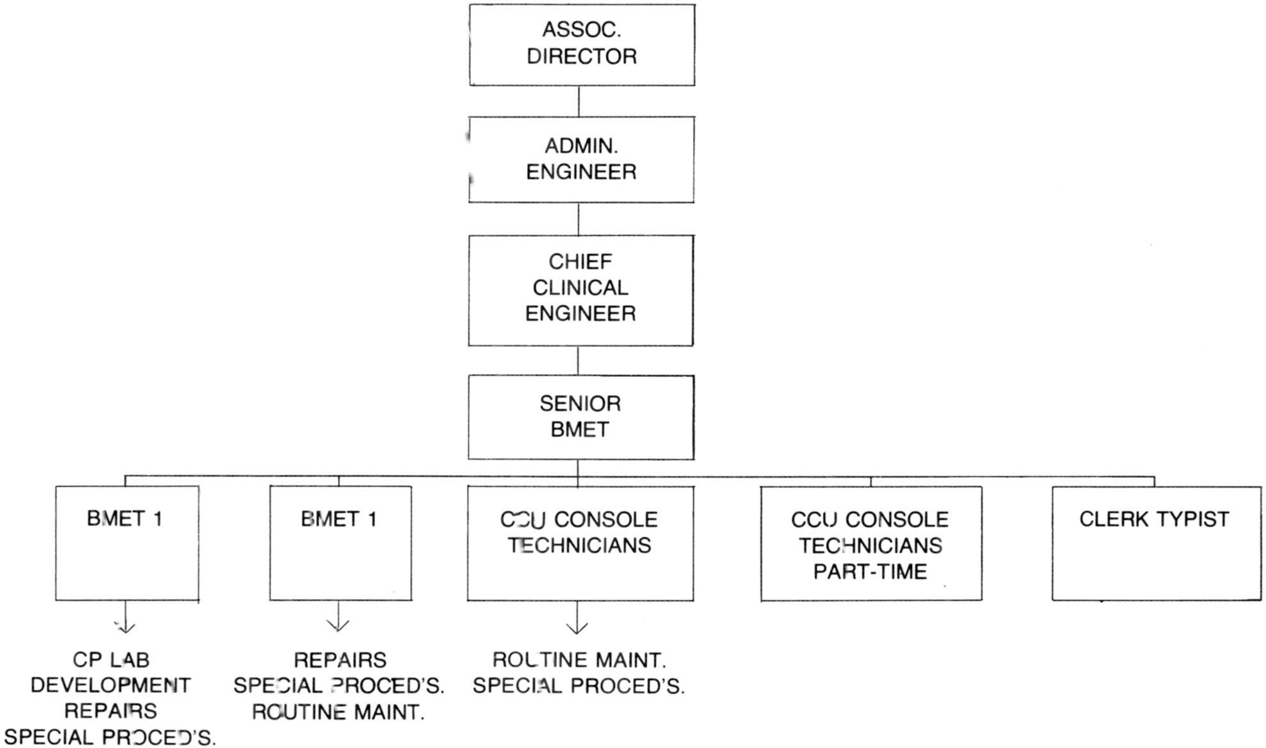

Figure 1

3. Perform as a consultant for biomedical engineering problems. If a member of the medical staff has or suspects a problem with electromedical equipment, the division head must give him advice and guidance. For example, problems with cardiac pacemakers are common. It is often difficult to determine if a pacemaker is malfunctioning, a catheter electrode is not placed properly or the patient's condition is not compatible with the pacemaker. Similar problems occur with other equipment, and the head of this division is often asked to make a judgment that will affect the treatment of a patient.

4. Design and develop new electronic instrumentation and circuits for biomedical applications. The chief of the division is required to occasionally design and develop circuits or instruments. These may be devices that are not available commercially, or if they are commercially available, it has been determined that they can be made in-house at less expense. In addition to devices used for medical applications, there is also a need to develop instruments for maintenance and testing. Some of the equipment that has been developed by this division includes the analysis system for long-term ECG tape recordings; the automatic transvenous defibrillator; pressure monitor; constant-current stimulator for ulcer healing; nerve stimulator; pacemaker tester; ECG recorder tester; and fetal heart rate monitor.

5. Evaluate requests for procurement of electromedical equipment. He must provide procurement advice on all instruments being considered for purchase. He should provide this advice particularly with regard to safety, state-of-the-art design, compatibility with existing equipment, and power requirements. He must evaluate the needs of the user to determine the selection of the right equipment.

6. Evaluate specifications and performance of new electromedical instrumentation. As the hospital needs to update and procure new equipment, he must be familiar with new devices. Similar devices made by different manufacturers often have significant variances in their characteristics. The clinical engineer must evaluate those characteristics to determine which is the best instrument. This often requires actual performance testing of the equipment.

7. Design and develop medical equipment systems, for example, the design of CCU and ICU monitoring systems. The clinical engineer designs instrument systems, arranges for their purchase, supervises the installation, performs acceptance tests and arranges the servicing.

8. Prepare maintenance and test applications for each instrument and define inspection cycles. The chief of the division establishes the routine maintenance protocol. He determines what maintenance procedures are performed and how often.

9. Develop training programs for the medical staff on the use of instrumentation. It is essential to continually train the medical staff in the proper use of instrumentation. This division consistently holds training seminars for the medical staff on the use of pacemakers, defibrillators, ECG recorders, and monitors.

10. Attend professional meetings and work on committees developing standards for electromedical instrumentation. It is necessary for the clinical engineer to

keep up to date with the latest equipment and techniques. He does this by attending important meetings and conventions. Also, he participates on standards committees so as to be in a position to help formulate favorable standards and gain knowledge about the most important features to look for when selecting equipment.

11. Write technical reports and articles. He must share his experiences, findings, and ideas with the rest of the bioengineering community.

The senior BMET has the following duties and responsibilities.

1. Supervise the CCU console technicians. The senior BMET must supervise seven full-time and six part-time technicians. He determines what projects they should work on and gives them advice and guidance on the repair of equipment. He also schedules their holidays and vacations and on-call emergency duty for weekends.

2. Train CCU console technicians. He is responsible for training all new console technicians. This training is also extended to experienced technicians when the need is indicated. This training includes fundamentals of electrocardiography, equipment operation, equipment maintenance, and principles of safety.

3. Schedule maintenance and servicing of instruments. It is the responsibility of the senior BMET to arrange the routine and emergency maintenance schedule. He assigns specific instruments to individual technicians for routine maintenance.

4. Instruct and train ECG technicians in the operation of ECG recorders. The senior BMET instructs all new ECG technicians in the principles of taking electrocardiograms. He teaches them the operating principles of the recorder, proper lead placement technique, and safety principles related to the use of electromedical devices on patients.

5. Modify new and existing instrumentation. It is often required to modify the electrical circuits of an instrument to either improve its performance or change its characteristics to suit a particular application. The senior BMET will either perform the modification personally or supervise a technician doing the work. The chief clinical engineer will prescribe the modification.

6. Maintain inventory of replacement repair parts. It is the responsibility of the senior BMET to maintain a stock of crucial replacement parts. This includes electrodes for monitoring, patient cables, isolette sleeves and filters, power plugs and cables, writing arms for recorders, and many miscellaneous parts that are likely to fail in equipment.

7. Maintain, service and calibrate test equipment. The division has a variety of test equipment that is used to service and maintain electromedical instruments. The list includes oscilloscopes, volt-ohm meters, leakage testers, signal generators, ECG simulators, capacitance meters, transistor testers, and frequency counters.

8. Perform incoming inspection tests on new equipment. Under the direction of the clinical engineer, the senior BMET will perform incoming inspection tests on new instruments. These tests are necessary to determine if the equipment is operating properly and whether it meets specifications.

9. Instruct nurses in the proper use of equipment. The senior BMET holds regular training seminars to teach nurses the operating principles of defibrillators, ECG recorders, and patient monitors.

The CCU console technicians have the following duties and responsibilities.

1. Complete operation of the patient monitoring console at the CCU central station. For 4 hours of their 8-hour tour, each console technician monitors the patients in the CCU. During the other 4 hours, they perform maintenance on equipment in the hospital. While on the console their duties include:

a. Observe each patient's electrocardiogram as displayed on the monitor screens
b. Detect and inform appropriate members of the medical staff of significant changes in a patient's electrocardiogram or if the patient enters an alarm situation
c. Record and file rhythm strips of the patient's electrocardiogram. This is a short record of the patient's ECG. The technician takes measurements from these records and discusses them with the nurses
d. Informs this division when equipment malfunctions
e. Takes diagnostic ECGs of patients. Full 12-lead ECGs are taken on every patient each morning and when they are admitted to the unit. A special three-channel recorder that records three simultaneous leads on patients for studying certain arrythmias is also used

2. Perform operator-level maintenance of console and bedside equipment.

a. Replace recorder paper and tape loops.
b. Adjust controls when necessary.
c. Determine if electrodes are attached properly.

3. Performance evaluation of coronary-care monitoring equipment.

a. Calibration of ECG recorders at operator level.
b. Calibration of heart rate—alarm modules at operator level.
c. Calibration of monitors at operator level.
d. Testing of defibrillators.

4. Assist in pacemaker operations. The technician performs the following duties during pacemaker insertions. He checks to see that the operating environment and equipment are electrically safe. He monitors the patient's ECG during the procedure and measures the pacemaker's stimulating and R-wave sensing thresholds.

5. Assist with patient monitoring during open-heart surgery. During open-heart surgery, the technician is required to set up the ECG and pressure monitoring equipment. He also checks the electrical environment for safety. During the surgical procedure, he monitors the blood pressure, keeps the transducer lines flushed, and draws blood samples.

6. Assist with pressure monitoring in the CCU and ICU. Whenever intraarterial or intravenous pressures are monitored in these areas, the technician assists in setting up the equipment. He again ensures that the instruments are operating

properly and that the environment is electrically safe. These procedures may occur anytime and are frequent.

7. Assist with cardiac catheterization procedures. A technician is required to operate the pressure and ECG recording system during these procedures. He again must check the electrical environment for safety. During this procedure, the technician is observing the ECG on the monitor and making recordings.

8. Fabricate high-quality power cords and extension cords for use in patient treatment areas. All electrical instruments are usually supplied with a poor-quality power cord and plug from the manufacturer. They are replaced with high-quality material by this division during incoming inspection or when observed on an existing instrument. The use of extension cords in this hospital is a problem and should be discouraged. However, where a genuine need is established, this division furnishes high quality extension cords.

9. Repair defective instruments. The technicians attempt first-line repairs of defective equipment. However, supervision is often needed for these repairs. An attempt is made to limit in-house time spent on repairs to 1 day. Sometimes, but not often, it is necessary to send the equipment to the manufacturer for repair.

The part-time CCU console technicians have the following duties:

1. Complete operation of the patient-monitoring console at the central nurse's station.
   a. Observe each patient's electrocardiogram as displayed on the monitor screens
   b. Detect and inform the appropriate member(s) of the medical staff of significant changes in a patient's electrocardiogram
   c. Notify appropriate member(s) of medical staff when a patient goes into an alarm situation
   d. Record and file rhythm strips on each patient
   e. Inform the division when equipment malfunctions
   f. Take diagnostic ECGs of patients
2. Perform operator-level maintenance of console and bedside equipment
   a. Replace recorder paper
   b. Adjust position and gain controls if necessary
   c. Determine if electrodes are properly attached

48

PERFORMANCE TESTING FOR SAFETY

M. Shaffer

Much has been written during the past 4 years on safety in hospitals, and, specifically, on microshock and macroshock hazards developed far from the offending equipment. Countless case histories have been reported of the dangers in hospitals throughout the country, where it is estimated that between 1200 and 1500 patients are electrocuted yearly. Strong recommendations have been made for the development of safety programs and the training of personnel to test for such hazards and to be on the alert for frayed wires or broken ground leads.

On the surface, this sounds as though, in the words of the courts, all reasonable precautions are being taken, and the present use of the ''part-time technician'' for such programs is still acceptable.

Unfortunately, it would seem that the testing for shock hazards is not adequate, shock hazards being only part of the problem. A far more dangerous situation exists when the actual data from the instrumentation is misleading. Such a situation arises when equipment failure, miscalibration, or misalignment causes a wrong reading to be monitored. It is believed that this is more dangerous because the hospital rarely has people available with sufficient electronic background to recognize performance anomolies in their early stages. A recent malpractice suit against a hospital in Washington, D.C., resulted in an award of over $550,000 against the hospital, one of the grounds being that the patient was at a different temperature than that indicated. This is not an isolated case; the corridors of hospitals are filled with instrumentation of questionable performance, and it is expected that more like cases will occur as the trend for more complex equipment continues.

It therefore seems mandatory that the performance of each instrument be checked at regular intervals. That this is not done must be attributed to both the instrument manufacturer and the hospital. In the former case, most equipment seems to be designed with a complete hands-off approach to in-place testing, specifically in such areas as procedures, access points, and reference material.

For instance, the test procedures provided usually require the use of comparatively complex equipment, including oscilliscopes, pulse and vector generators, simulators, and counters. They also involve considerable time expenditure. Neither of these conditions can be tolerated in patient-care areas, so either a remote test laboratory is set up, or the instrumentation is simply not tested; the latter condition usually subsisting.

For example, the 24-bed special-care unit at the George Washington University Hospital has 102 patient-monitoring instruments located at the bedside. Testing in accordance with the manufacturers' recommended procedures is estimated to take approximately 2 hours/bed and 2 weeks for the complete unit; this is completely unacceptable in a busy area.

Regarding access points, these are required to allow simulated input signals to be introduced and the outputs to be measured easily without disassembly of the unit and its interface connections, both bad practices leading to a higher fault incidence. Such externally accessible test points are absolutely necessary for performance testing if the normal operational configuration at the bedside is not to be disrupted.

Finally, the reference material supplied by the manufacturer is usually limited to nurses' operating procedures. Schematic diagrams needed for developing a test program or performing first-level maintenance are treated almost as proprietary information.

The hospital's part in this shared responsibility lies in not accepting the fact that, with the advances in medical instrumentation over the past 10 years, we are in a different ball game, being confronted with an estimated 5000 types of instruments produced by more than 1300 manufacturers. Complex equipment in hospitals is the rule rather than the exception, and we are doing little to close the gap between our "part-time technician" syndrome and the equipment suppliers' reluctance, because of economic and personnel problems, to provide competent direct-factory or dealer representation.

A pilot program has therefore been initiated by the George Washington University Hospital Anesthesiology Department to monitor the performance of 200 instruments in the ORs, recovery room, and special-care unit. The program has as its specific objective the development of an adequate level of testing within the very limited time constraints of under 5 min/unit and 3 days for all program instrumentation. Within these time constraints, the tests are designed to apply a simulated (1 mV or 1 V as appropriate) pulse input on a unit basis; measure the outputs with the sensitivity and other front panel controls, which are varied between their maximum and minimum positions; and compare these outputs against values previously obtained. Any variations in these readings are a good indication that something has changed and a bench checkup may be needed.

Figure 1 shows the type of test form completed by the safety technician for each unit. The program is now in its third month of operation and has identified three units with changed performance, two due to changes in component values and one due to a misalignment.

George Washington University Hospital
Anesthesiology Department
Instrumentation Performance Checklist

TEMP/VENOUS PRESS AMP
Hewlett-Packard Type 780-10 (LO TEMP) Serial No. 1207A01408
Test equipment
Resistance (simulated temperature) box
Voltmeter (across remote plug pin 6/7 to 3)
Pressure shorting plug (pins A-C)
Leakage current meter
Procedure
Plug in resistance box, vary resistance, and note temperature, reading, and voltage (pin 6 to pin 3).
Check alarm lights.
Check leakage current.

	18°		21°		31°		42°		Leakage Current
Date	Temp	Volt	Temp	Volt	Temp	Volt	Temp	Volt	
11/27	18	.25	21	5	31	1.45	42.5	2.5	0
12/08	18	.25	21	5	31	1.40	42.3	2.4	0

SYSTOLIC/DIASTOLIC PRESS AMP
Hewlett-Packard Type 780-9 Serial No. 1206A1692

Test equipment
Pressure shorting plug (pins A & C connected)
Voltmeter
Leakage current meter

Procedure
Set zero.
Vary sensitivity control and measure voltage at remote plug pins 6 and 7 to pin 3 (ground with 200 mm cal button pressed).
Check alarm lamps light.
Check leakage current.

	Systolic (pin 6 volts) Sensitivity			Diastolic (pin 7 volts) Sensitivity			Leakage Current
Date	Min	Max	200 mm	Min	Max	200 mm	
11/29	1.12/130	4.3	1.75	1.12/130	4.3	1.75	0
12/11	1.1/130	4.3	1.75	1.1/130	4.3	1.75	0

Fig. 1.

49

RECORDING OF PERFORMANCE AND HAZARDS

F. I. Gilbert, Jr.

There are about 8000 different medical devices in use today. Physicians, nurses, administrators, and, more recently, federal lawmakers are expressing increasing concern over both the safety and efficacy of clinical equipment. Attempts are being made by the American Society of Internal Medicine (ASIM) to gather information on injuries, complications, and deaths associated with the improper design, manufacture, maintenance, or use of all types of medical devices by individuals or institutions.

ASIM members and others are urged to contribute information to support this continuing effort. Reports will be mailed to the ASIM office where staff will transmit all information to appropriate study groups. Contributors may be assured that each problem will be appropriately referred for investigation and that they will receive a report regarding the problem.

If one encounters unsatisfactory performance, servicing, maintenance, or failure of a medical device that may be directly or indirectly responsible for injury to either a patient or the user, ASIM can be notified by letter or telephone. Only information related to the device is necessary.

The required information includes:

1. Type of device (e.g., electrocardiograph, oxygen-powered resuscitator, heart valve, wheel chair, blood pressure apparatus, coronary- and intensive-care monitoring equipment)
2. Mode of injury and effect on patient or user (e.g., laceration of hand by sharp-edged equipment housing, tissue reaction to implanted pacemaker, ventricular fibrillation, and death due to electric shock by patient monitors, thrombosis, and infection due to venous catheter)

3. Cause of problem if identified with reasonable certainty (e.g., operator error in using defibrillator, broken plug and frayed electrical cord, component or circuit failure, calibration difficulty, unknown)
4. Name of manufacturer, model number, and serial number of the device, if possible
5. What action, if any, was taken to correct the problem or prevent future injuries (e.g., replaced with new equipment, rewire electric cord and plug, unknown)

A standard Health Devices Problem Reporting Form can be obtained directly by writing to the American Society of Internal Medicine, 525 The Hearst Building, Third at Market, San Francisco, California 94103.

The basic procedure involved after one submits a health devices problem reporting form consists of the following: The form is first subject to board approval and then forwarded to the editor of the *Internist*. The report sent from the user proceeds to the staff where photocopies are made and sent to: (*a*) AAMI—are there standards on this device; and (*b*) ECRI—has this device been evaluated? Does it meet the accepted standards? When the staff receives the information from AAMI and ECRI, it is forwarded to the individual reporting the problem. Finally, the health-care technology committee reviews the preceding correspondence to ensure that the individual has received an adequate response. If the response has not been adequate, more information will be gathered and transmitted to that individual.

FDA Medical Device Experience Monitoring Network

In the past, the FDA has not had explicit legislative authority to require that medical devices and diagnostic products be proven safe or effective prior to marketing. While awaiting new amendments to the Food, Drug, and Cosmetic Act, which will mandate a new regulatory program for medical devices, the FDA established a voluntary reporting system to monitor device performance in actual usage.

At present, the FDA has reports of adverse experiences with these products stored in computer-retrieval form. It is necessary, however, that physicians and other health professionals continue to report usage problems so that the information remains current and reflects the type of difficulties being experienced. Although the FDA has particular interest in serious, life-threatening, and fatal device experiences, the range of reportable material may include any problem, unacceptable condition, or performance difficulty.

The United States Pharmacopeial Convention, Inc, which operates a reporting program funded by the FDA, receives the reports and forwards them to both the FDA and the manufacturer for appropriate action. Practitioners are invited to participate in this program.

50

EMERGENCY REPAIRS

M. Shaffer

Many articles have been published emphasizing the difficulties in maintaining hospital instrumentation from the viewpoints of both the instrument manufacturer and the hospital. On the one hand, the manufacturer seems to adopt an almost hands-off approach, providing few access points for testing the instruments, inadequate manuals, and complex maintenance procedures that made in-place testing almost an impossibility. These shortages are justified on the basis that the average hospital does not have the necessary maintenance expertise; consequently, a proprietary approach is probably the best. In line with this, the hospital has been inclined to play down the expertise needed to maintain the equipment, assuming that the work is on a part-time technician level and has indeed failed in the past to provide qualified personnel who can develop the maintenance programs and procedures necessary. Between these two approaches, as with an ostrich with its head in the sand and suffering from psychological impotence, little has been achieved.

The hospitals for their part are now showing distinct signs of correcting their side of the problem, employing higher-level professionals such as clinical engineers and certified biomedical electronics technicians to develop their internal capability. However, the personal relationships created by the introduction of a newly claimed specialty are too often neglected, and it is timely that they be evaluated realistically on a generic class basis. This is essential if the clinical engineering staff is to assert itself as an integral part of the health-care team and is to develop its full potential.

Reducing the problem to its basic form, emergency maintenance is always in critical demand by the hospital, and it is in this area that the clinical engineer is invaluable. Thus, the first and almost natural inclination of the medical staff is to see the clinical engineer as a repairman whose function is directly equivalent to that provided by the manufacturer or independent service representative. This impression inevitably leads to a psychological separation of the instrumentation responsibility into a ''we have a sick patient and your equipment has broken down'' relationship.

Furthermore, the association of clinical engineering and outside servicing together should in itself create potential competition. In emergency repairs, the clinical engineer must cover a wide spectrum of diverse instruments from many manufacturers, with limited spare parts, manuals, and technical instruction for any one specific instrument. He is, however, in a good position to reduce equipment breakdowns by preventive maintenance. Conversely, the manufacturer's service representative can specialize in a limited line of equipment and so should have an abundance of spare parts, manuals and experience on his specific line; thus, he should be expected to do a more expeditious job of emergency servicing. This is a reasonable expectation, as it costs the hospital about $150 per call. Accordingly, the advantages for in-house clinical engineering maintenance have to be based on reducing the number of emergencies by preventive measures and on the savings accrued. For example, one 450-bed hospital spent almost $150,000 for 960 service calls during one year; their in-house clinical engineering group, taking over the maintenance function and providing additional consultation services and safety inspections, is currently costing the hospital $72,000 per year—the savings is quite obvious.

From the timeliness aspect, the in-house clinical engineer during normal working hours can provide an almost instantaneous reaction to emergencies. Outside working hours, he is in a vulnerable position if his reaction time is not within the limits expected by the medical staff. The danger signal is ''we have a sick patient, your equipment does not work, and we need it now.'' Experience has shown that the in-house clinical engineer should not attempt 24-hour-a-day coverage unless there are qualified personnel or standby equipment available. If the standby units are not available for instant substitution, considerable thought should be given to putting such maintenance under contract with the manufacturer's service representative.

Finally, the overall work level must be appreciated so that the clinical engineer is acknowledged and respected as a specialist. Unfortunately, the presently accepted classifications are not meaningful enough; the title ''repairman'' is not appropriate, and the titles ''engineer'' and ''technician'' tend to bring to the minds of the uninitiated the vision of hospital boiler repairmen and the electrocardiograph operators.

It is therefore mandatory that good communications be organized to inform the medical staff that clinical engineering encompasses more than maintenance and should be considered a technical specialty. Since hospital administration is the head of the nonmedical support personnel, it must assume the leadership in setting up such communications, including educational programs, presentations, and cost analyses to show clearly the value of the full service. The theme should be that the instrumentation belongs to the medical departments, it is their responsibility to operate and maintain the equipment, and the clinical engineering group is more than willing to assist in maintenance if, by so doing, hospital money can indeed be saved.

51
SYSTEMS CONSIDERATIONS

M. Shaffer and B. S. Dunbar

Medical instrumentation has progressed over the past two decades from the single-unit, self-contained entity to the multiple-unit conglomerate. As in the commercial equivalent, the instrumentation conglomerate demands a high level of management integration to ensure full potential. This integration has been inadequate; far too little effort has been applied toward making the systems properly cost effective. The type of work needed falls within the scope of clinical engineering.

First, all hospital systems to some degree or other require space, heat, air conditioning, power, operating and maintenance staffs and equipment, all to be provided within some funding restrictions. These elements are variables and must be integrated. Space, heat, air conditioning, and power are already at the rationing point in some hospitals and may require augmentation. Furthermore, individuals comprising operating and maintenance staffs seldom conform to any predictable pattern in their desires for instrumentation needs.

Second, the cost of equipment from a manufacturer is itself a variable depending on the demand for certain equipment, with standard production-line items relatively inexpensive and special items comparatively expensive. In view of all the variables involved, it may well be that the requirements may not be met by the standard equipment of one manufacturer. Thus, there may be economic advantages in using the standard items from a number of different manufacturers, thereby compounding the integration work.

In some cases, a compromise or trade-off between user requirements and the capabilities of the manufacturer's standard equipment may be possible so as to avoid the need for special items. In attempting this compromise, the hospital, on the one hand, may not be aware of all the available technology and its support problems. The manufacturers, on the other hand, may not be able to define clinical requirements, especially in those cases extending the state of the art; they usually opt to sell standard products. A relationship may indeed develop in which a deadlock occurs between an inability to define requirements and an inability to recommend needs.

Thus a new system may well turn out to be an expensive technological marvel that both fails to meet hospital needs and fails to be widely saleable by the manufacturer. With this in mind, the hospital clinical engineering group must structure itself to act as the intermediary. It should be able to present to the user a system balance sheet showing a credit side with income and subjective advantages as well as a debit side containing the equipment and operating costs. The user can then evaluate worth. The clinical system engineering work should be in four main parts, namely, to define functions, features, interfaces, and values.

The definition of a system by its functions rather than by equipment configuration establishes what the system is to do. With such a definition, the manufacturer knows what the user expects in the way of objectives, has the flexibility to develop how the system may function with as many standard items as possible, and is better able to establish and demonstrate acceptance criteria. For these reasons, this definition can act as an ideal basis for developing a system specification in which both user and manufacturers may document mutually acceptable practical objectives rather than an unattainable wish list.

The system functions are best identified by starting with a broad definition, progressing down with increasing detail in logical levels, and establishing the input and output requirements for each level. As an example, an instrumentation system may have data gathering, data processing, and data display as its top-level functions. The data-processing function might then be broken down into common subfunctions such as complex calculations, logical analyses of multiplex parameters, data logging, and therapeutic processes.

An arrhythmia detector will use complex calculations for pattern recognition, with functional inputs and outputs that include both the criteria for sounding the alarm and the alarm indication itself. On the other hand, long-term trend detection of vital signs might well involve all of the first three subfunctions, and the expected inputs and outputs for each of these subfunctions require definition. In this case, particular attention will have to be paid to the people interface, covering the manual and automatic data to be fed in and the parameters to be displayed for each subfunction.

These details can be used to initiate the system specification that will list, as shown in Table I, the functions and subfunctions and ultimately the actions, the parties responsible, and the schedules for each subfunction. Costs may be included as a classified appendix. This specification must be viewed as a living document, to be updated as the subsequent three parts are developed, so that in its final form it is a valuable adjunct to the purchase order.

The second part of the work identifies the wanted system features, and so, to some extent, the equipment. A list of typical features for consideration is given in Table II. Here a number of compromises may be necessary as the features and the available hardware are reconciled. Portability and low weight provide advantages

TABLE I
System Specification Typical Main Headings

1. Functions
2. Actions required
3. Responsibilities assigned
4. Schedules
5. Funds

but usually coincide both with materials less able to withstand the rigors of constant hospital use and with restricted dimensions making maintenance more difficult. An instrument should be bought only if it can be maintained. For this reason, the manufacturers' recommended maintenance procedures must be given a detailed review to determine the balance between laboratory and in-place testing. Rapid, simple in-place testing is preferable, particularly for critical patient areas, and its potential value must therefore be established. The adequacy of available test points and the quality of the manufacturers' maintenance instruction books, procedures, schematic diagrams, along with the parts lists, may point out difficulties that could develop in this area. The local support that can be provided by the manufacturer for emergency repairs is also pertinent and should be defined.

The system must operate under the worst conditions, remembering that hospitals have large turnovers among personnel. Sometimes fewer controls with less accuracy and simpler procedures are best if less accuracy can be tolerated.

An idea of the reliability of the system must be obtained. Technically, a reliability figure is usually calculated from the probable number of component

TABLE II
Features

1. Portability	5. Adaptability
Size	Standards
Weight	Input levels
Strength of materials	Output levels
2. Maintainability	Interchangeability
In place	6. Safety
Bench	Leakage
Documentation	Grounding
Spares	Dangerous materials
3. Operability	7. Environment
Data inputs	Noise/vibration
Data outputs	Corrosion
Displays	Electrical interference
Accuracy	Storage
4. Reliability	Cleanliness
Calculated	
Expected	

failures expected in a given time and is expressed as the "mean time between failures." Since this figure represents component quality only, it does not reflect the dynamic system reliability, which depends largely on the effectiveness of the maintenance and user interfaces. Poor system reliability can be obtained both by too little or too much maintenance, as well as by frustrated operators. The comments of other actual users of the equipment provide the best subjective evaluation of this measure.

The system should also be adaptable; consequently, it should comply with commonly accepted standards so that its components can, without undue modification, be interfaced with other equipment, including unexpected additional equipment. Many of the electrical inputs, outputs, levels, and codes for equipment are now standardized. By way of example, most stand-alone data terminals and printers now use the Electronic Industries Association Standard RS-232 levels and the American Standard Code for Information Interchange code. Equipment compatible with these standards is easily obtained. Equipment made up of separate modules, each with convenient inputs and outputs complying with the standards, gives even greater flexibility.

Compliance with safety regulations is mandatory in critical patient areas. Attention must therefore be given to instrumentation patient isolation, leakage currents, grounding, isolated power systems, and floor conductivity. In the event of a safety incident, a hospital could well find itself having to defend itself for purchasing equipment from manufacturers who have not previously supported the medical market and so are allegedly inexperienced in the rigors of medical procedures.

The effects of the environment on the system and vice versa must also be weighed. Special precautions may have to be taken against noise, vibration, electrical power, and radiated interference, corrosion, pollutants, and the dangers of toxic and explosive materials. The features decided on as a result of this review will be a further input to the system specification that should now be forming the sound basis for a meaningful contract between supplier and user.

The third part, the interface task, as listed in Table III, takes the established features and identifies the major software and hardware blocks needed for the overall system.

In a data-processing system, the algorithms, those equations used in the computations, will determine the data to be collected, which in turn will affect the memory storage capacity and speed of the system. In considering personnel, the mode of operation is pertinent. As an example, special data entry and display units at each bedside will develop interface problems not encountered with a single central nurses' station and will affect communications and personnel procedures. Perhaps maintenance can be made more effective by remote monitoring and testing from a central control desk. Standby equipment needed to continue emergency operation in the event of a breakdown must not be overlooked; uninterrupted service can be provided with 100% standby equipment. However, partial degraded performance may be acceptable with something less than complete duplication. Therefore, the degree of acceptable degraded performance must be defined and should be a factor incorporated into the system specification.

TABLE III
Interface Definitions

Algorithms
Software
Hardware
Communications
Man/man
Man/machine
Emergency provisions
Facilities
Space
Air conditioning/heat
Light
Power
Water/drainage
Furniture
People
Formats
Procedures
Training

The space, air conditioning, heating, power, lighting, furniture, and even the floor-loading requirements are similarly affected and should now be estimated. In addition, the often neglected task of integrating people and equipment can be assessed. This can include developing the most suitable displays, operator/ maintenance procedures, training lessons, and accompanying visual aids for both the normal and the emergency conditions. This total interface effort will result in establishing for the system specification the operations required to be completed and the consequent assignment of responsibilities for them.

The fourth part of the work now becomes an assessment of the real value of the system. The debit measurements shown in Table IV include the hardware and software costs amortized over the expected lifetime, the expendables, and labor. These figures will reflect relatively finite system advantages such as reduction in numbers of people, reduction in operative and maintenance skills required, and

TABLE IV
Balance Sheet

Debit	Credit
Amortization of hardware and software	Income
Purchase	Intangibles
Holding/storage	Better procedures
Installation and checkout	Accuracy
Operating costs	Communications
Facilities	Availability
Expendable materials	Skills mix
Labor	

reduction in paperwork. On the credit side, both the earned income, which is finite, and the more intangible subjective advantages, such as improved clinical procedures, accuracy, person-to-person communications, response, and maintenance time may be placed. The decision as to whether or not the debit side is indeed exceeded by the credit side will rest with the user.

In summary, a system, to be fully effective, requires some evaluation and definition of its functions, features, interfaces, and value. Hospital systems will have more potential and be more economical if clinical engineering provides such a service.

52

THE DEVELOPMENT OF INSTRUMENTATION STANDARDS

J. J. Riordan

There was a time, not long ago, when policy and methodological problems in product standards and specifications were considered the specialized and largely exclusive province of engineers and technicians. That day has passed. Events of the past 5 years, and the foreshadowing of events to come, have generated a lively interest in standards along the executive hallways of industry and of professional and trade associations.

These events, amply reported in the public press, are largely manifestations of an amorphous but powerful social force that is generally identified as the consumer movement. It has spawned numerous governmental actions—administrative, legislative, and judicial— to protect consumers and users against deficient products and to recompense them for injuries sustained as a result of product deficiencies. It is understandable, therefore, that the standards by which products of various kinds are defined, controlled, and evaluated should become a focus of interest among manufacturers, buyers, users, and consumers. Standards are of particular concern to psysicians, dentists, and other professionals in health services who daily make critically important decisions regarding the utilization of the many new devices and diagnostic products offered in the medical product marketplace.

This concern is not merely academic. In the background looms the possibility of civil lawsuits. In the case of manufacturers of conventional consumer products, there is the further threat of criminal liability. Public Law 92-573 (the Consumer Product Safety Act of 1972) is a symptom of a current trend. It requires (Section 15) that manufacturers, distributors, and retailers report to the Consumer Product Safety Commission products that "create a substantial risk of injury to the public." If noncompliance with this requirement persists after notification by the Commission, a manufacturer is subject to criminal penalties (Section 21). This law—as well as developments related to warranties and liability, and pending legislation for control of medical devices—accents the need for rational, objective, and efficient methods for drafting product standards and for establishing programs to assure compliance with such standards. This need is particularly urgent in the medical area. Very likely the government will soon establish standards for numerous—if not most—medical devices. Then, too, standards are becoming increasingly necessary to protect ethical manufacturers and the public from less-than-ethical competitors in the burgeoning medical products industry. Standards that are fair and objective serve the interests of patients, doctors, hospitals, and manufacturers.

It is rarely the informed person who is insensitive to the social, economic, and legal imperatives for standards. But many manufacturers, users, buyers, and consumers are perplexed and confused in attempting to organize or participate in projects for developing and implementing standards.

There is no dearth of *ad hoc* techniques and methods for drafting standards. But there is a dearth of managerial principles and strategy for utilizing and marshaling these techniques, efficiently and effectively, in an organized system of standards preparation.

Among the many problems that militate against expeditious standards preparation is the anarchistic semantics that surround logical confrontation of standards problems. Many agencies of the government and private standards-preparation organizations have tried, for example, to define and to distinguish between the words "standard" and "specification." Even the most casual review of these efforts indicates that there is little agreement on exactly what these words mean and how one differs from the other. Both standards and specifications have as their central function the identification and description of physical phenomena, products, materials, devices, tests, processes, programs, and services. Considerable time and effort can be saved and confusion avoided by using the word "standard" as inclusive of (or synonymous with) "specification."

There are other semantic quagmires that trap the wayfarer in the wilderness of standards. What, for example, is a "performance" standard? Contrariwise, what is a "detail" or "design" standard? As the word "performance" implies, a performance standard defines a product in terms primarily of function—mechanical, electrical, physiological, chemical, etc. A hearing aid, for example, transmits and amplifies sound. A performance standard for a hearing aid should delineate quantitatively its sound transmission and amplification properties. A "detail" standard would specify materials used to fabricate the device and other specific characteristics such as configuration and color. It is possible to write performance standards for relatively simple items. Nonetheless, it would be difficult to write a standard for, let us say, a common pencil without specifying materials. It is illusory to assume that "performance standards" alone can adequately define and describe complex products such as medical devices. Ordinarily, performance standards must be augmented by some requirements related to materials, design, and testing. A standard should identify and describe a product to the degree necessary to achieve its stated purpose (e.g., to assure the usability, safety, and reliability of the product) without a preemptive restraint that it be a "performance standard" or otherwise.

Finally, there is a need for distinguishing the term "standard" from "standardization." In a strict sense, all standards result in some degree of standardization. However, the prime purpose of a standard is not necessarily product standardization. It is probably true that most standards have, as one of their purposes, assurance that all items of a particular identity are replicas of each other for specified characteristics and, in some cases, that their parts are interchangeable. However, a standard may have a very limited function. For example, a drop or vibration test might be prescribed for a packaged medical device. This is hardly "standardization" as that word is commonly understood in the context of product uniformity. The reason for making this difficult and somewhat elusive distinction between "standards" and "standardization" is to help allay age-old anxieties that cling like barnacles to the word "standardization," including the notion that standardization, and therefore standards, are roadblocks to innovation.

The Purpose of Standards

Standards are really compacts between producers and users, or buyers and sellers, that define what constitutes a satisfactory device or product, including requirements for effective manufacturing. These compacts may encompass a wide and diverse range of provisions regarding configuration, performance, reliability, maintainability, and other characteristics, depending on the character of the product. Whether standards are mandatory, voluntary, performance, detailed, or otherwise, all share a common core—namely, a description of the "thing" or service and an explanation of how the product or service will be evaluated for conformance to prescribed requirements. The purpose of a standard is to effect clear and precise mutual understanding between those who produce and distribute products and those who buy, use, or consume them regarding a "satisfactory" entity.

The question that now presents itself is at once elementary and complex. By what administrative chain of events does one draft a document—a standard—that describes a "satisfactory" product?

The Satisfactory Product—Prerequisites

Whether a product is a complex diagnostic instrument, or a simple tongue depressor, there are four prerequisites that must be satisfied if a product is to be satisfactory, i.e., if it is to fulfill a specified need. These prerequisites are:

1. The product must be clearly identified and its function(s) precisely delineated.

2. The product must be effectively designed in the light of the product's prescribed function(s).
3. The product must be manufactured, distributed, stored, repaired, and logistically supported under conditions that prevent degradation of the original design.
4. The product must be inspected and tested to prescribed criteria before delivery to users and consumers.

If this generalized list of prerequisites is accepted as reasonable by both manufacturers and users of medical devices, the stage is set for a rational strategy for drafting standards that conciliate their respective interests. Whether the resultant documentation is considered "mandatory" or "voluntary" is a secondary issue that can be administratively resolved by reasonable people. The central problem is to draft needed standards efficiently and expeditiously. Current practices are too slow, too expensive, and ineffective. To add insult to injury, the time, energy, and money expended on standards not infrequently results in documents satisfactory to nobody.

Standards Preparation—Administration

At the risk of pedantry, the strategy of standards preparation might best be discussed on a step-by-step basis.

Step I. Verification of Need

Before attempting to draft a standard, its need must be clearly established. In some instances, this need can be readily documented—for example, experience data might demonstrate that a particular medical instrument is unreliable or potentially dangerous. Experience data, however, are not the sole basis for establishing need. Reasons of prudence and good judgment may be adequate. Understandably, of course, it is important that problems associated with medical devices and instruments, particularly product failures, be researched as thoroughly as possible. In some instances, governmental agencies will identify and describe the product for which a standard is needed. In other instances, professional organizations, consumer groups, or trade organizations may play this role. It is assumed that the role of need identification is played by a governmental organization, a professional society, or a private standards-setting organization. In any event, it is essential that adequate staff work verifying that a need exists be accomplished before embarking on the turbulent seas of standards preparation.

Step II. Project Initiation

As a purposeful act, a responsible person in government or elsewhere must make an authoritative decision to establish a project to prepare a standard with scheduling and budgeting restraints.

Step III. Project Assignment

The aforementioned project must now be assigned formally to a person, a department, or an activity, public or private, for execution. In general, it is highly advisable that the project be assigned to one person—a project officer. That person must be given authority and responsibility for managing the project.

Step IV. Project Definition

As his initial responsibility, the project officer must fully "define the project." This means that he must spell out the objectives of the project and how he intends to fulfill these objectives within assigned budgetary and schedule limitations. The project definition is submitted to the agency or organizational director for his approval. Now the project officer is ready to move out, to go public, so to speak, and assemble the resources of people, information, and facilities necessary to fulfill the promises implicit in the project definition.

Step V. Appointment of Task Group

The time has now come for the project director, acting in accordance with guidelines established in the project definition, to nominate a task force or advisory committee to guide the development of the standard or to write the standard as a working group. The task force should be composed of persons most qualified to contribute to the project. In the case of some medical products, the advice of physicians and other health specialists, and of design and production engineers, should be augmented by the advice of representatives of consumers—particularly if the medical product is used directly by consumers. Not all members of the task force need to be professionals to contribute to its effectiveness. Depending on the original provisions of the project definition, the task force may have either an advisory or directive function. In the latter circumstance, the project officer must be responsive to the task group rather than vice versa. Therefore, the technical excellence of the final draft of the standard is the responsibility of the task force. Administrative considerations of this kind are ordinarily addressed in the project definition phase of the operation. That, again, is why thoughtful project definition is so necessary—it serves to anticipate and resolve issues that otherwise become time-consuming and possibly contentious "housekeeping" problems as a project evolves.

Step VI. Project Objectives

The project officer, in collaboration with the appointed task group (by whatever name) must now define precisely the purpose(s) for which a standard is being drafted. These purposes may include assurance of product usability, reliability, safety, or others. The purpose might be economic—to cut costs by volume production of a standardized product. The purpose may be legal—to make sure a product conforms to a safety regulation or other rules established by law, by judicial decision, or by administrative fiat. In some instances, the objective is limited—for example, to assure product safety. Unless the group agrees on the purpose (or purposes) it is not likely that an effective standard will be written. These purposes should be stated as exactly and as clearly as possible and should be incorporated into the previously mentioned project definition as an amplification or revision of the original as mentioned under Step IV above.

Step VII. Preparation of Prototype Standards

For the purposes of saving time, money, and wear and tear on the human psyche, the single most useful action the project officer can take—at the direction of the task force—is to prepare or arrange for the preparation of prototype (model) standards for subsequent task-force consideration. Standards preparation is a demanding, difficult, and frustrating task. The task can be enormously expedited by staff preparation of prototypes or working drafts. If personnel are not available, it may be possible to assign *ex parte* tasks to members of the group or to contract for their preparation. In any event, the project officer retains responsibility for the quality and completeness of prototype documents. Prototypes help to clear away minutia related to phraseology and format and other factors as well as hasten resolution of substantive technical issues. It is almost impossible for a committee to draft a standard. A committee can, however, improve, augment, amplify, or otherwise cause a standard to be truly responsive to previously agreed objectives.

Step VIII. Analysis, Revision, and Approval of Prototype Standards

Assuming that prototypes have been developed, it is now the business of the task force to analyze them, specify revisions, augmentations, or deletions, and finally, to approve the completed standard(s) for coordination among specified persons and organizations.

Step IX. Coordination

The standard is now coordinated by the project officer in accordance with the guidance of the task force. Subsequently, he collects and collates comments for presentation to the task force for acceptance, rejection, or revision. Schedules must be rigorously enforced. Otherwise, the standard will be outdated before it is printed. No standard will satisfy everyone.

Step X. Issuance

Standards may be issued by government agencies, private standards-setting organizations, trade associations, and by corporate activities for their own use. These may be mandatory or voluntary. The basic strategy and methodology of standards preparation is similar under either circumstance. The measure of the standard's effectiveness and usefulness is the degree to which it fulfills its own stated purposes. Since standards are usually under constant surveillance and revision, the issuing agency should devise an arrangement for users to propose corrections and revisions. Incidentally, the provisions of a standard may be both voluntary and mandatory. They may be voluntary in the sense that a manufacturer has the option to accept or reject them, but once having accepted standards, they become mandatory.

Preparation of Standards for Medical Products

General

Apart from essential formalities of product identification, selection of references, editorial and format decisions and other prerequisites, for a complete standard, the three bedrock questions that standards groups must answer are

1. Requirements: What characteristic, including function, should be specified and how?
2. Testing: How shall conformance to these requirements be evaluated?
3. Risks: To what characteristics should risks apply and to what degree?

While these questions, as posed, are quite general, they suggest the flavor of the problems confronting those who bravely attempt to write a "good" standard. In more conventional words, we might say that the heart and soul of a standard consists of requirements, testing, and risk delineation. Requirements pertain to "what." What is expected of the product? What functions must it perform to what degree of safety and reliability? What must be its shape, size, and weight? These, of course, are questions that merely indicate the scope of requirement provisions. The "shape," for example, of a device is usually defined in the design drawings. However, a standard may include amplifying requirements; for example, with respect to the smoothness of edges that may affect usability or safety. In short, the requirement provisions of a standard should set forth whatever needs to be said in amplification of design data regarding a product's expected performance, safety, reliability, configuration, cosmetic qualities, and other parameters, depending on the character of the product

When requirements have been established the next question is: How can we make sure the product conforms to these requirements? This question is answered under the heading of "Inspection or Testing," "Product Assurance," or merely "Testing." As is so often true in writing standards, the word "testing" has no fixed definition. Some agencies of the United States government, for example, use the word testing as inclusive of inspection. This makes sense because it is not practical to draw a sharp line between inspection and testing. Inspection is conventionally identified with the visual examination of a product, whereas testing is assumed to mean that the product is instrumented for purposes of measuring certain product characteristics. Actually, "inspection" frequently necessitates instrumentation, as, for example, in the microscopic examination of high-precision electronic devices. The word "testing" is used, therefore, in this paper as inclusive of inspection. Both editorial convenience and technical accuracy are thus well-served.

The testing provisions of standards must complement preestablished requirements. If these requirements are ambiguously defined, it is difficult, and possibly impractical, to conduct an appropriate test. A requirement, therefore, is a "paper tiger" if its incorporation into the product cannot be confirmed. Unhappily, it is not unusual for standards to include requirements that are saintly aspirations rather than of the real world. For a test to be practical, it must be planned to include: (*a*) statement of its purpose; (*b*) exact identification of the characteristics or properties to be tested including assigned tolerances; (*c*) identification of the instrument, device, or tool by which the test is conducted; (*d*) description of procedure for performing the test; (*e*) qualifications of the person conducting the test; and (*f*) arrangements for recording test results. Procedural details, however, need not be incorporated into the body of the standard. This would "clutter up" the document and discourage its utilization. Frequently, details of testing practice are described in reference standards. If a test is unique, it must, of course, be explained fully in the text of the standard.

Finally, a standard must address the question of risk, that is, how many units of the product must be tested, how often, and at what stage in the product design, production, or distribution cycle? Happily the mathematical statisticians have provided many easy-to-use guides for specifying risks and related sampling plans, with built-in decision rules, for use when good judgment suggests that sampling is advisable. There are circumstances, however, when sampling should be avoided. The literature of sampling theory and technique is quite ample.

Formulation of Requirements

It is no easy task to develop a logical scheme for specifying requirements without under- or overstatement. To expedite formulation of requirements, it is suggested that they be classified into clear and self-defining categories. These may be:

Functional (Performance) Requirements. A medical device can be defined with respect to its physiological, mechanical, physical, chemical, or other functions. For example, a suction apparatus must produce "intermittent suction at 70 mm or 100 mm mercury." This is a simplified and abridged illustration. But the point is that the function(s) must be defined in explicit measurable terms.

Configuration Requirements. These specify the static characteristics of the product with respect to shape, size, weight, density, labeling, and packaging. Design drawings augment the standard in defining these properties.

Reliability Requirements. Reliability, by definition, necessitates specification of a time frame (seconds, minutes, hours, days, months, years, cycles) and an environment within which the device must perform without (*a*) breakdown; (*b*) adjustment; or (*c*) repair, as the character of the product dictates. Reliability is a critically important requirement for medical devices and instruments. Reliability requirements must be stated quantitatively as a probability. The reliability requirement for a lamp used in a common medical device might be stated as follows: "The lamp shall be a 2.5 volt, 0.4 ampere, single-contact type, close-coiled tungsten-filament, prefocused and precentered. It shall have an average life of 9 hours with a 95% probability when tested as specified below (i.e., under 'Testing')." It may be advisable to also specify the MTBF (mean time between failure). Similar provisions may apply to maintainability. This refers to the need to specify the maximum time it would take to repair a device (or instrument) and return it to its normal functional capability. Obviously, such a requirement can be critical for life-related devices and instruments.

Safety. It would be idle to suggest specific safety provisions, considering the diversity of medical devices. Typically, however, limits of radiation leakage, if any, must be specified for radiological devices. For a conventional hypodermic needle, safety requirements would relate to resistance to breakage, elasticity, freedom from contamination or foreign matter, and fluid tightness, to identify the more obvious safety prerequisites.

These categories of requirements—function, configuration, reliability, and safety—are mere indicators of how requirements can be categorized. There are others. Specialists in various fields of medical devices and instrumentation would, no doubt, devise an alternative categorization. What is important is that these categories provide a structure for logical and systematic itemization of those requirements that are needed.

Testing. The range of tests, procedures, and equipment is so extensive that it serves little purpose to explore the subject further than discussed above. It is emphasized, however, that testing provisions should be restricted to identification of the purpose of the test and the property to be tested, the procedures and equipment to be used, and the qualifications of the test specialist. An extensive literature of standards and guidance for testing is available from government and private standards organizations.

Risk. Ordinary "risk" is assumed to be exclusively a statistical dimension. It is commonplace to ask: "What is the probability that this product will fail?" For standards-preparation purposes, the concept of risk might be broadened somewhat beyond the purely statistical. In this way, we can develop a practical plan for integrating requirements, testing, and risk into an easily understood arrangement by which the relationship of these topics, each to the other, is clarified. Let us ask, then, this question: How much testing is necessary, for which parameters, and where and when should tests be conducted? The manner in which this question is answered determines the risk—statistical or nonstatistical—that a product will not be satisfactory.

Let us consider the "where and when" question. We know that a product comes into existence as a result of progression from concept, through design and production, to distribution and consumer utilization. Where and when should tests be imposed during this cycle? While this question is not amenable to a categorical answer, here are some options:

After Design. This is design verification. At this time all functional and other tests are conducted on the product to determine its conformance to design requirements.

After the First Article Is Produced. This is, as we would expect, usually called "first article inspection." Its purpose is to ascertain that the manufacturing process is capable of producing a product in conformance with the design and that the design itself is practical. This is a "must." In this way "design degradation" is prevented at the very beginning of production. Downstream problems are thus largely precluded.

During Production. This can be called "production testing." Tests are conducted weekly, monthly, or at other time intervals to assure that the product is continuously manufactured in accordance with design requirements. These periodic tests are not statistically designed procedures. An item is simply "pulled off the line" at specified or random intervals and thoroughly scrutinized by design, quality control, or other specialists. The standard should specify intervals of such testing or frequency, with schedules to be determined randomly. Other tests must be conducted during production if the characteristic to be tested is not accessible after the final product is assembled.

Postproduction Testing. This is, as previously mentioned, final inspection. For this purpose, the standard should include a complete final inspection plan containing identification of characteristics to be inspected, their categorization into different levels of significance (critical, major, and minor), specification of measuring instruments, sample sizes, and decision rules.

If the task force has a clear vision of "where and how often" certain tests are needed as generated by the requirements, it is now possible more explicitly to confront the statistical problem of risk. At the outset, it may be well to assume that it is not likely that a manufacturer can, over a period of time, produce a consistently perfect product. Perfection is always an objective, rarely a reality. Perfection, however, can be "approached" by use of automated, in-line testing procedures. Even so, deficiencies are occasionally to be expected.

To a degree, the assignment of risk is a subjective decision. However, to inject as much objectivity as possible, it is suggested that the significance of each required functional and other characteristic be evaluated by some reasonable and practical set of criteria. With no claim to virtue greater than attachable to other criteria, it is suggested that each characteristic of the product be judged in terms of likely unfavorable consequences were it deficient as measured against specified requirements. All potential deficiencies that are classifiable under Category 1 must be prevented by maximum testing—ordinarily by testing each unit of product. Deficiencies in Categories 2 and 3 may be risked to whatever degree is tolerable for a particular product. Sampling procedures describing these risks are readily available in the literature as previously indicated.

Categories of Medical Device Deficiencies

Category 1. Safety Hazards. Any condition of a device that causes a substantial risk of injury or death by reason of design, production, or other defects or because of hazards resulting from interactions of the device with the user or the circumstances under which the product is used.

Category 2. Usability Deficiency. (*a*) A condition that is not likely to cause personal injury or death but could cause the device to be nonusable in a device man/environment context. (*b*) A condition that is not likely to cause personal injury or death but could reduce the usability or effectiveness of the device.

Category 3. Cosmetic Deficiency. A condition that does not affect personal safety or usability but detracts from the appearance of the device.

These categories are suggested merely to help establish a vantage point, a way of looking at things, that may help rationalize standards preparation. There are more refined techniques available for this purpose, including fault-free analysis, failure-mode analysis, and others. These are recommended for utilization when products have critical applications. In that event, of course, these techniques should be specified for use with other procedures (e.g., researching failure and experience data) in the project definition alluded to earlier.

Product Standard—Overview

The following is an outline of a standard that incorporates some of the concepts discussed above. It is not intended to suggest format, but merely identifies the content of a reasonably complete document.

Medical Device Standard

1. Product Identification: This must be exact and complete.

2. References: This identifies applicable supporting standards and other documents.

3. Scope: This is a summary of the provisions of the standard, an exploration of the purpose of the product to which it applies and, if necessary, advice regarding how or under what circumstances the product will be used.

4. Requirements: (*a*) *Function:* This defines the physiological, mechanical, physical, chemical, or other functions of the product. (*b*) *Configuration:* This is a delineation of all static characteristics (e.g., color, finish, dimensions, weight, packaging, labeling, etc.) considered of such significance as to merit explicit description. (*c*) *Reliability:* This specifies how long the product is expected to perform in a specified environment without breakdown. (*d*) *Safety:* This is a statement of potential hazards that must be guarded against by appropriate actions such as testing. (*e*) *Environment (i)* Biological. This relates to man/device compatibility, including *in vivo* product applications. (*ii*) External. This relates to stresses (e.g., pressure, heat, shock; vibration, radiation, humidity) that the product must withstand.

5. Testing. (*a*) Schedules and sequences; after design, first article, production, and postproduction. (*b*) Properties (and related tolerances) to be tested. (*c*) Designation of test equipment and procedures. (*d*) Sampling and decision rules or 100% testing. (*e*) Record-keeping practices.

6. Notes: This covers incidental information—administrative or otherwise—that does not fit into previous sections.

It is again emphasized that the above is a skeletal outline intended to suggest an orderly categorization of ideas. It is by no means inclusive.

In the long run the effectiveness of a medical device, instrument, or product depends, as previously stated, on (*a*) good design; (*b*) disciplined manufacturing; and (*c*) testing to real-life needs spelled out in a product standard. A function of a product standard is to test the efficacy of the product design and to verify, by testing, that performance and other required characteristics are incorporated into the product. However, testing has limitations. A device might pass a test—the most carefully formulated test—and fail in service. Thus, testing does not provide adequate protection against product deficiencies. The reason is that many deficiencies have their roots in bad manufacturing practices whose consequences manifest themselves only with the passage of time. For example, the design of a device may specify a particular material for use in product fabrication. By inadvertence or otherwise, a superficially similar but technically different material may be substituted for what was specified. In a circumstance of this kind, there is a strong probability that testing will not disclose such a deficiency. The consequences can be extremely serious when the product is used in service. This is not a mere opinion. Experience data substantiate this fact.

The same observation might be made regarding other elements of manufacturing processes. As a general theory, it is reasonable to propose that product effectiveness is significantly a function of manufacturing discipline.

System Standard

With rare exceptions, it is necessary for originators of standards for medical products to issue not only a product standard but also a system standard identifying the elements of good manufacturing practice. Such a system standard complements the related product standard. Apart from serving an essential technical function, the system standard simplifies preparation of the product standard. It obviates the need for details that are not appropriate for inclusion in the product standard. Frequently, it is possible to reference available systems standards. Thus, the drafting of new system standards may not be necessary. System standards in current use are identified by various titles such as "quality program requirements" (Mil-Q-9858). It would be erroneous, however, to assume from the aforementioned title that a manufacturing system standard is the equivalent of a quality control document or vice versa. Actually, a system standard includes numerous quality control provisions, plus others.

There are two features of a system standard that are important. The first is that the standard must be addressed to the executive management of industry. It is the responsibility of management to implement its requirements by any organizational or other arrangement most practical for a particular facility. Second, the standard identifies "what" rather than "how." For example, the system standard may specify that measuring instruments be properly calibrated. Scheduling and procedural details are the responsibility of the manufacturer subject to verification for effectiveness by the buyer. If the buyer lacks an enforcement capability and the manufacturer fails to implement the system standard in good faith, there are legal avenues for buyer redress. Not all products must be subjected to equal degrees of manufacturing control. Without attempting a discussion of the provisions of system standards, the following are typical topics included in such documents.

Elements of a System Standard for Manufacturing Effective Medical Devices and Instruments

1. Applicability
2. Policy
3. Planning
4. Organization
5. Training
6. Design review
7. Documentation and change control (configuration control)
8. Purchase product control
9. Production control
   (*a*) Materials
   (*b*) Work instructions
   (*c*) Facilities
   (*d*) Special processes
   (*e*) Work environment

10. Quality control
  (*a*) Facilities (including labs)
  (*b*) Testing techniques and equipment
  (*c*) Sampling
  (*d*) Segregation of defectives
11. Measurement and calibration
12. Labeling
13. Packaging
14. Handling and storage
15. Repair
16. Recall
17. Corrective actions
18. Records
19. Audits
20. Consumer services

Understandably, not all of the above topic-elements are applicable to all devices and instruments. This list is intended merely to invite the attention of the reader to considerations related to manufacturing that impact directly on the safety, reliability, and usability of products used for medical purposes. More detailed discussion of the above topics may be found in a publication entitled "Handbook and System Standard for Manufacturing Safe Consumer Products," available from the US Consumer Product Safety Commission, Washington, D.C. 20207. That publication is addressed to the safety of consumer products in general. However, its substance, with some retailoring, could be used to draft a system standard for products in the medical field.

The central premise is that current practices for preparing standards for medical devices, instruments, and products is too slow, too expensive, and too cumbersome. Many manufacturers, users, buyers, and consumers are perplexed and confused in attempting to organize or participate in projects for developing and implementing standards. The preceding suggests a step-by-step system for drafting a standard, identifies three basic questions that a standard-preparation group must answer, and provides an outline of a standard to suggest an orderly categorization of ideas. Application of these basics will result in the establishment of administrative mechanisms to expedite standards preparation, and the development of concepts and techniques from which rational, orderly, and less-expensive standards-preparation programs can be derived. The application of the administrative, conceptual, and methodological aspects of standards preparation presented and actions suggested might contribute to improvements in the effectiveness of standards and in the methods of their preparation.

53

STANDARDS AND THE CLINICAL ENGINEER

G. S. Hammer, II

Introduction

Standards are the means by which the clinical engineer communicates with industry, government, and the profession about technical recommendations or requirements that are essential to safety and effectiveness. Technical recommendations or performance requirements are found in voluntary consensus standards, whereas regulatory requirements are contained in federal mandatory standards.

Another aspect of standards is the complex problem of reconciling the economic limitations of the industry, knowledge of the professions, state of the art of technology, and government regulatory authority to serve the patient.

Some individuals observe standards as an impediment to the benefits of a dynamic state of the art of biomedical engineering technology. Others observe standards as a means by which the state of the art may be made static enough to assure safety and effectiveness.

Most individuals agree that both voluntary and government standards are an ever-increasing contribution to innovation, investigation, maintenance, and use.

For purposes of simplification it is convenient to view clinical device standards as a three-tier model.

Level 1 Research recommendations identify those areas of future innovation that should not be restricted by the development of standards. Sometimes, however, they exceed generally available technology and are therefore not acceptable as minimum standards but are valuable as educational tools.

Level 2 Consensus standards address primarily the areas of safety and efficacy. They may include requirements that are set for convenience, to facilitate communication, and they may contain recommendations for use. These are minimum standards that are often specifications in the area of materials but are performance standards in the device area.

Voluntary standards promote understanding of the products of biomedical technology and provide a basis for ensuring the quality and safety of medical devices in the clinical environment.

Level 3 Regulatory performance standards are expected to be based on clinical experience and established data and address only safety and efficacy considerations. Regulatory standards are not expected to address areas of convenience, areas without demonstrated need, or push the fringe of the state of the art as do research recommendations. They are expected to contain minimum requirements for a safe and effective medical device.

Regulatory standards are often accompanied by disagreements that could be diminished if it were recognized at the outset that two distinct standards problems are usually posed, one primarily technological and the other primarily political. Consider, for example, a governmental agency that is called on to regulate the amount of chassis leakage current acceptable for a medical device. The technological task is that of developing reliable, reproducible standard methods for measuring the leakage current. This technological problem, in common with all other standards problems, yields best to the combined attack of all affected parties, in this case, the government, the manufacturers to be regulated, and any other analytical talent that can make a contribution. Measurement standards should be full consensus standards.

Setting a limiting value of leakage current for chassis leakage, however, is and must be a unilateral act by government. In making this decision, the government must consider medical data on the effects of the leakage current on patients and users and the economic effects of its proposed regulation. In the final analysis, the promulgation of such a standard is a political decision that is reached through a process whereby the public makes a trade-off between a benefit and the degree of hazard it is willing to tolerate in order to enjoy the benefit. Setting such a standard is a regulatory action, and regulatory action is the province of government, an authority that it cannot delegate.

Benefits of Standards

The use of standards can greatly simplify commerce in a highly industrialized society. Their absence would greatly complicate the tasks of the user in specifying his needs and of the manufacturer in meeting them. Standards also provide improved communication between buyer and seller.

In any evaluation, there are criteria that are used in the decision-making process. These criteria are, in essence, personal standards. The disadvantage of this personal-standards approach is that the standards lack uniformity, are arbitrary and unwritten. When standards have been established by prior agreement, both the clinical engineer and manufacturer will have a higher level of confidence in the performance of the device.

In some areas, it is in the interest of patient safety to standardize certain components of devices. An example of this is in the area of patient/device interface. If a patient is being monitored in the OR by one type of equipment and is moved, after the operation, to an ICU utilizing a different type of monitor, it is in the interest of the patient's safety to have compatible connectors for both types of devices. Equally important is the necessity for uniformly different connectors on powered devices so that inadvertent mating of an electrically energized connector with an intimate patient-electrode connection may be prevented. In the area of implantable cardiac pacemakers, there is a demonstrated need for a standard connector between the pulse generator and electrode lead. This would eliminate the present need for adapter inventories to accommodate the increasing variety of pacemaker connectors.

It is more important, however, to realize that it is not in the interest of the patient to standardize any of the parameters or components of a medical device other than those that have been identified as having a bearing on safety or effectiveness. In the process of developing "purchase specifications" for a particular hospital within the clinical engineer's areas of responsibility, it is important that this concept of minimum requirements be kept in mind. Each specification that relates to standardization but that is unneeded will narrow the field of competitive bidders for that product. The development of performance standards or requirements for clinical medical devices provides the most reasonable assurance of quality products with minimal cost to the purchaser. This is especially important when the actual purchase is made by a department that is isolated from the individual writing the purchase request.

Design Versus Performance Standards

A standard that defines the boundaries or limits of the characteristics of a product or material may be one of two kinds: It may be a design specification or a performance requirement. A design specification imposes limiting values on the design of a product or the constituents of a material. A performance requirement imposes limiting values on how the product or material will behave under a given set of conditions. Those who criticize the idea of standardization frequently charge that it inhibits innovation and leads to undesirable uniformity In the case of design specifications, this may sometimes be true; they may inhibit innovation, but the uniformity may be desirable. Performance requirements, on the other hand, that set goals for performance and leave to the designer's ingenuity the method of achieving those goals promote innovation.

Establishment of Priorities

Clinical medical device standard requirements address the attempt to protect the public against unreasonable risk of injury or illness from medical devices. A scheme for grouping medical devices by risk into the three following categories has been developed: (*a*) Those devices subject to general regulatory controls but exempt from standard setting and scientific review; (*b*) those devices for which standards should be set and enforced; and (*c*) those requiring scientific review. There are approximately 8000 different medical devices in the United States. In order to determine which devices shall be put into the standards category, *ad hoc* committees composed of experts from medical-specialty areas were organized to develop and recommend general procedures and criteria that could be used to formulate a system for the classification of all medical devices. The recommendations of these committees were reviewed and revised with the assistance of the health professions and the regulated industry. These efforts resulted in the development of a classification logic system for determining one or more appropriate levels of control for any medical device. The resulting device-classification system included a series of questions relating to a device's characteristics, which determine its appropriate classification. These questions have been incorporated into a classification logic system, which is the central element in the classification process.

The classification process itself was initiated by dividing all devices into 14 separate categories, generally based on medical specialities: orthopedics; cardiovascular; dentistry; anesthesiology; obstetrics and gynecology; gastroenterology and urology; radiology; neurology; ear, nose, and throat; ophthalmology; general and plastic surgery; physical medicine (physiatry); diagnostic products; and general hospital and personal use.

Fourteen classification panels were established, comprised of experts skilled in the use of, or experienced in the development, manufacture, or utilization of, medical devices and corresponding with the medical specialities just listed.

Each device subject was sequentially carried through the device classification logic system to determine which of the following controls would apply: general controls, performance standards, or scientific review. The determination was made after consideration of 18 logic system questions relating to the safety and effectiveness characteristics of the device under consideration. All human medical devices would be subject to the minimum level of general controls; some such devices also would be subject to other controls. The 18 classification logic system questions were designed to differentiate which devices require additional controls and which do not. The least restrictive level of control would be determined consistent with the overall objective of ensuring that the device is both safe and effective. The level of control selected for a particular device must be the most practical means of materially reducing whatever risk is associated with it, consistent with appropriate public-health considerations. Although experts in the use and application of the device under review can best utilize the classification system, it is designed so that anyone generally familiar with a particular device can classify the device by using the system.

Classification Logic System

Question 1: Is the device custom made?

Answer: Yes— Go to question 2. No— Go to question 3.

Question 2: Although the device is custom made, can standards be applied?

Answer: Yes— Appropriate and applicable standards apply; go to Question 17. No— Go to question 17.

Question 3: Is the device life sustaining or life supporting?

Answer: Yes— Go to question 5. No— Go to question 4.

Question 4: Is the device or diagnostic information derived from use of the device potentially hazardous to life or good health when properly used?

Answer: Yes— Go to question 5. No— Go to question 7. Do not know— Go to question 5.

Question 5: Is the device of such a nature that: (*a*) sufficient scientific and medical data exist from which adequate standards governing the device safety and efficacy could now be established; and (*b*) development and application of such a standard would be adequate to control the device?

Answer: Yes— Go to question 7. No— Go to question 6. Do not know— Go to question 6.

Question 6: Is the device currently in use and marketed in the country?

Answer: Yes— Scientific review and general controls apply; go to question 7. No— (Assuming that the device is ready for and will be introduced into full-scale marketing.) Scientific review and general controls apply. Go to question 7.

Question 7: When the device is used, is it remote from the body? (Remote means no physical or energy connection to the body, nor is it used as a part of or a delivery system for gases, fluids, or other materials to or from the body.)

Answer: Yes— Go to question 14. No— Go to question 8. (Device is not remote if it is: (*a*) associated with the body through some form of energy transmission or conduction or used as a delivery system for gases, fluids, or other materials to or from the body; (*b*) used on surface of the body; (*c*) used in contact with internal body surface or cavity or used as a short-term implant; and/or (*d*) used as a long-term implant that is designed to be inserted into the body and reside indefinitely within the body.) Do not know— Go to question 8.

Question 8: Is the device powered by a nonmanual external or internal source (such as electrical, pneumatic, nuclear, etc.)?

Answer: Yes — Go to question 9. No— Go to question 13.

Question 9: Will the use of device or failure of power or device power source present a potential hazard to the patient?

Answer: Yes— Electrical, mechanical, or some other safety standard that reflects the powered nature of the device will apply. Go to question

10. No— Go to question 10. Do not know— Electrical, mechanical, or some other safety standard that reflects the powered nature of the device will apply; go to question 10.

Question 10: Does the device emit and/or inject any form of energy to or into the body?

Answer: Yes— Go to question 11. No— Go to question 13.

Question 11: Have the energy levels used been shown to be acceptable?

Answer: Yes— Go to question 12. No— Energy level standards apply. Go to question 12.

Question 12: Will malfunction of the device result in safe energy levels?

Answer: Yes— Go to question 13. No— Energy level standards for the device apply; go to question 13.

Question 13: Does the device use material for contact with the body that is generally acceptable or has known and acceptable properties that can be provided with no additional control requirements?

Answer: Yes— Go to question 14. No— Standards for material applicable for that portion of the device that comes in contact with the body, body fluids, or materials delivered to the body; go to question 14. Do not know— Standards for material applicable for that portion of the device that comes in contact with the body fluids or materials delivered to the body; go to question 14.

Question 14: Does the device have any known hazards, limitations, or shortcomings that can be avoided by promulgation of regulations applicable to the device in question?

Answer: Yes— Go to question 15. Proscriptions apply (limitations, hazards, difficulties, problems of a device or class of devices that can be controlled by specific regulations concerning the devices in question). No— Go to question 15.

Question 15: If the device performs some measurement function, should the accuracy, reproducibility, or limitations of the information supplied be clearly indicated in the labeling so this information is readily available to the user). No— Go to question 16.

Question 16: Does the device have performance characteristics that should be maintained at a satisfactory level, such level having general agreement among the user groups?

Answer: Yes— Specific performance standards apply. Go to question 17. No— Go to question 17.

Question 17: Is the device used with other devices in such a way that the system in which it is used can be hazardous if the system is not assembled, used, or maintained in a satisfactory fashion?

Answer: Yes or do not know— System considerations and general controls apply. (Systems considerations, as a control category, at present is beyond the jurisdiction of the law but should be encouraged by working with outside organizations that may have more jurisdiction and authority.) No— General controls apply.

Question 18: Is the device potentially hazardous to the fetus or gonads when properly used?

Answer: Yes or do not know— The device will be reviewed by classifying panels for further classification.

Classified Devices

The medical experts, using the above classification logic scheme and their own judgment, have determined that performance standards are required for certain medical devices. In addition, these devices have been categorized, in order of priority, into three groups. The first group with the highest priority includes:

Aneurysm clips/devices
Arterial grafts and vascular prostheses
Cardiac monitoring systems
Defibrillators
Electroconvulsive therapy devices
Electromagnetic diathermy (shortwave)
Emergency ventilators and resuscitators
Endoscopes
ETO sterilizers
Gas anesthesia machines and breathing systems
Hand driving controls
Hearing aids
Hip implants
Infant warmers/incubators (mobile and permanent)
Internal shunt assemblies
Intraoral X-ray machines
Knee prostheses
Medical gas supply and vacuum systems
Ophthalmic lasers
Respirators and breathing machines (all types)
Tracheal and tracheostomy tubes and cuffs
Ultrasound diathermy
Uterine suction devices (abortion)
Vacuum devices

The second priority group includes:

Cryosurgical apparatus and accessories
ECGs
External cardiac compressor
External transcutaneous cardiac pacemakers
Finger joints
Hard contact lenses
Heart-lung resuscitator
Hypothermia/hyperthermia devices/systems
Withdrawal-infusion pumps
Intraaortic balloons and balloon pumps
Intrauterine catheters
Nursery apnea monitors
Pacemaker batteries, electrodes, and lead adapters

Proximal femoral devices
Sorbent hemoperfusion apparatus
Spectacle lenses
Surgical lasers
Wheelchairs

The third priority group includes:

Artificial shoulder implants
Auditory impedance testers
Autoclave sterilizers
Automatic gas furnaces
Beta radiation units
Compressed gas cylinders
Dental casting machines
Electromagnetic diathermy (microwave)
Fixation screws
Fetal vacuum extractors
Foley catheters
Foot-ankle assemblies
Intermedullary rods
Inductively coupled implanted neurostimulator
Internal prostheses and mesh
Knee units
Nystogmograph
Ophthalmalic photocoagulators
Paracervical anesthesia sets
Perineural nerve stimulators (i.e., facial)
Transcutaneous electronic nerve stimulator
Uterotubal insufflators, CO_2
Anesthetic jet injectors
Therapeutic X-ray collimators
Therapeutic X-ray generators

Legal Considerations

The importance of having a calibrated instrument is self-evident. A diagnosis can be no better than the information from which it is derived, and faulty information will contribute to a faulty diagnosis. In addition, proposed legislation regarding medical technology is expected to place the burden of proof on the hospital for ensuring that instrumentation and equipment is performing as expected at all times. While not yet considered, the "traceability" of the standards used to verify instrument calibrations may become relevant. Traceability means the ability to trace back along the path of successive instrument calibrations, from the instrument under test to the primary standards of measurement held by the National Bureau of Standards, in order to establish the uncertainty of a given measurement.

The courts will be seeking persons in the hospital environment who are unbiased and knowledgeable to act as neutral parties in bringing to the attention of those engaged in the judicial process information concerning a medical device in question. Because the clinical engineer is one of the most knowledgeable persons in the hospital in respect to medical instrumentation, it is logical that he should find himself involved in matters concerning instrumentation in the courts. This situation will increase his responsibility. With this responsibility will come the authority to assure that the hospital is meeting its obligation to the patient and the visability that he has sought for so long. However, there are certain disadvantages that will accompany this long-sought visibility. The manufacturers of medical instrumentation are seeking someone to assume the responsibility for the equipment in the hospital. The physicians are seeking someone to assume the responsibility for equipment they use and over which they have no control. The logical choice to satisfy both of these needs is the clinical engineer.

The development of federal standards focuses attention on the legal aspects of the use of medical equipment in the hospital. The very existence of these standards affords the clinical engineer the opportunity to get an authoritative answer to the question: "What is the standard for this particular piece of equipment?" For example, the AAMI Pacemaker Standard developed under contract with the US Food and Drug Administration was a joint effort of doctors, manufacturers, and clinical engineers. This standard promotes the reliability of the clinical engineer in determining whether a pacemaker is functioning properly at the time of implantation. The clinical engineer might be the person to test each medical device before implantation. This would make his position that of front-line determination as to whether or not standards are met. In this situation, he is provided with information that may be required as testimony regarding compliance with standards. Manufacturers have, in the clinical engineer, the means to determine if there has been any change in device-operating parameters between the time of shipment and the time of use. Of course, the regulatory authorities have also expressed an interest in this type of information. The clinical engineer is in a position to intercept faulty devices, which also allows for retrieval of the device in question for observation in an investigational laboratory to determine whether the problem is likely to show up in other devices or not.

Some manufacturers in the past have been reluctant to publicize widely their failures due to the adverse reaction of the general public. On the other hand, one physician has stated that regulations that attempt a "no-risk state" are neither desirable nor beneficial to the public. Too stringent regulations, he claims, may stiffle innovation and research, and the medical profession may experience a "medical device lag" similar to the "drug lag," which, it is said, presently deters safe and effective drugs from reaching the marketplace.

The medical-device industry has few consumers among the general public. Hospitals are the main consumers of medical devices, and hospitals only want standards that are necessary, relevant, clear, and unambiguous. Hospitals do not want standards for everything they use, and they do not want standards that are difficult to change. It is hoped by many clinical engineers that standards will provide the needed technical information for physicians, operators, engineers, and, when necessary, patients as well. Hospitals also require better prepurchase information in order to deal with the complex marketplace. Concern has been raised, however, that the rationale behind the standards address safety and effectiveness, and it should be further related to the practical application of the device in the clinical setting.

Confirmed data illustrate that many, perhaps the most serious, problems associated with medical devices are not under the control of the manufacturer. This is one reason why the manufacturer welcomes the employment of a competent clinical engineer in the hospital. The problems, in order of increasing incidence, are usually the result of operator error resulting from inadequate training; deficiencies in repair, maintenance, and control of the device in the institution; design deficiencies; and deficiencies in manufacturing quality control. The question of where the legal responsibility lies may be answered by observing that most of the problems occur in the hospital. User education and the selection and maintenance of the device in the hospital environment are important problems in which manufacturers, users, and patients have a vested interest in helping to solve. Although there is no single user of any medical device in a clinical setting, it seems that the clinical engineer will have the ultimate responsibility for the status of medical devices in the hospital. It is hoped that standards will help define his responsibility and assist him in determining whether this responsibility has been met.

The Development of Standards

Standards developing bodies are professional organizations through which clinical engineers can further develop their professional capabilities and contribute to the advancement of patient care.

Standards organization members represent a broad spectrum of professionals who provide the depth and diversity necessary to implement their programs. Current members include physicians, hospital personnel, clinical engineers, technicians, nurses, manufacturers, government officials, purchasers, researchers, and developers.

Committee members are recognized leaders in their fields.

A multidisciplinary standards organization assists professional and industrial organizations interested in furthering standards' development in the following ways: (*a*) by assuming full responsibility for a standards-development function upon request; (*b*) by acting as the secretariat of an organization permitting the organization to develop the standard, with follow-up on its refinement; or (*c*) assisting organizations in their standards activities as an educational function.

Voluntary consensus standards' objectives are to develop standards with representation and participation by all relevant and affected disciplines and interests. The concept of *consensus* involves reconciling the limitations of medicine, engineering, and industry with safety and effectiveness. This is not a process of perfection; it is a process of conciliation and compromise.

Consensus on a standard is achieved when those individuals having a direct and substantial concern with the scope and provisions of the proposed standard achieve substantial agreement according to the judgment of a duly appointed authority. Consensus implies much more than the concept of a simple majority but not necessarily unanimity. Consensus is defined as substantial agreement on a standard by a committee, by letter ballot and subsequent approval with final public review.

A standard is a product of many considerations and viewpoints; it is a product of many trade-offs. It must not be written or evaluated on the basis of whether it will be liked by a user-expert who may desire a level of sophistication that may not be possible by a standard or by industry representatives who greatly fear restriction on innovation but by those who can take into consideration all factors relevant to the establishment of a reasonable level of safety and effectiveness. A standard should not be written or reviewed on the basis of whether it is an ideal document from the viewpoint of the individual clinical engineer, physician, researcher, or industry and government representative or the consumer representative. Few individuals will completely accept a standard since it does not adopt any individual viewpoint; it reflects an accommodation of viewpoints.

A consensus standard is a voluntary standard. The word *voluntary* implies two things: First, the standard is developed with the voluntary cooperation of all concerned; second, the use of the standard by those affected is voluntary. The voluntary standards system of the United States, like most other systems, is pluralistic. Standards are developed in many different types of organizations: in companies, trade associations, governmental agencies, technical and professional societies, etc. There is, therefore, a broad spectrum of possible degrees of consensus that can underlie the development of a voluntary standard. By no means must all standards be developed in the full-consensus system: Some are intended for use only within a company, an industry, or a governmental agency. A standard for a commodity in the marketplace, however, or one that addresses a characteristic of the physical environment, should be developed by a full-consensus procedure in which all parties interested in either its development or use are fairly represented in the committee writing the standard. Such a standard enjoys the highest credibility in the marketplace for three reasons:

1. With a broad input into the standard during its development, the result will be technically valid.
2. A standard being developed in a committee room in which all parties at interest are present and voting will enjoy the highest level of immunity from charges of anticompetitive behavior on the part of those present.
3. Having all interest present in the committee at the outset is more likely to produce a standard. Often overlooked is the fact that standards committees decide what is not going to be included in a standard.

Often no standard will be developed without a stimulus from those whose need for it is most urgent, and the stimulus is most effectively applied from within the committee.

Once the need for a standard is identified, the next step should be to make a judgment on the breadth of consensus required in its development. Two questions should be asked: Who will use the standard? How will it be used? The answers to these questions should identify all of the various parties that have interest in the development and use of the standard, that is to say, the breadth of consensus required in the development of the standard.

This process is based on the premise that standards must be written (developed) by small groups and exposed to larger groups to assure all valid viewpoints have been heard and reflected in the standard (consensus). By the time a standard is ready to be considered as a national standard, it should have been (or will be) exposed to all relevant groups for consideration. The initial standards writing or development process, unlike the consensus process, requires a limitation on the number of participating experts. As the standard proceeds toward national acceptance, it will require broader exposure. All individuals with competence in the subject of a proposed standard should be allowed membership on a standards committee, subcommittee, or working group. All other interested parties should be given the opportunity to express their views. There must be appropriate representation of all interests, but no single interest should have a majority. Membership on a standards committee or subcommittee must be balanced as equally as possible between manufacturers and users. The word "user" includes consumer representatives.

Standards contain requirements that address essential or critical characteristics of a material, product, or system. The following are the different types of requirements:

1. A glossary or standard definition of terms establishes a common language for a given area of knowledge to facilitate communication.
2. Labeling requirements that address safety or performance that are essential for a device to perform as intended or represented by the manufacturer. This also includes information that is important to the clinical engineer, physician, or other user for proper application of the device.
3. Performance requirements define the boundaries or limits on the characteristics of a product or a material by imposing limiting values on how the product or material will behave under a given set of conditions. Performance requirements leave to the designer's ingenuity the method of achieving goals established by the requirements.
4. Design requirements impose limiting values on the design of a product or the constituents of a material. Those persons who criticize standards frequently charge that they inhibit innovation and lead to undesirable uniformity. In the case of design standards, this may sometimes be true: They may inhibit innovation, but in some cases the uniformity may be desirable.
5. Referee test methods provide a means of verifying the labeling and performance requirements of a standard. A test procedure should be a referee test method giving the user the option of using the suggested test method or one of his own that is equivalent.
6. Standard classifications establish categories in which objects or concepts may be grouped.

Device Definition. The terms *device, instrument,* or *system* mean instruments, apparatus, implements, machines, contrivances, implants, *in vitro* reagents, and other similar or related articles, including their components, parts, and accessories (*a*) recognized in the official National Formulary, or the US Pharmacopeia, or any supplement to them; or (*b*) intended for use in the diagnosis of disease or other conditions or in the cure, mitigation, treatment, or prevention of disease in man or other animals; or (*c*) intended to affect the structure or any function of the body of man or other animals; and (*d*) which do not achieve any of their principal intended purposes through chemical action within or on the body of man or other animals and are not dependent on being metabolized for the achievement of any of their principal intended purposes.

The development of a standard requires an understanding of the chronology of development and the format, which are related. A suggested order for standards development and a format is as follows:

1. Scope
2. Glossary of terms
3. Labeling requirements
4. Performance requirements
5. Test methods
6. Appendix, which includes rationale (as standard is developed) and other information not considered an integral part of the standard.

The suggested steps in the development of a standard are as follows:

Determination of Need. This can be determined by the committee, another professional organization, or by a government agency. This should ultimately be a committee determination.

Standard Requirements. A subcommittee or working group should determine precisely the critical characteristics of devices that can and should be subjected to standards requirements. This involves an understanding that many safety and performance parameters can be more appropriately handled by other means (i.e., good manufacturing practices, clinical or product development protocols, etc.) In many instances, specific information is not available to write standards. It should also be noted that many device characteristics do not pose any unreasonable risk to the patient or user and do not require standards. Standards should not be written based on personal preferences or convenience.

First Draft. If it is determined that a device standard is necessary and the essential characteristics have been determined, a first draft should be prepared by an expert designated by a committee or working group. It is very difficult for more than one or two individuals to prepare the first draft of a standard. It is better for one group to develop portions of a standard rather than attempt to write a comprehensive standard unless many experts are available to work and coordinate work. The first draft of a standard will very likely be a crude but necessary beginning. Experience has shown that the most difficult part of the standards writing process is getting a first draft on paper.

The first draft of a standard should be reviewed and edited by a working group of about five experts. Much of the review work can be handled by mail. For example, one person can assume responsibility for coordinating comments on the first draft and reflecting the comments in the second draft. Successive drafts should be submitted, commented on, and reviewed until a draft standard is ready for committee review.

The "Draft Standard Guidelines" in Appendix I outline a step-by-step procedure for the development of a draft standard, with space provided for actual drafting of requirements, test methods, and rationale. Experience in using these guidelines has shown that the process is an efficient and effective means of overcoming the inertia in the development of the first draft.

US Standards Organizations

The American Dental Association (ADA), ADA, 211 East Chicago Avenue, Chicago, Illinois 60611, ANSI Committee Z-156: Dental Materials and Devices has 25 standards completed that range from alloys to zinc phosphate cement.

American Heart Association (A.H.A.), A.H.A., 44 East 23rd Street, New York, New York 10010. The more than sixteen A.H.A. standards and criteria include blood-pressure determination, nomenclature, cardiovascular and renal clinics, cardiac diagnostic and surgical centers, cardiac catheterization labs, emergency services section of Accreditation Manual for Hospitals, CPR and emergency cardiac care, and many standards for electrocardiography.

American Medical Association (A.M.A.), A.M.A., 535 North Dearborn Street, Chicago, Illinois 60610. The A.M.A. has five standards, which include two terminology standards.

American National Standards Institute (A.N.S.I.), A.N.S.I., Inc., 1430 Broadway, New York, New York 10018. The A.N.S.I. is the American representative to the International Organization for Standardization (I.S.O.) as well as to the Pan American Standards Commission (COPANT). A.N.S.I. has more than 62 standards, which concern medical devices or hospital facilities. Most of these standards are prepared by other organizations in the United States. A catalog may be obtained by contacting the address above.

Compressed Gas Association (C.G.A.), Compressed Gas Association, Inc., 500 Fifth Avenue, New York, New York 10036. The C.G.A. lists over 30 standards, which concern testing, labeling, use, and specifications for compressed gas. Information can be obtained from the address shown.

Federal Communications Commission (FCC), FCC, Washington, D.C. 20554. The FCC is a source of information concerning regulations governing the use of diathermy and telemetry devices as well as other equipment that radiates energy into the environment.

Food and Drug Administration (FDA), FDA, Silver Spring Plaza, 8757 Georgia Avenue, Silver Spring, Maryland 20910. The FDA is a source of information concerning regulations governing medical devices. All regulations are published in the Federal Register, US Government Printing Office, Washington, D.C. 20402. Standards have been published for biological products, nonsterile devices, recalls, X-ray and many standards that are under contract.

Health, Education and Welfare Department (H.E.W.). The Public Health Service has published standards for hospital electrical facilities, electronics for hospital patient care, operation of generators, construction, and prevention of shock injury. They are available from the US Government Printing Office.

American Society for Artificial Internal Organs (ASAIO), ASAIO, 3600 Spruce Street, Philadelphia, Pennsylvania 19104. ASAIO has worked in conjunction with the Association for the Advancement of Medical Instrumentation during the development of four standards, three of which are available from AAMI.

American Society for Testing and Materials (ASTM), ASTM, 1916 Race Street, Philadelphia, Pennsylvania 19103. ASTM has over 40 standards completed that are primarily material specifications for orthopedic implants. A catalogue is available from the address above.

American Water Works Association (A.W.W.A.), A.W.W.A., 2 Park Avenue, New York, New York 10016. The A.W.W.A. has published a policy statement on the grounding of electric circuits water pipe.

Association for the Advancement of Medical Instrumentation (AAMI), 1901 N. Fort Myer Drive, Suite 602, Arlington, Virginia 22209. AAMI is the principal organization for the development of performance standards, with over 14 standards published and over 10 in committee. The standards include such devices as pacemakers, safe current limits, EO-sterilization, hemodialysis, ECG connector, intraaortic balloons, blood gas exchangers, neurostimulators, and catheters. A catalogue is available on request.

Institute of Electrical and Electronics Engineers (I.E.E.E.), I.E.E.E., 345 East 47th Street, New York, New York 10017. The I.E.E.E. has published more than seven standards, which include: terminology, measurement methods, grounding, electrical systems, and emergency power systems.

Instrument Society of America (ISA), ISA, 400 Stanwix Street, Pittsburgh, Pennsylvania 15222. ISA has published more than 10 standards, including: electrical instruments, hazardous locations, terminology, and identification plates and manuals.

Joint Commission on Accreditation of Hospitals (J.C.A.H.), J.C.A.H., 645 North Michigan Avenue, Chicago, Illinois 60611. The J.C.A.H. publishes the Accreditation Manual for Hospitals, which is one of the most important standards in clinical engineer's practice. A hospital survey questionnaire is also published by the joint commission.

National Bureau of Standards (NBS), Institute for Applied Technology, Engineering and Product Standards Division, Washington, D.C. 20234. NBS published "An Index of U.S. Voluntary Engineering Standards," covering those standards, specifications, test methods, and recommended practices issued by national standardization organizations in the United States.

The "Standards Information Services" provides a technical library and referral activity. Inquirers may write or visit the center, which is located in the Technology Building, Rooms B151–B159, NBS Gaitherburg, Maryland. Although the NBS does not write standards, it does develop standard test methods. Examples of standards activities are concerning use and testing of sphygmomanometers, laser parameters measurements, ultrasonic standards for medicine and industry, neutron personnel monitoring, medical thermometry, linac medical applications, materials for synthetic implants, clinical standard reference material, calibration techniques, and hearing-aid testing.

National Committee for Clinical Laboratory Standards (NCCLS), NCCLS, 2525 West Eighth Street, Los Angeles, California 90057. Most of the many NCCLS standards do not involve devices; however, they have published a standard for preparation of manuals for installation, operation, and repair of laboratory instruments

National Council on Radiation Protection and Measurements (NCRP), NCRP, Publications Dept., P.O. Box 30175, Washington, D.C. 20014. NCRP has published more than 18 standards concerning radioactive materials, procedures, protection, precautions, and specifications of sources.

National Electrical Manufacturers Association (N.E.M.A.), N.E.M.A., 155 East 44th Street, New York, New York 10017. NEMA has published more than four standards concerning X-ray equipment and electronic power connections.

National Fire Protection Association (N.F.P.A.), N.F.P.A. Publications Service Dept., 470 Atlantic Avenue, Boston, Massachusetts 02210. NFPA has published the "Basic Library of Healthcare Safety," a compilation of 12 standards and the "Supplemental Library of Healthcare Safety," a compilation of 13 standards, in addition to the "Manual on Hospital Emergency Preparedness." Information is available by writing to the above address.

National Sanitation Foundation (NSF), N.S.F. Building, Ann Arbor, Michigan 48105. NSF has three standards for hospital and laboratory furniture, respiratory equipment, and laminar air flow equipment (in preparation).

Underwriters' Laboratories, Inc. (UL). UL was founded in 1894 and is chartered as a nonprofit organization without capital stock, under the laws of the state of Delaware, to establish, maintain, and operate laboratories for the examination and testing of devices, systems, and materials. UL standards are "standards for safety" and do not include diagnostic features. Offices: 1285 Walt Whitman Road, Melville, New York 11746; 207 East Ohio Street, Chicago, Illinois 60611; 333 Pfingsten Road, Northbrook, Illinois 60062; 1655 Scott Boulevard, Santa Clara, California 95050. UL has published more than 32 standards concerning such areas as: electrical circuits and equipment, therapeutic lamps, conductive floorings, cord sets, lighting fixtures, medical equipment, ground fault circuit interrupters, line-isolation monitors, and nurse-call equipment. Information is available from the addresses above.

US Department of Labor, Occupational Safety and Health Administration (OSHA), US Department of Labor, Washington, D.C. OSHA has published the 326-page "Occupational Safety and Health Standards in the Federal Register, Vol. 39, No. 125, Part II, June 27, 1974. In addition, bulletin #216, "Control of Electric Shock Hazards" rev. 1968, has been published.

Veterans Administration (VA). The VA has developed two standards: Specification X-1414 for biomedical monitoring systems and X-1432 for medical electrical safety. For copies of VA specifications write to: Special Equipment Requirements Division, (134A), Supply Service, Veterans Administration, 810 Vermont Avenue, Washington, D.C. 20420.

National Standards Organizations

There are many organizations around the world that are developing standards for medical devices. The following organizations may be contacted for further information concerning standards for specific devices or current status of draft standards:

Albania: Byroja e Standarteve, Prane Komisionit te Planit te Shtetit, Tirana.

Argentina: Instituto Argentino de Radionalizacion de Materials, Buenos Aires.

Australia: Standards Association of Australia, Standards House, 80–86 Arthur Street, North Sydney, N.S.W. 2060.

Austria: Osterreichisches Normungsinstitut, Leopoldsgasse 4, Postfach 130, A-1020, Wein 2.

Bangladesh: Bangladesh Standards Institution, 3-Dit(Extenstion), Motijheel Commercial Area, Dacca-2.

Belgium: Institut Belge de Normalisation, Avenue de la Brabanconne 29, B-1040 Bruxelles 4.

Brazil: Associacao Brasileira de Normas Tecnicas, Caixa Postal No. 1680-ZC-00, Rio De Janeiro.

Bulgaria: Committee for Quality, Standardization and Metrology at the Council of Ministers, 21, 6th September Street, Sofia.

Canada: Canadian Standards Association, 178 Rexdale Boulevard, Rexdale, Ontario M9W 1R3.

Ceylon: Bureau of Ceylon Standards, 53, Dharmapala Mawatha, Colombo 3.

Chile: Instituto Nacional de Normalizacion, Plaza Bulnes 1302, Of. 62, Casilla de correo 995, Santiago.

Colombia: Instituto Colombiano de Normas Tecnicas, Apartado Aereo: 14237, Bogota D.E.

Cuba: Instituto Cubano de Normalizacion, Metrologia y Control de la Calidad, Reina 408, La Habana.

Czechoslovakia: Urad pro normalizaci a mereni. Vaclavske namesti 19 113 47 Praha 1.

Denmark: Danish Standards Association, Postbox 77, Aurehojvej 12, Dk-2900 Hellerup.

Egypt: Egyptian Organization for Standardization, 2 Latin America Street, Garden City, Cairo.

Ethiopia: Ethiopian Standards Institution, P.O. Box 2310, Addis Ababa.

Finland: Suomen Standardisoimislitto r.y., (Finnish Standards Association), P.O. Box 205, SF-00121, Helsinki 12.

France: Associaton Francaise de Normalisation, Tour Europe, Cedex 7, 92080 Paris-la Defense.

Germany: Deutscher Normenausschuss (German Standards Association), 407, Burggrafenstrasse, Postfach 1107, 1 Berlin 30; or Verband Deutcher Electrotechniker (VDE), Stresemannalle 21, 6000 Frankfurt/Main 70, Germany.

Ghana: National Standards Board, P.O. Box m, 245 Accra.

Greece: Ministry of National Economy, Industry Sector, Standardization Division, 13 Xenofon Street, Athens 118.

Hungary: Magyar Szabvanyugyi Hivatal (Hungarian Standards Office), Postafiok 24, 1450 Budapest 9.

India: Indian Standards Institution, Manak Bhavan, 9 Bahadur Shah Zafar Marg., New Delhi 110001.

Indonesia: Jajassan "Dana Normalisasi Indonesia," Bjalan Braga 38 Atas, Bandung.

Iran: Institute of Standards and Industrial Research of Iran, Ministry of Economy, P.O. Box 2937, Teheran.

Iraq: Iraqi Organization for Standardization, Ministry of Industry, P.O. Box 11185, Baghdad.

Ireland: The Standards Division, Institute for Industrial Research and Standards, Ballymun Road, Dublin o.

Israel: Standards Instituteion of Israel, 42 University Street, Tel-Aviv 69977.

Italy: Ente Nazionale Italiano de Unificazione (Italian National Standards Association), Piazza Armando Diaz 2, 120123 Milano.

Jamaica: Bureau of Standards, 6 Winchester Road, P.O. Box 113, Kingston 10.

Japan: Japanese Industrial Standards Committee, Ministry of International Trade and Industry, 3-1 Kasumigasekil, Chiyoda-ku, Tokyo.

Korea: Committee for Standardization of the Democratic People's Republic of Koarea, Pyongyand.

Korea: Korean Bureau of Standards, Industrial Advancement Administration, Youngdeungpo-ku, Seoul.

Lebanon: Lebanese Standards Institution, P.O. Box 3118, Beirut.

Malaysia: Standards Institution of Malaysiz, Fourth Floor, Wisma Damansara, 5 Jalan Semantain, P.O. Box 544, Kuala Lumpur 23-03.

Mexico: Direccion General de Normas, Avenida Cuauhtemoc No. 80, Mexico 7, D. F.

Morocco: (General Direction of Standards) Service do Normalisation Industrielle Marocaine, Direction de l'Industrie, Sous-Secretariat d'Etat a l'Industrie et aux Mines, Rabat.

Netherlands: Nederlands Normalisatie-Instituut, Polakweg, 5, Rijswijk (ZH) 2106.

New Zealand: Standards Association of New Zealand, Private Bag, Wellington.

Nigeria: Federal Ministry of Industries, Nigerian Standards Organization, 11 Kofo Abayomi Road, Victoria Island, Lagos.

Norway: Norges Standardiseringsforbund (Norwegian Standards Association) Haakon VII's gt. 2, N-Oslo 1.

Pakistan: Pakistan Standards Institution, 39 Garden Road, Saddar, Karachi 3.

Peru: Instituto de Investigacion Technologica, Industrial y de Normas Tecnicas, Avenida Abancay N°1176-2° piso, Apartado N°145, Lima 1.

Philippines: Bureau of Standards of the Philippines, Sixth Floor, Manufacturers Building, Plaza Station, Cruz, P.O. Box 3719, Manila.

Poland: Polski Komitet Normalizacii Miar (Polis Standards Committee) U1. Elektoralna 2, Warszawa 00-139.

Portugal: Reparticao de Normalizacao, Avenida de Berna 1, Lisboa-1.

Rhodesia: Standards Association of Central Africa, Coventry Road, Workington, Salisbury.

Romania: Institutul Roman de Standardizare, Casuta Postale 10, Bucarest 1.

Saudi Arabia: Saudi Arabian Standards Organization, Airport Street, P.O. Box 3437, Riyadh.

Singapore: Singapore Institute of Standards and Industrial Research, P.O. Box 2611, Singapore.

South Africa: South African Bureau of Standards, 191 Private Bag X191, Pretoria.

Spain: Instituto Nacional de Racionalizacion y Normalizacion, Serrano 150, Madrid 6.

Sri Lanka: Bureau of Ceylon Standards, 53 Dharmapala Mawathaa, Colombo 3.

Sudan: Sudanese Organization for Standards Specifications, Ministry of Industry and Mining, P.O. Box 2184, Kartoum.

Sweden: Sveriges Standardiseringskommission (Swedish Standards Commission), Box 3 295, S-103 66 Stockholm 3.

Switzerland: Association Suisse de Normalisation, Kirchenweg 4, Postfach 8032 Zurich; or Schweizerischer Elektrotechnischer Verein (SEV) Seefeldstrasse 301, 8008 Zurich.

Thailand: Centre for Thai National Standard Specifications, Applied Scientific Research Corporation of Thailand, 196 Phahon-yothin Road, Bangkhen, Bangkok.

Turkey: Turk Standardlari Enstitusu, Necatibey Caddesi, 112 Kakanliklar, Ankara.
United Kingdom: British Standards Institution, 2 Park Street, London W1A 2BS.
United States: American National Standards Institute, 1430 Broadway, New York, New York 10018.
Uraguay: Instituto Uraguayo de Normas Tecnicas (Uraguayan Institute for Technical Standards), Montevideo.
USSR: Gosudarstvennyj, Komiet Standartov, Soveta Ministrov S.S.S.R., Leninsky Prospekt 9b, Moskva 117049.
Venezuela: Commission Venezolana de Normas Industriales, Piso 6 Torre Sur, CS.B. Of. 653, Caracas, 101.
Yugoslavia: Jugoslovenski zavod za Standardizaciju, Cara Urosa ul. 54, Post pregr. 933, 11001 Beograd.
Zambia: Zambian Standards Institute, P.O. Box RW 259, Lusaka.

International Standards Organizations

The following organizations are responsible for activity in international standards development:

Coordination Committee of the Radiological and Electromedical Industries (C.O.C.I.R.). C.O.C.I.R., Secretary General, 13 Nassaulaan, The Hague, The Netherlands.

International Commission on Radiological Protection (I.C.R.P.). I.C.R.P., 4 & 5 Fitzroy Square, Pergamon Press, London, WC1, England.

International Commission on Rules for the Approval of Electrical Equipment (CEE). CEE, General Secretary, Urechtseweg 310, Arnhem, The Netherlands. The CEE deals with the same kinds of products that, in the United States, are listed by Underwriters' Laboratories. CEE Specifications are used as the basis for the regulations that control approval of electrical products for sale throughout most of Europe.

International Electrotechnical Commission (IEC). The IEC was founded in 1904 and has National Committees in 41 countries. Central Office of the IEC: 1, rue de Varembe, 112 Geneva, Switzerland. IEC working documents may be obtained from: US National Committee of the IEC, American National Standards Institute, Inc., 1430 Broadway, New York, New York 10018.

International Organization for Standardization (ISO). ISO Central Secretariat, 1, rue de Varembe, 1211 Geneva 20, Switzerland. The ISO is the specialized international agency for standardization, comprising the national standards bodies of more than 80 countries. ANSI is the American member body of ISO. ISO covers virtually every area of technology, with the exception of electrotechnical questions, which are the responsibility of ISO's sister organization, the International Electrotechnical Commission (IEC). Recently, a third body, the Pacific Area Standards Congress (PASC), was formed by ANSI in cooperation with the national standards associations of Canada, Japan, Australia, and New Zealand. The purpose of PASC is to strengthen ISO and IEC and the ability of the nations on the Pacific rim to participate in these organizations.

Appendix I. Guidelines to Develop Standards*

Step 1: Determine Title. It should be as short as possible for ease in referencing the standard, preferably two or three words.

Step 2: Write Abstract. It should describe the nature of the document in a way that the reader will be able to decide whether or not the information he is seeking is contained in the document. It should contain less than 50 words.

Abstract: This standard contains labeling requirements, performance requirements, test methods, and terminology for ______________________________.

Step 3: The foreword should include a history of the standard; a description of its purpose; and, if it is a revision, an explanation of the principle changes between the current and earlier edition. A list of the committee representatives at the time of publication should also be included. Fill in the blanks.

This standard was developed by the ____________________ standards committee. The objective of this standard is to provide labeling requirements, performance requirements, test methods, and terminology that will help establish a reasonable level of safety and performance for ______________________________.

The concepts incorporated in this document should not be considered inflexible or static. This standard, like any other standard, must be reviewed and updated periodically to assimilate progressive technological developments. To remain relevant, it must be modified as advances are made in technology and new data come forward.

This standard reflects the conscientious efforts of concerned physicians and clinical engineers, in consultation with manufacturers, to develop a standard for those performance levels that could be reasonably achieved at this time.

1. Scope

Step 4: The scope should explain what is and is not covered by the standard or its application. Fill in the blanks. Add terminology with definitions to Glossary.

1.1 General. This standard establishes requirements for ____________________.

1.2 Inclusions. Examples of devices included: ____________________.

1.3 Exclusions. Examples of devices excluded: ____________________.

2. Applicable Documents

Step 5: This section should contain a numerical listing of documents used in the preparation of the standard and/or referenced in the text or appendix. This list may include articles in periodicals, books, standards of other organizations, studies, etc. The following are examples:

2.1 Style Manual for Preparation of Proposed American National Standards, SR5 HSM872. New York: American National Standards Institute, Inc., 1972.

2.2 AAMI Draft Standard Guidelines, AAMI DSG 5/76. Arlington, Va.: Association for the Advancement of Medical Instrumentation, 1976.

2.3 ______________________________.

3. Requirements

3.1 Labeling

Step 6: Identify requirements affecting safety and essential for a device to perform as intended. Fill in the blanks. Add supporting rationale to Appendix A as requirements are developed. Add terms to Glossary.

3.1.1. Device Labeling. ______________________.
3.1.1.1. Minimum Information. ______________________.
3.1.1.2. Legibility. ______________________.
3.1.1.3. Content and Design. ______________________.

Step 7: Identify information concerning the device that is important to the user for proper application of the device. Fill in the blanks. Add supporting rationale to Appendix A as requirements are developed. Add terms to Glossary.

3.1.2 Information Manual. ______________________.
3.1.2.1 Minimum Information. ______________________.
3.1.2.2 Content and Design. ______________________.
3.2 Device Performance

Step 8: Identify those characteristics which would represent unreasonable risk to the patient through some failure mode and that have a history of failing to function properly, thereby causing the device to become unsafe and/or ineffective. Fill in the blanks. Add supporting rationale to Appendix A as requirements are developed. Add terms to the Glossary.

3.2.1 ______________ Requirement. ______________.
3.2.1.1 Stability. ______________________.
3.2.1.2. Tolerance. ______________________.
3.2.2 ______________ Requirement. ______________.
3.2.2.1 Stability. ______________________.
3.2.2.2 Tolerance. ______________________.
3.2.3 ______________ Requirement. ______________.
3.2.3.1 Stability. ______________________.
3.2.3.2 Tolerance. ______________________.
3.2.4 ______________ Requirement. ______________.
3.2.4.1 Stability. ______________________.
3.2.4.2 Tolerance. ______________________.

4. Tests

Step 9: The requirements of Section 3 must all have objective test methods developed to serve as referee methods. Fill in the blanks. Add supporting rationale to Appendix A. Add terms to the Glossary.

4.1 *Referee Test Methods.* This section contains test methods to provide a means of verifying the performance of______________. The test methods and procedures of this section are for use in order to determine compliance with the requirements of Section 3. These referee test methods and procedures are not intended for design qualification purposes or for quality-assurance inspections.
4.2 ______________ Test Method. ______________.
4.2.1 Apparatus. ______________________.
4.2.2 Test Sequence. ______________________.
4.2.3 Acceptance Criteria. ______________________.

5. Glossary

Step 10: The glossary should contain an alphabetical listing of terms used in the standard which have technical meanings or are unique to the field of study of which the standard is a part. Defining terms used in the draft at the time they are introduced will provide a common basis for communication among members of the committee and users of the standard and should minimize the amount of confusion during discussion.

This section contains nomenclature and associated definitions to be used in applicable written and verbal communication, such as manufacturers and users literature and specifications, technical papers, periodicals and texts.

________________. ______________________________

Appendix A

RATIONALE FOR THE DEVELOPMENT OF THIS STANDARD

Step 11: A complete rationale must be written to support the conclusions of steps one through nine. The rationale should be developed during the standards writing process rather than at its conclusion.

A1. *Labeling Requirements* Requirements of this section assure that the medical community has available sufficient product information to assure safe and effective use of the products. It is the intent of these requirements to furnish the physician with reliable information concerning those parameters that ordinarily must be taken into account during a procedure.

A2. ________________. ________________.

A3. ________________. ________________.

A4. ________________. ________________.

A5. *Performance Requirements.* The specific parameters addressed in this requirement are those believed to be significant to the physician when using the device in its intended manner. Other parameters of interest from a purely engineering point of view have been omitted. Some of the requirements are conventional to achieve uniformity of measurement and hence, communication.

A6. Rationale for those items not conventional in nature is as follows ____________.

A7. ________________. ________________.

A8. ________________. ________________.

A9. Test Methods. ______________________________.

Appendix B

TECHNICAL RECOMMENDATIONS

Step 12: This section contains recommendations that address safety or performance concerns for which there is insufficient information on which to base standards.

B1. Because there is insufficient knowledge of ________________, definitive standards cannot be written in this area at this time. It is therefore the responsibility of the ________________ manufacturer to use his best judgment to meet the intended performance characteristics.
It was determined that neither government nor industry standards have been written that could be used as a basis for the proposed ________________ standard. Published data were not found on this subject during an extensive survey of the literature.

B2. Guidelines for ______________________________.

B2.1 Recommendation. ______________________________.

B2.2 Performance Requirements. ____________________.
B2.3 Test Procedure. ____________________.
B2.4 Definitions. ____________________.

Appendix C
GUIDELINES FOR USE

Step 13: Since voluntary consensus standards do not normally address user requirements, they are included in a separate section as guidelines. If applicable, fill in the blanks.

C1. Guidelines for use of ____________________.
C1.1 Recommendation. ____________________.

PART VIII

INDUSTRY AND THE CLINICAL ENGINEER

54

THE MARKET FOR HEALTH-CARE EQUIPMENT AND SUPPLIES

C. Berkley

The total size of the health-care product market is quite large. For example, Stanford Research Institute has estimated that health-product sales, which were $30 billion in 1971, would rise to $65 billion in 1980. The market absorbs large quantities of product sales. For example, Modern Plastics states that United States consumption of medical plastics alone is 90 million pounds. The general field is growing from 10 to 15% per year and may surpass the pharmaceutical industry in demand. The market for health care medical instrumentation is not limited to the United States. In a survey of eight European countries (Belgium, France, Germany, Holland, Italy, Spain, Sweden, and U.K.) by R. S. First, Inc., a market studies firm of New York City, sales of major health products in 1971 totaled $521 million. It is expected that this figure will triple by 1980.

At the stage of their first introduction into the health-care system, individual new products may result in large dollar volumes. For example, C. H. Klein, a management consulting firm in Fairfield, New Jersey, estimates that equipment and medication used for inhalation therapy will result in an expenditure of $100 million in 1972 and $200 million by 1977. It has been estimated that surgical equipment (which includes medical instrumentation), which had a dollar value of $500 million in 1967, is expected to approach $3 billion in 1973. It also states that the total medical-care market in 1973 was $95 billion. The ''Health Care Industry Information Bulletin,'' published by Paine, Weber, Jackson and Curtis in 1972, indicated dollar volumes for the entire health-care industry for 1971 of $75 billion, $115.4 billion for 1975, and $172.5 billion for 1980. Only $1.9 billion was spent on research.

Size of Medical Instrumentation Sector

Medical instrumentation, as such, obviously occupies only a portion of the larger health-care market. The Midwest Research Institute in Kansas City, Missouri, estimated that annual sales of medical electronics in 1965 totaled $250 million. In 1971, Lab Management stated that the instrumentation area "will spend $865 million during 1971 on new instrumentation and expendables." Frost & Sullivan, a management consulting firm in New York City, estimated that by 1976–1977, the United States market for instrumentation would reach $1 billion and that it would reach $500 million in Europe. Individual instruments sometimes reach large dollar volumes because of their general utility. For example, Dumont Oscilloscope Laboratories in Caldwell has recently been awarded a United States government contract for $5.5 million for cathode-ray oscillographs.

Specialized transducers reach volumes of millions of dollars. For example, optical sensors consisting of light-emitting diodes and photocells reached a dollar volume of $40 million per year in 1973. Companies are constantly starting up new divisions in the instrumentation and control field. For example, Esterline, Inc., in New York, has founded a division to manufacture and market liquid-level and related control instruments for the petroleum, chemical, shipping and similar industries, which are strongly represented in New Jersey.

Exports of medical electronic equipment from the United States reached a level of $24 million in 1968. Individual types of instrumentation will reach large volumes, depending on particular public needs or interest. For example, by 1980, air pollution analysis instrumentation is expected to reach a level of $60 to $80 million, according to Arthur D. Little, Inc. Electronic Design indicates a medical electronics market ranging from $101.6 million in 1954 to $895.5 million in 1975. In 1968, Merrill, Lynch, Pierce, Fenner and Smith, Inc., indicated a volume of $300 million per year.

Arthur D. Little, Inc., in a study conducted in 1969 that included the instruments listed above as well as such instruments as blood-flow meters, audiometers, phonocardiographs, electromyographs, electronic sphygmomanometers, aerospace medicine devices, defibrillators, diathermy, pump oxygenators, resuscitators, etc., indicated a market ranging from $221 million in 1963 to $810 million in 1973. The annual growth rate for this period was 15%. Arthur D. Little, Inc., predicted a continuing growth rate from 1968 to 1973 of 12%. It has actually been approximately 15%. It is clear that this is an exponentially growing market.

Manpower Estimates

It is also clear that the field of medical instrumentation is currently approximately a $1-billion-a-year market. If we use as a basis the estimate that the sale of $100,000 worth of equipment creates at least two jobs, one in the manufacturing/marketing field and the other in the institutions using the equipment or in the ultimate consumer, this results in a job market of approximately 10,000 in the production end and 10,000 in the utilization end.

55

THE CLINICAL ENGINEER—AN INDUSTRIAL PERSPECTIVE

J. Donahue

Future trends point to health outlays growing faster than GNP on a worldwide basis. Although sales of most conventional nonpharmaceutical health products will grow steadily, the major impetus will come from newly developed products. In 1970 some $700 million was spent for nonpharmaceutical products (prosthetic devices, biomedical supplies, and equipment). By 1980 sales of these products will reach about $18.4 billion, or nearly 30% of total outlays for health products. On a broader scale, total health expenditures in the United States will claim about 10% of GNP by 1990, up from 7.5% in 1970. As one of the most rapidly growing fields in the United States, contributions by engineering to health and welfare may well surpass any other activity of engineering science and art.

These data portend a strong need for educational programs in the engineering sciences that will serve to accelerate the process of technological innovation, especially in the area of devices. Signs of solutions to the problems inherent in the accelerating need for doctor/engineer interface are just now emerging. Organizations with representation from doctors, biomedical engineers, and hospital administrators—are opening up avenues of communication. Some interns are taking courses that cover medical electronics. The gamut of complementary approaches aimed at meeting this growing need also includes better and simpler devices, training of specialists in bioengineering, providing continuing education for physicians, and developing and broadening the role of the clinical engineer.

In the hospital, the clinical engineer can be an effective communication bridge between the medical team and industry. He can be instrumental in bringing about significant cost savings to the hospital. In bridging the technology gap between the medical and physical sciences, he can often eliminate the need for a paid medical assistant in the operating room, assist in training of the medical staff, which in turn should result in fewer patient-care problems and less cost; bring about proper maintenance and effective use of devices in the hospital; and help prevent the recurrence of common technical problems with respect to placement of devices in patients (e.g., loss of "capture" after implantation of a pacemaker or premature replacement of the device). However, many hospitals do not have a clinical engineer or staff, so some commercial concerns provide them so that they can supply the necessary technical/paramedical services to meet the physician's needs. In the area of pacemakers, for example, the engineers can

1. Assist the physician with the technical, nonsurgical aspects of implantology. These representatives often go into the operating room with the medical team
2. Provide patient education pre- and postoperatively (e.g., films and patient booklets)
3. Provide for effective control and maintenance of the devices in the hospital
4. Distribute statistical reliability studies to help the physician gauge the safety and effectiveness of various devices
5. Provide data on a quarterly basis to the doctor on each of his device patients to minimize the record-keeping function
6. Participate in educational seminars for the physician regarding devices and their application, as well as conducting in-service training programs at the hospital (such as film presentations of surgical-implant procedures)
7. Work with the physician in research facilities to clinically test devices and/or prepare for human implant

What kind of person can provide these services to the medical specialist? He is generally someone with a good engineering or medical-science background and communications skills.

Some commercial concerns hire biomedical, electrical, mechanical, and chemical engineers, as well as 2-year electronic school graduates and those with backgrounds in the medical and biological sciences. Others who are hired come from device and instrumentation firms and the pharmaceutical industry, often joining as field service representatives.

Training in formal classroom settings, in the laboratory, and under supervised job conditions in the hospital is usually provided. In addition to a technical staff, medical consultants to assist with education and training are made available for such training. Such training varies with the individual and his job requirements, and refresher courses are periodically needed to keep the staff abreast of the state of the art.

Primary efforts in industry are directed toward research and manufacturing of device systems. Some typical engineering functions include packaging (packaging design, performing and evaluating tests to determine shock, vibration, temperature, and sterility ranges), engineering electrode development (providing expertise in chemical materials and processes to aid in mechanical stress analysis, impedance factors).

Dependent on product areas, certain specialized activities may be carried out, for example, in designing, developing, and testing pain control devices and rehabilitative devices that provide therapy: cardiovascular systems (electromechanical packaging and design of external and implantable devices, project planning, coordination, and technical direction of support personnel).

Some industries are developing teams of people composed of experts in quality control, reliability assurance, standards and protocol, and clinical testing. Some teams can be marshaled within a medical affairs division, whose responsibility is the assurance of safety and effectiveness of the company's devices. Physiological research centers help in the long-term documentation and reliability studies that may eventually be required by federal device legislation. One manufacturer plans to establish a nonprofit medical research institute in which it will be possible to work closely with the medical community on research projects. Such research could focus on such major factors as the product acceptance cycle and how it can be shortened.

To bring about proper use of increasingly sophisticated life-improving devices, more specialists are needed to work with physicians in such areas as patient selection and management, documentation of results, and interface with the manufacturer. These specialists would be present during the surgical implantation to work with the doctor on interference control, sensor placement in those devices with feedback mechanisms, calibration of the instruments for a particular patient, and titration to suit the patient's particular conditions and life style. It is felt that more of these specialists must be trained and take up their role in hospitals. Their role must mature to that of peer status with other medical specialties.

The Wall Street Journal has reported that many hospitals are now hiring engineers for the first time; many hospital administrators are predicting that the hospital industry will have the greatest growth in engineering employment of any industry in the country over the next 3 to 7 years.

However, this is not enough. More physicians who are acquainted with the hard sciences and can apply engineering technology to the hospital setting are needed.

An active role must be taken in the education of the physician if he is to use the devices and technology available to him. We must work with medical teaching institutions in developing and implementing an engineering science curriculum for medical students so they will grow to understand the technology of devices as they do the biochemistry of drugs.

In the near future, there will be vast changes in the way that health care is delivered to the patient. We should be preparing to meet those changes. When engineering technology is fully integrated into clinical medicine, medical device products will help improve the quality of life for even greater numbers of people. We want to be instrumental in bringing about this integration, which will mean effective clinical engineering in the hospital.

56

INDUSTRY: THE KEY TO TRANSFER OF TECHNOLOGY TO THE PHYSICIAN'S HANDS

M. Eden and S. Padwo

This chapter concerns the transfer of technology to the clinical area and means that can be used in the implementation of medical-engineering advances.

The word *agency* can be selected to denote and encompass the agents and means responsible for the transferral. In this chapter, a federal group concerned with transferral was the model for the study. However, any group, federal or nonfederal, can develop its own agency, following the guidelines given that suggest various means that in total or in part can be used for the transferral of technology from a laboratory to the routine health-care setting. The future cost-effective development of health-service delivery depends on an appropriate mechanism. It is perhaps because the public is not aware of the feasibility of procedures that agencies, federal or otherwise, have not developed in greater numbers.

It is necessary to delineate ways in which the national resources of engineering manpower and industrial capability in modern engineering theory and practice can be turned to be solution of problems of health care. It is necessary to show how industry can better interact with government research, development, and service programs in order that their resources might more effectively be used for the solution of urgent health problems in this country. Two things can be attempted:

1. Identify the critical factors that influence the rate of progress from the time that the need for a clinical device is recognized to the entrance of a manufactured product into the commercial market
2. Suggest ways in which adequate coordination among government, the industrial sector, the academic community, and the health-care system can be achieved

Historically, medical needs have been recognized first in the clinic or research laboratory, and the initial steps to devise techniques to satisfy these needs have been taken there. The role of industry has been to bring products developed from these beginnings into the health-care market. The high-speed dental drill, the cardiac pacemaker, the artificial larynx, and the sophisticated monitoring systems for patients in intensive-care units are examples of the many advanced technological products that have been produced by industry and have gained a substantial measure of acceptance by health-care professionals and the public.

Students of the current health-care system have raised several questions. Is the current rate of progress in providing commercial devices for the great variety of health-care needs adequate? Are there enough safeguards to ensure reliable performance? Critics have suggested that industry has been slow to introduce an important number of effective and reliable components, devices, and systems that are deemed necessary for providing modern health-care services of high quality to all Americans.

While it is true that today's overall costs for health care are much higher than they were a decade ago (primarily due to hospital cost increases), the use of products of technology *per se* have rarely tended to increase the expense of medical service. The products of technological innovation have, in some instances, decreased individual service costs by increasing productivity. Routine automated laboratory tests are a case in point. At the same time, technological products have made it possible to provide certain important diagnostic and therapeutic services that had been performed inadequately or not at all, for example, radioactive tracer scanning, mammography, and ultrasonic visualization. Perhaps most striking, one may include the development of artificial blood dialyzers that can substitute for malfunctioning or nonfunctioning kidneys on a long-term basis. Clearly, these devices add to the cost of health-care service but at the same time provide a potentially more beneficial health service.

Interviews were conducted with technical and managerial personnel in several companies representative of the biomedical industry to determine what factors were felt to be serious obstacles to vigorous growth of the field. One factor raised in interviews is that of patient policy in the biomedical field. A more general issue raised centers on the problems of coordination and collaboration among government, industry, the research laboratory, and the clinic in carrying an idea through the several stages of development to a marketable product.

In order to gain further insight into these issues, several ways can be examined in which agencies can best stimulate technical development and participate in guiding the course of the development.

It is necessary to focus on a specific development as a model. The development chosen for study, sponsored by the Medical Systems Development Laboratory (MSDL) of the Public Health Service, Department of Health, Education and Welfare, involved the transmission of a patient's electrocardiogram over telephone lines to a central station in which the signals of the heart's electrical activity could be analyzed by computer and the subsequent diagnosis retransmitted to the original sender in a matter of minutes. (MSDL was a government agency whose purpose was to promote the development of products and methods with a particular application to health-care delivery.)

MSDL thus serves in this chapter as a model for an agency that acts as a catalyst, was a source of some financial support and provides coordination in carrying out the development of a specific technological system intended for wide use in national health care.

In review of a mode, various viewpoints must be obtained from members of government groups, hospital administrators, medical practitioners, the academic community, and industries in the communications, data processing, and instrumentation fields. Various topics must be included for consideration:

Industry-agency interaction
Research and development
Market evaluation
Production and profit
Patents and product liability
Safety and standardization
Point of application
Communication and user education
Merchandising
Maintenance and service

There is a strong consensus on the pivotal importance of the coordination function in carrying through such complex development programs. Thus, the chapter deals largely with the role of an intermediary, referred to as the agency, which mediates the interaction of the industrial and the medical-care communities.

The agency need not be considered as purely an arbiter but as an active participant in the triparties collaboration of industry, government, and the medical-care system. For example, personnel of the MSDL worked as professionals in the electrocardiography program. They contributed to market analysis, preparation of specifications, clinical trials, etc. At the same time, the organizational structure, form, and level of participation exemplified by this federal laboratory were not optimal for all technical projects. Accordingly, agency is used in the generic sense and not in the specific sense of a subdivision of the federal government.

The basic premise can be that properly functioning "agencies" can be the dynamic forces in accelerating the rate of technological progress toward the goals of higher productivity, more uniform distribution, and lower cost in the delivery of health care with no diminution in quality of care.

No explicit recommendations are made regarding the organization, structure, and financing of such an agency or, indeed, whether one or several entities are to be preferred. Rather, it is hoped that by concentrating on the operating characteristics of the "agency," the chapter is useful to those responsible for establishing such agencies, whatever form they might take.

The Model "Agency"

There were many forces and interests that brought the industrial participants and the staff of the former Medical Systems Laboratory together. Each was influenced by the other. Among the questions to consider are: What are the forces that cause industry to seek government subsidy and the government to seek industrial development? What are their mutual interests? How are decisions made with respect to the division of responsibilities? What are some of the pertinent motivations, such as profit considerations, public image (of both industry and government), as well as humanitarian impulses? What role can a public agency (governmental or non-governmental) best play?

The recent history of interaction between industry and the medical professionals in the development of devices for use in health care has shown that an agency or individual can act effectively as a catalyst to establish an active working collaboration. The mechanism of interaction can be formal or informal. The agent has sometimes been a practicing physician who approaches an industrial company, an official or laboratory worker in a local hospital, a municipal government health department, or a nonprofit corporation. (In Illinois, for example, the nonprofit Biomedical Engineering Resource Corporation was established to fulfill this function.) In the case study considered by the workshop, the agency was an arm of the federal government, with a specific mission in the health-care field.

At times, humanitarian purposes—an aspect common to virtually all health-oriented projects—will motivate management in both the medical field and in industry to the point of constructing a device and offering it for sale. This can happen before a detailed analytical review of business considerations and the ways in which the device actually enters into medical practice is made. These tasks fall to the agency, and the more nearly representative the agent or agency is of the *total* medical environment, the more realistic are the assessments of the medical value of the device, the potential market, and the evaluations of other business criteria. As a consequence, the chances for success also are improved. Conversely, the narrower the medical specialty or range of medical understanding of the developer, the more likely it is that the device will be idiosyncratic and the smaller the chance of widespread acceptance and business success.

In order to increase the likelihood of success, the agent or agency should be national in scope and should bring a systems approach to the task of integrating a proposed medical device into the health system. The emergent agency between industry and the medical professions is concerned with the national interest. It must maintain a reputation of medical and administrative competence in order to assure acceptance of its activities in national health care.

The Agency. An agency can serve to link industry and medicine by providing a number of valuable services to each. The agency can be of service to the community physician, attempting to evaluate his requirements and integrate them with other requirements of medical practitioners in rural and urban environments. It can translate the requirements into a specific and concrete form to mesh with the requirements of industrial decision makers. Experience in the telemetered electrocardiographic diagnosis program has shown that the detailed organization of the service should be tailored to the locality or region, the availability of expert cardiologists, the size and density of the patient population, etc.

An agency need not engage in basic research and development, but it will be actively involved in promoting the *application* of technology and in determining the feasibility of certain medical devices and systems, first under controlled experimental conditions and then in field use. It follows that such an agency would maintain its own competence in both medical practice and engineering. It must also be knowledgeable and sensitive to the considerations of good business practice. The agency can act as a catalyst for projects that are often so advanced conceptually that industry's management might be loath to approve the financial investment to carry out the development without the initiative, consideration, and understanding of the agency.

The agency can be responsive to the ideas of research workers and individual innovators, as well as to industrial entrepreneurs who intend to find other uses and, perhaps, new markets for a product. It will also keep a door open for new industrial entrants who have neither the experience nor acquaintance with the field but who have ideas, energy, and ability. It may want to refine systems and devices or modify specifications after carrying out evaluative field trials under optimal, real-life conditions involving typical and unique users.

An agency can act as an intermediary in the process of introducing technology by way of new products and also in the areas of training, safety, and maintenance in the field use of these products. It will not only stimulate innovation, but it also will help assure that systems and devices are reliable in every area of use over extended periods of time. Its concern would include education in the proper use of the device and education leading to the acceptance of the product's value to the ultimate user. Activities of this nature conducted by an agency would be well received by industrial participants.

Industry. Although the health-care field has special attractions to industry (e.g., the possibility of contributing a positive social image), industrial companies will continue to be guided by the same general criteria that have governed their decisions toward direct investment and commitment of resources to product development in other fields.

Industry's prime objective is, of course, to produce a reasonable volume of products or service transactions at a reasonable profit. In addition to and in pursuit of that goal, industry uses its expertise to:

1. Establish specification for a product and make projections of the expected market and future market capacity
2. Visualize additional benefits, spin-offs, and opportunities for product-line expansion
3. Advance its competence in the state of the art of its own particular products or services
4. Create interest and offer a stimulating challenge to its own engineering staff
5. Obtain competence in areas with which it is not immediately identified by participating in programs coordinated by an agency

Research and Development

Research and development initiate the process of commercial innovation. The first steps in exploring a problem and demonstrating the feasibility of a new method to solve it are usually taken by an academic or medical team. In this workshop case study, the basic research on electrocardiography had already been completed, but development of suitable methods of telephone transmission, automated diagnosis, and logistics were required before the program could be implemented. Contributions were made by academic, government, and industrial sources.

What are the stimuli and the sources for stimulating industry to do research and start development of a particular product in the medical field? What are the dividing lines between basic research and engineering application? How important are the expressions of interest, contributions, and opinions of potential users such as physicians, hospital administrators, and medical insurance groups? Are companies interested in advancing their state of the art as well as expanding their product line?

Only after an extensive research and development process can most devices be manufactured. The medical scientist, the research engineer, and the industrialist do not necessarily understand research and development in the same way, and their goals and priorities are often different. The medical scientist is primarily concerned with medical utility, and he regards research as work directed toward that end; the engineering scientist is concerned with the technical feasibility of a device; and the industrialist must see that the process of research and development is carried out to produce an adequate return on investment.

The medical scientist is likely to underestimate the extent, scope, constraints, and substantial costs of research and development for economic return. Administrators in government who allocate research and development funds are often scientists unfamiliar with the problems of industrial development. This is particularly true in biomedicine, in which experience has been limited; only recently have federal agencies recognized the need to foster technological innovations in the health-care field.

The experience of the electrocardiography project demonstrates that an intermediary agency can sponsor a project initially, before it becomes clear to industry that the specific project objectives can, in fact, be realized.

If a feasibility study provides evidence that the proposed device can be developed into a profitable and marketable product, and when a working model has been demonstrated, industry will respond quickly to take an aggressive investment position. Companies have differing policies with regard to participation in government-sponsored research and development projects, however. Some are eager to collaborate because they stand to gain an opportunity to take an early position in the market. More conservative companies believe that active collaboration with government-supported laboratories may prevent them from developing a strong patent positions. They place less emphasis on early market entry and prefer to depend on superior product design, merchandising, and strong sales efforts.

Persons in industry and the agency obviously share several goals in research and development: the humanitarian and public-service motives underlying work in the health-care field, as well as an interest in technological products or services. The participants also have various incentives and will undertake different tasks within a coordinated program. The scientist or clinical research worker is likely to find intellectual stimulation in a complex technical problem. The freedom to publish technical results in the open literature is an additional incentive to him. Some organizations will want to undertake fundamental research and developmental tasks; others are more interested in entering programs at an advanced stage of development.

Research and development are costly, the market capacity for the end product is likely to be fairly small in the health-care field, and the necessary time for the product to penetrate the market can be very long, comparatively speaking. Nevertheless, companies will undertake research and development, especially if the financial investment is minimized by government subsidy or partial support, because it provides a convenient, natural way to enter the field of medical devices and systems and to begin to establish a position in the field. The attributes of the three components of the interacting system are summarized in Table I.

TABLE I
Characteristics and Needs of Involved Groups

1. The Agency

The agency plays an important role in research and development by:

a. Providing an evaluation of current national needs based on objective data and the judgments of specialists

b. Striking a balance between the theoretical, intellectual, investigative pursuits and the achievements of programmatic goals

c. Furnishing a meeting ground for the exchange of ideas

d. Establishing incentives for participation

e. Offering technical help and background information to industrial firms

f. Assuring continuity of effort

2. Industry

The industrial participation will undertake research and development

a. After the market is well-defined and shown to be sufficiently large

b. When research and development provide an opportunity to extend the company's professional stature and competence

3. Medicine

The health-care professional or the academic medical research worker has several requirements regrading research and development programs. He will want

a. To have his ideas translated and presented to the technologists and industrialist

b. To continue his participation in the research and development program and to contribute to decisions governing its direction.

Market Evaluation

Market evaluation is a key requirement for industry. Companies place great importance on accurate and informed estimates of the market potential. At the same time, the estimates are among the most closely guarded industrial secrets.

How is market research conducted in the biomedical field? What are the special difficulties of completing market research in this field? What is the cost to the company? Are biomedical consultants to be brought in, and who are they? Would an advisory council be helpful? What are the engineering and merchandising considerations?

Sound analyses of the market for biomedical engineering devices and systems are difficult to make, and several companies have found that commercial market reports have been faulty. Because there is a great diversity of products and users, the market experience gained in one product line is often misleading when used to project the market for another product, particularly one intended to meet the requirements of a different medical specialty. For example, experience in the well-established X-ray equipment market does not seem to offer very much guidance in assessing the market for hospital automation systems.

In a number of instances, the potential user (i.e., the physician) is slow to recognize the relevance of a new product to his professional needs. The average physician is properly very conservative in his attitude toward possible change in his manner of diagnosing and treating patients. This conservatism may be illustrated by commercial experience with electronic stethoscopes and automatic or semi-automatic plethysmographs. Neither type of device has had demonstrable impact on the market, although a variety of models are available. It is clear that until the physician is convinced that new ways are significantly better than old, he will not use them. The participants in the workshop agreed that this type of conservatism is highly desirable, although some commented that resistance among physicians to the automated electrocardiography program was less than they had anticipated. This was interpreted by the companies to mean that the nonspecialist appreciated the value of specialty services that would otherwise not be available to him and his patients.

Many companies share the general feeling that the biomedical-device field represents a very large potential market. However, because market evaluation is difficult and product acceptance uncertain, some companies emphasize the importance of correct timing. They believe it would be too risky to market a product or service before it has (*a*) been accepted by recognized medical luminaries; (*b*) had some successful clinical trials that are reported in the medical literature; or (*c*) obtained some form of certification by responsible medical or public bodies. One company representative remarked that his company preferred to be second to enter the field in order to profit from the pioneering experiences of the first. On the other hand, some companies believe that very early entry into this highly competitive field can "shake out" the market and diminish the number of potential competitors.

The consensus of industry is that one cannot create a market by aggressive salesmanship as can sometimes be done in other sectors of the consumer and industrial fields. At present, a number of company representatives feel that a conservative corporate policy is safest. If a company, especially the small company, limits its entry into the biomedical market to individual products adapted to the medical need from its current product lines, it is in a better position to absorb the penalties of errors in judgment. Large and diversified companies determine the extent and type of participation in the biomedical field by the same criteria they use for other product lines. In many instances, the corporate threshold for minimal gross yearly sales is so high (one company indicated that it expected a minimum of $20,000,000 annual gross sales for a new product) that they will not enter the limited biomedical-technology market even if the projected product is profitable.

Industry depends heavily on councils of advisers to evaluate reports of trade researchers, to formulate specific product requirements, and to criticize the practical user aspects of system operation. Many industrial organizations employ medical specialists either as part-time consultants or, more rarely, as staff members. The companies are much less likely to call on the consultant services of biomedical engineers, in part because the engineers (even though they may be advisers to potential equipment buyers) are, themselves, not responsible for purchasing decisions and therefore do not adequately reflect the desires of the marketplace.

Companies prefer to consult several physicians who represent different points of view during the product identification stage. All too frequently, the companies find that physician consultants express very strong biases toward a particular product or design philosophy. Several consultants are almost always used prior to actual marketing; industry prefers to test its products clinically in a number of different places. The Medical Systems Development Laboratory program helped by furnishing important data relevant to market evaluation and also by making available expert opinions not only of physicians but also of hospital administrators, biomedical engineers, and biomedical computer specialists.

The agency can help industry sharpen market projections by interpreting and clarifying the needs and practices of medical specialists whose current procedures and requirements are varied and may be poorly defined. The agency can be a forum for criticisms of the existing technology and can take an active part in bringing to the attention of the industry informed opinion on the needs of the biomedical market.

The industry should recognize that sound market evaluation will depend on extensive interviews with users in different markets. In particular, market evaluation should not only be based on the needs of large, urban hospitals but also on the preferences and experiences of rural and small health-care units.

The health-care professional should recognize the costs of maintaining individual choice in diagnostic and therapeutic procedures and should consider the advantages of following uniform and standard procedures based on objective needs, with the resulting gains in productivity and savings in costs. The physician can assist in market evaluation by calibrating his judgment against the judgment of his colleagues. He also can assist by learning to express his requirements in well-defined and, when possible, quantitative terms.

Production and Profit

In a well-managed company, an investment policy, a system of inventory management, and a program for continuous production over a specified period of time are established at the outset. There is an understanding and a plan for manufacturing and marketing the product. There also is an understanding of the product's design and performance specifications, which will be advertised to the public and inevitably will become available to other manufacturers. Industry has a philosophy toward the problems of production and profit in the biomedical field. The objectives and criteria used by business can be related to those of governmental agencies and the public.

Planning for production, like market evaluation, is a difficult area within the field of medical instrumentation. Manufacturing for this field at this time, and probably in the immediate future, is a "job shop" business. The required numbers of a product or device with a special function are frequently quite small. For example, a device for monitoring flow of an anesthetic may have a fair market price of about \$500 and a nationwide market size that is limited to the hospitals performing major surgery, about 1000. Virtually every medical specialty may require sophisticated diagnostic equipment, but the potential market for each device may be limited to relatively few specialists in medical schools.

To industry, it often seems that there are too many companies in the field. Although no statistics are available, it is the general impression that the number of small companies entering and leaving the field each year is higher than for comparable industrial sectors.

Frequently, the manufacturer will need 5 years or more following the introduction of the product into the market before he can recover his original investment, which must include the costs of research and development, product design, clinical trials, and other preliminary expenditures. In other industrial lines, the time span is closer to 2 years.

Among the other troublesome aspects of the biomedical field encountered by manufacturers are the following:

1. The time schedule may be erratic. Even after device feasibility is demonstrated, the time for product development is difficult to project because the original performance definition provided by the medical consultant often is imprecise. Similarly, clinical trials may be inconclusive and may uncover medically relevant design errors. For example, insufficient attention was paid to effective grounding and shielding of the patient from stray currents in the development of electrocardiographic devices.

2. The user (physician or nurse) and the public may not have an adequate understanding of the potential value of the system, its limitations, and its operating requirements. For example, the stringent operating and formating requirements of some hospital information systems seem to have evoked hostility or apathy, particularly among more senior hospital personnel. Ironically, enthusiastic users of hospital-information systems sometimes are frustrated by what they regard to be the limited capabilities of the system.

3. There is likely to be little flow into inventory units or spare-parts inventory because total production is low.

4. A projection of service and maintenance requirements is difficult to make. In most industries, the manufacturer has greater knowledge of the conditions under which his device is being used. As with automobiles, some users are hard on a device, others are careful. Biomedical devices may be used by personnel who do not understand the requirements of care and maintenance; the level of technician training is felt to be quite variable.

Profit is an obvious consideration for the supplier. It also is a consideration for the user. The user (hospital, physician) must recover the cost of supplying its services whether from the patient, third-party payment, or government subsidy. Industry should examine carefully its definition of profit, including consideration of the value of public-service identification for the company and other possible socioeconomic returns on the investment. It should look at all costs associated with the product aside from the direct costs of production, including hardware and software required to interface the product with other devices in the user's system.

Production for profit is fundamentally the responsibility of industry. It would seem to be wiser for the user to concentrate on establishing the definitive requirements of a medical device or system and to allow industry to work out the specific details by which the requirements are satisfied. The agency can assist the user in this task of defining the need and the performance objectives. It also can consider health-care requirements that cannot be met because the market is too small or the preproduction costs unacceptably high to industry. In such cases, an agency, with the collaboration of users and industry, may be able to promote government subsidy in the public interest.

Patents and Product Liability

Traditionally, many industrial concerns have placed great importance on patent protection to safeguard their market position. To some extent, this view is held by companies in the biomedical field. Does the industry feel a strong need for patent protection? What rules govern patenting when the government has participated in development? How do companies assess the legal and financial risks relative to product liability?

It is the general view of many of the industrial firms participating in the medical-instrumentation field that patents are not very important. The notion that patent policies of the federal government are a deterrent to industry participation in research and development contracts has been overemphasized. If the device is used by recognized experts who have participated in the development, their publications can gain quick, authoritative recognition in the medical community. Professional recognition is considered by many to be a much more valuable asset than patent protection.

In technological industries today, it often takes an aggressive competitor no longer than 6 months to 1 year to build a device that will bypass existing patents. The rate of technological improvements is so great that the major protection is in company know-how. Furthermore, when the product is to be used in a system, the competent devices must be compatible. Corporate profit, then, hinges on expeditious solutions within the total systems problem.

Firms manufacturing automated or instrumental systems used in health care should be cognizant of their liability for negligent operation and design. The law provides for redress from professionals for a victim's injuries sustained as a result of malpractice. It also offers the plaintiff the opportunity to establish claims against negligent designers, manufacturers, and operators of equipment and their professional superiors. Some sources of liability include

1. Direct physical injury to a patient as the consequence of a diagnostic or therapeutic procedure
2. False test information (either false positive or false negative), which leads to detrimental action by or on the patient
3. Invasion of privacy by unwanted or inadvertent disclosure of medically privileged information

It is the practice of organized medicine to recognize that the physician is the responsible agent in making medical decisions; hence, he is the one who should be sued by the patient claiming malpractice. The physician can, in turn, bring suit against a manufacturer in the event that negligent design or faulty operation by the equipment was a cause of the physician's error in diagnosis or treatment. In order to win a malpractice suit, a plaintiff must provide that the practitioner failed to perform the duties of a professional. These duties are ordinarily not expected to extend beyond those standards of care exercised by the professional's peers.

Safety and Standardization

Medical instrumentation and its relation to patient safety are attracting widespread public attention. This is particularly true of devices that are physically connected to the patient's body and provide life support (e.g., artificial kidneys) or that monitor a critical condition, as in ICUs and CCUs. Public awareness will continue to grow because of the increasing need for these services, their dramatic and emotional impact, and the exceptionally high costs associated with them. It is widely agreed that federal medical safety legislation is inevitable and necessary.

There are many factors governing safety regulations and design standardization for normal function, defective performance, and device failure. In a complex system, special attention must be paid to the safety and reliability properties of the interface between each component product and the operating system. The safety and reliability of an interface device, such as the electrical system into which a complicated and life-sustaining machine is plugged, must be as close to infallible as possible. A back-up system, such as an emergency generator in the event of an electrical blackout, may need to be added to the original design.

There are many difficulties in defining safety requirements. For one thing, human responses to electrical and other physical or chemical stimuli are incompletely understood; sick people are likely to have a heightened sensitivity to such stimuli. The problems are becoming more complicated because of the increase in the number and complexities of electronic and electrical devices connected to the patient simultaneously. Poor outlet wiring in the hospital rooms, inadequate grounding, conducting surfaces that are or can come in contact with the patient, transient phenomena induced by other equipment operating in the vicinity, stray fields, etc., further compound the problem. Some feel that with the exception of users in major research hospitals, operating personnel are insufficiently sensitive to the problems of safety and lack an adequate knowledge of the technical aspects of medical instrumentation.

In view of the uncertainties associated with product liability, the manufacturer's safest course is to be very conservative in the design of equipment. This policy will be reflected in substantially increased costs. Even with extravagant precaution in design, however, equipment will not always remain in calibration and can be subject to misuse. In some cases, the manufacturer may be liable if his equipment can be modified easily and misused as a consequence, for example, if a safety interlock can be easily circumvented.

Within the field of biomedical instrumentation, a comprehensive set of standards is available for the safe use of sources of high-energy radiation. Experience in the field of radiation safety has shown that a cooperative effort on the part of the medical profession, radiological societies, the manufacturers, and the government can lead to a mutually acceptable set of standards and operating procedures. Standards development is far less advanced in the other areas of biomedical instrumentation. At the present time, a number of professional and industry associations, for example, the AAMI, the American National Standards Institute (ANSI), and the National Fire Protection Association (NFPA), have prepared safety standards and are attempting to draw up further guidelines for establishing safety and performance standards. The federal government, primarily within the FDA, is also addressing itself to this task of enforcement.

Some individuals in industry are apprehensive that government controls will be too stringent, although there is universal awareness of the need to protect the public. They fear that specifications and rigid standards would be unrealistically constraining, especially if they require premarketing clearance, and that they would stifle industry's desire to innovate in this field. A mutually satisfactory resolution requires informed collaboration among the concerned parties.

Participants in the industry are faced with a major challenge to establish standards of care for circumstances in which devices are being used. They want to participate in formulating safety and performance standards together with criteria and guidelines governing the requirements of product design and testing. Guidelines also are needed on the limits to which safety design should be carried to guard against the hazards of misuse. Such guidelines and standards can be established by publication of pertinent limitations, precautions to be taken, and contraindications to the product use, as well as by presentations of evidence of efficacy.

Health-care personnel can help themselves as well as industry by instituting uniform device safety controls for hospital and specialized services. These would include procedures for periodic inspection and compliance with manufacturer's safety instructions, codes of good practice in instrument setup and operation, certification of technical personnel and supervisory committees for safety review.

The federal government has the primary responsibility for regulating the safety and efficacy of medical devices. The workshop participants agreed that the several interested sectors (industry, medicine, the public, instrumentation scientists, and the government) need a forum to resolve the issues. This forum could assure an equitable representation of all interested parties and could assist in various ways, including:

1. Establishing safety and standardization specifications for field operation, taking into account the variety of users and operating conditions
2. Verifying that the equipment peforms as represented and reviewing and evaluating modifications, alternative approaches, and new concepts with reference to safety
3. Publishing information on system capabilities, constraints, precautions, desirable modifications, upgrading, etc.

Agencies actively engaged in promoting the development of a biomedical system may have a special role in interpreting the technical and medical characteristics of the system to the regulatory branches of government.

Points of Application

A critical determination in the application of a medical-instrumentation system is the point in time at which the equipment and its software are likely to be sufficiently reliable in the hands of the average user to be efficacious in ordinary clinical use. In order to be useful to the medical profession, equipment must be designed for the user, who is usually not one with engineering competence and training. Frequently, the laboratory model of an instrument will have more switches, dials, and calibration points than are to be found on the back panel of a home color television set. The production product designer will try to minimize the number of controls and the complexity of calibration protocols. The needs of the user cannot be ascertained from surveys or short interviews; the user and his environment must be studied in depth.

The key to a product's application may lie with the problem of validation; can the product satisfy the needs of the field? The likelihood is that improvements and modifications in software and hardware will always be required. Different value analysis criteria can be expected, and provision for these changes must be planned. Workshop participants felt that if an agency were responsible for evaluating changes in the system and validating them, the user would accept the system more readily.

There are at least two points of resistance to the acceptance of new systems in a hospital environment. First, technicians prefer to use existing systems with which they have had experience and are familiar. Second, experienced doctors often feel that they do not need the new equipment. They may not have used the new system enough to have confidence in it, they are threatened by methods they do not understand, and the diagnostic information provided by the new system may not agree with individual judgment preconceptions.

There is agreement that the conservative attitude of physicians is proper and valuable. The physician is responsible for human life, health, and well-being. He should not be expected, nor would it be ethical, to modify his attitude toward his practice until it is clearly demonstrated that a new procedure is superior to the best currently accepted practice.

Companies intending to introduce new devices or systems must learn to live with special characteristics of the health-care industry. If they introduce too many types of equipment into the market at an early stage of development, the health-care professional will have difficulty knowing which are best for his applications. In this situation, one can expect heightened sales resistance and purchased devices will stay on storeroom shelves. If companies act conservatively and hold back commercial selling until after full field trials and extensive clinical evaluation, they obviously lengthen the time for putting their equipment into volume production.

Those in the medical profession can help to reduce the uncertainty in deciding on the point of application by learning to translate their judgments of diagnostic factors or therapeutic results into terms that can be used to establish analytical and quantitative measures.

The agency can help by periodically bringing together the users and suppliers to talk about problems, changes, and other factors affecting overall system operations. The agency could also provide the meeting ground on which all participants can seek better understanding of the other's language and problems.

Communication and User Education

One theme that recurs in all discussions with industry is the need for good communication with the health-care professional and the difficulties in achieving it.

This communication is necessary to choose useful, marketable products, to effectively develop and evaluate them, to sell them (discussed more fully below), and to train purchasers in proper use of the products sold. The lack of effective communication between the scientific or technical side and the medical side comes about because the physicians are often not able to express clearly their needs and requirements to the engineer; in turn, engineers often misunderstand and misinterpret what they hear from the medical professional. As a consequence, there is uncertainty at every decision point in the process of introducing and marketing biomedical devices. Whose advice should be heeded? Is there an organization that speaks authoritatively? Who can help to evaluate divergent opinions?

Some individuals believe that the problem is due in part to a difference in professional standing or perceived professional standing between the physician and the engineer. The doctor is alleged to look down on the engineer and to regard him as a technician rather than his (the doctor's) professional equal. Further, there is a philosophical difference between the two professions. The medical profession tends to look on itself as trying to solve an immediate human problem (after all, the doctor's job is to help the patient), whereas the engineering profession tends to look on itself as trying to solve a technological problem. For instance, an oncologist may propose thermography as a clinical procedure because he wants to be able to diagnose early tumors; diagnosis is his problem. For the engineer who works on developing a suitable device, measuring small temperature differences is the problem.

The physician carries out much of his work with the aid of qualitative, descriptive terminology. In large measure, it is efficient and parsimonious. A patient is judged by the pallor of his skin, the appearance of his eyes, what he says to the doctor, and so on. On the other hand, the technologist knows that his devices can only work if the sensing element is defined in physical or chemical terms; the output is usually a number. He must deal with quantitative measures.

Some companies are supplementing their engineering staffs with people who have some background and experience in the life sciences. A few are hiring biomedical engineers in order to translate medical needs and requirements more ably. In the marketing area, companies have tried to hire personnel who have spent some time in attendance at medical schools because they should be able to approach problems in a way similar to that of a physician rather than with the technological orientation of the engineer. A few firms are beginning to offer on-the-job training, which includes exposure to a medical environment (e.g., operating monitoring equipment on animals in laboratory studies).

In preparing its educational material, the industry should be aware that the user is likely to be untrained in the fundamentals of engineering on which products and systems are based. He is interested in knowing the capabilities, limitations, and methods of interpretation rather than in the details of design. A case history approach and comparison of alternative techniques is suggested as being particularly valuable. Industry believes that the ideal dialogue is between the user and a respected member of the medical community; the user will give less credence to the manufacturer's claims than to the experiences of a knowledgeable colleague.

Education must also extend to the technicians working in the medical setting. All too frequently, unskilled or inadequately trained personnel will unknowingly abuse and misuse equipment. Since the medical supervisor may know little more than the technician about the inner workings of the equipment, blame for failure will fall on the manufacturer.

Industry wishes to establish direct contacts with medical centers, and increasingly its representatives attend medical and biomedical engineering meetings. Manufacturers should consider the publication practices of the pharmaceutical industry, which commits a substantial portion of its advertising budget to educational literature for distribution to physicians. However, industry's ability to support extensive educational programs is limited. About 80% of the companies currently manufacturing medical instrumentation have annual volumes of less than $1 million each.

The agency can contribute to user education by preparing case histories and comparisons of innovations in instrumentation with accepted existing techniques. It also can help to identify individuals or groups who can best present the engineering point of view to the medical profession.

The medical profession should become acquainted with engineering philosophy and the criteria guiding industrial decisions. Company representatives at the workshop indicated that their firms would welcome visits by health-care professionals to their industrial plants in order that the physicians might meet with engineering staffs and in this way come to understand the engineer's role more thoroughly.

Merchandising

The biomedical-instrumentation industry, in common with virtually all other American industrial sectors, must find ways to sell its product to a wide range of users. Emphasis can be placed on industry's need to understand better the requirements of the health-care system so they could manufacture medically efficacious devices. The problem peculiar to merchandising medical products and systems centers about the converse, namely, the need for industry to communicate the value of its technologically complex devices to the health-care professional in terms that are relevant to his tasks. Medical professionals are concerned primarily with the product's potential benefit in treating the patient. In addition, both physicians and hospital administrators are sensitive to the desirability of the economic savings that can come from increased productivity.

Selling a medical product requires the education of the salesman as well as the physician, hospital administrator, medical technician, and, perhaps, the patient and his family. Advertisements and brochures are directed toward these audiences, but an engineer may be required to teach nurses, clinicians, and technicians to use the machine. There may be special manpower qualifications for educating and communicating with users. It is important that these issues be considered beyond the narrow context of technology and with the interest of the patient in mind.

Merchandising practices must also show how the system will affect the quality, efficiency, and operating patterns of the health-care personnel, the organizational arrangements within the hospital, the interpersonal relations in the place of work, etc. Health-care providers are likely to place less importance on a product's initial cost than to savings in manpower and the ease with which the product fits into the existing hospital operational patterns.

In order to carry out a merchandising policy effectively, the industrial firm needs sales personnel who can communicate correctly and knowledgeably with the user; they must understand the human and medical problems as well as the engineering virtues of the product. The salesman's underlying orientation should be that of a problem solver whose goal is to improve health care by the proper use of medical systems. For example, the sales person of intensive-care-unit instrumentation will have to concern himself with problems of compatibility with equipment already used in the unit and how his product line can decrease congestion in the unit, eliminate the hazards of stray wires, simplify the nurse's task of observing instrumental displays and the patient directly, etc. This approach suggests that field personnel need to be backed up by scientific and engineering personnel who are readily available for consultation.

Industry finds that although there is a growing group of personnel who are sufficiently knowledgeable in engineering and medical problems to bridge the communications gap, the number of such people is still small. People in this category usually have been trained in engineering and have acquired their knowledge of biomedicine either by formal medical study or more often by employment in a laboratory or hospital. A few have been trained in formal biomedical engineering programs. Most companies, however, have had little or no experience with biomedical engineers. The companies contend that the major university programs in biomedical engineering educate students who are geared to careers in academic research rather than clinical instrumentation technology.

The buyer-seller relationship is different from other trade situations. The industrial user of equipment will make his decisions about purchasing instruments on the basis of a set of detailed specifications. The buyer of medical equipment depends much more heavily on a demonstration; each purchaser acts as his own judge and uses his subjective standards. Such demonstrations under realistic working conditions are found to be an effective means to promote medical systems. A working system or installation is worth more than all other merchandising efforts combined. Movies, slides, sales brochures, and advertising in professional journals are acceptable to the medical profession, but the presentations must be accurate and conservative in describing relevance to the exact medical circumstances the system is supposed to help and must indicate the benefits to the user in the language of his profession.

Since the provider of health services is likely to regard demonstrated performance as the *sine qua non* for any new biomedical product or system, prior to any demonstration there needs to be a clear understanding between industry and the health-care specialist of the criteria that will be used in deciding whether the medical system is functioning adequately. It is equally important to refrain from selling devices or systems before the problems associated with the user's particular application have been worked out to the point that adequate reliability is assured. Under most circumstances, the application problems are solved during the premarketing period of clinical trials and evaluation.

When a biomedical system is complex and relatively expensive (the automated electrocardiography system is a case in point), and when the constituent components are products of more than one company, the system can be sold effectively by a collaborative sales program. The merchandising also could include joint demonstrations, exhibits, and training programs.

Maintenance and Service

There are obvious differences between the criteria of reliability for devices for sustaining the life and health of a patient (e.g., the operating requirements of a blood dialyzer) and, say, a household washing machine. Preventive maintenance and service, both of the biomedical system and its components, are major points of concern to the field. Products can be designed to require less frequent service and repair, but as experience with space-life-support systems has shown, manufacturing costs are increased substantially if the system must not fail to function on demand. The current trend to modular construction of products and the standardization of connectors, voltage levels, software, etc., that modularity demands will also affect maintenance procedures.

The type of training and the level of technical education required for maintenance personnel are important aspects of the problem. The military hardware, aerospace, communication, and air-transport industries have found that highly skilled engineers and technicians are needed to maintain and repair complex systems. As a consequence, maintenance costs may be an appreciable fraction of operating cost.

Here, as with other functions of the biomedical-instrumentation industry, good communication between the parties must be assured. A hospital or other health-care service would be well advised never to close a contract for a medical instrument or a system without making provisions for adequate maintenance and service. In the hospital environment, all professional personnel, especially physicians, expect to make the most efficient use of their time. They expect equipment to work immediately on demand and to work faultlessly. If it fails, they expect it to be replaced or repaired quickly. The solutions to medical-instrumentation requirements that are developed by a manufacturer's engineering staff must take into account the maintenance problems as they are experienced and understood by the physician.

Physicians and paraprofessionals also must take into account the system requirements for periodic performance testing and for adherence to good operating practices. Workshop participants observed that the engineering concepts of preventive maintenance, marginal testing, and system reliability are often unfamiliar to health-care professionals.

At the present time, companies follow a number of approaches to maintenance and service, offering service by company personnel, contracting service requests to independent service companies, etc. Some hospitals have engineering maintenance groups of their own, while others depend on service companies or on the manufacturer.

Industry has certain specific areas of responsibility. Manufacturers must formulate maintenance policies that provide the user with choices that are suitable to the user's working environment, including his operating schedules, logistics, support personnel, and other operating equipment. The user needs details so that he can properly program and budget for maintenance before he buys the equipment. Manufacturers must arrange for competent training of system operators, both those in their employ and those in the employ of the hospital. This includes the preparation of carefully written operating-instruction handbooks, detailed trouble-shooting guides, and maintenance manuals. Manufacturers should supply any special maintenance tools required. They also should assure that long-distance servicing based on telephone or mail requests is competently staffed and supported. Manufacturers should formulate comprehensive service plans that can include an inventory of back-up equipment at the user's site, fast service calls from the factory, and company maintenance personnel immediately available to the user.

The agency can contribute in several ways. It can be a communication channel between user and manufacturer to establish system maintenance requirements. It can help to educate health-care personnel in the philosophy of preventive maintenance. It can help to evaluate the need for in-house instrumentation and software competence. It can facilitate the creation of training programs to assure competence of operating and maintenance technicians. This may include the establishment of a system of certification or licensure of this type of instrument technician.

An Overview of Transferal

The special problems of the biomedical instrumentation industry are both substantive and serious. Unless they are understood and faced, the widespread application of technology will be hampered and lag behind needs, product innovation will be slow, and the public expectation of a more equitable distribution of health care of high quality will continue to be frustrated. The manufacturing industry has the capability to act aggressively to produce components, devices, and systems for modern health care in accord with good business practices. To be successful, industry must (with the help of the "agency") have the ability to

1. Adequately define a product that will satisfy the majority of potential users
2. Introduce a product with a reasonable assurance that the time from design to market acceptance will not be prohibitively long

3. Forecast a market need
4. Produce a product in a sufficiently large quantity and plan the inventory requirements so that the sales price will provide a profit and an adequate return on investment.

The user in the health-care industry wants these new products, providing:

1. They are an adequate substitute for manpower and/or they improve on current procedure.
2. The product is not an additional burden to the staff and does not complicate further their working habits and relations.
3. The acquisition and utilization of the product saves money and/or time for the hospital or health professional.

Medical applications are attractive and challenging to the persons and companies who are interested in the advancement of technology. The attraction may influence a company toward entering the field even when the potential for growth and profit is smaller than usual. However, industrial organizations often find that a major problem exists in obtaining a consensus among users about product definition and acceptance. Often, too, companies have stopped initiatives because of unprofitable and frustrating experiences.

The background and experiences of the average physician or user of medical equipment have neither prepared nor predisposed him to the efficient use of technological systems. The modes of analysis employed by the user have been oriented toward the human body rather than toward machines. He may be suspicious of electrical, mechanical, or sonic measurements that are far removed from his direct sensory experiences, and he must be convinced of their relevance to solving human problems.

Manufacturers, in turn, know little about physicians' operating conditions. In general, they do not employ physicians on a regular basis, their engineering personnel know little biology, and they depend on the health-care professional to supply the special requirements dictated by human physiology and the condition of the patient. Too often, the manufacturer's representative and the potential user fail to understand each other's needs.

Tenacious and strong-minded individuals are required in a field with so many impediments, and the field has attracted a number. They must be committed to aggressive pursuit of their objectives. If their success is to increase, they will need the support of an action-oriented coordinating body (referred to as "the agency") with professional stature and a measure of power to assist in:

1. Bringing the medical and industrial interests to a common meeting ground
2. Creating an operational entity to show what can be accomplished on a laboratory level, particularly in systems applications
3. Developing uniform standards, especially for systems in which a number of products must function in a coordinated manner

4. Evaluating state-of-the-art advances
5. Finding supplementary funding when development costs are likely to be too high to be assumed by a manufacturer, and even for manufacturing costs if the product is important for human health but too specialized to justify profitable manufacture.

POSTSCRIPT: THE CLINICAL ENGINEER IN THE ADMINISTRATION OF TECHNOLOGY

D. Lubin

The conventional role of the clinical engineer has been defined and described by several authors. To participate fully in the application of technology—which is defined as "the totality of the means employed to provide objects necessary for human sustenance and comfort"—clinical engineering should include additional responsibilities of an administrative nature to help integrate the parts that add up to a "totality." The administrative clinical engineer should be recognized in this context. He must be alert to the need for a continuous search for facts on which to base his judgment and advice and be willing to express dissent in the name of accuracy, effectiveness, and efficiency.

This philosophy of clinical engineering is discussed and a case history presented to illustrate its workability and validity.

Clinical engineering is a profession embracing practitioners who, in many cases, are specialists. To delineate at least some of these, the title clinical engineer should include a designator such as C.E. [electronic]; C.E. [optical]; C.E. [radiology]; C.E. [respiratory therapy], and so forth.

Because the elements involved in the application of clinical engineering specialties must be integrated to obtain the most effective and efficient utilization of varied but related modalities, another specialist should be recognized, the administrative clinical engineer.

It is interesting to note that dictionary definitions of the words "engineering" and "administration" include the word *manager,* and a "manager" is defined as one "who controls and manipulates resources and expenditures." The dictionary also says an engineer is "a person who carries through an enterprise by skillful or artful contrivance." This definition is also applicable to an administrator.

The administration of health-care technology requires involvement in several areas. These include

1. Application of political pressure to achieve reasonableness in the administration of various requirements
2. Persuasion and cooperation in working with designers and manufacturers to keep the state of the art progressing
3. Involvement in the education and training process in working with administrators, department heads, and staff
4. Research to determine relevant parameters of safety and improvement of safety devices and systems
5. Cooperation with code and standard-making panels and committees and active committee participation whenever possible
6. Participation in the evolution of the profession of clinical engineering and in the certification of its practitioners.

To maintain cohesiveness in the application of state-of-the-art technology in health care, clinical engineering must be involved in the design and installation of equipment, systems, and areas that comprise the actual health-care setting. The administrative clinical engineer is logically the person to provide liaison with the manufacturer, the architect, and the various professional engineers (electrical, mechanical, and structural) hospital administration, and medical staff.

The acquisition, installation, and use of equipment do not in themselves provide the health-care facility with a technology because "technology" is the "totality of the means employed to provide objects necessary for human sustenance and comfort." The integration of resources that results in totality is an administrative and technical function of the clinical engineer.

It is axiomatic that the clinical engineer should adhere to the principles of professional engineering ethics. While he is obligated to conform—and recommend conformance—to codes and standards that have attained legal status, he is also obligated to consider and evaluate the real-world exigencies and special characteristics of the health-care environment and be willing to use his special competence to obtain the most suitable technology rather than be satisfied with exact compliance with a legal document. The clinical engineer must display a willingness to seek full use of waivers and exceptions, where permitted—or where they should be permitted—and to seek involvement in political and legislative processes, where they do not exist, in order to achieve necessary change.

The clinical engineer should always be aware of the possibility of using alternative methods that are sound and pursue activities that will make them legitimate. Intelligent administration of health-care technology makes the clinical engineer a strong supporter of performance standards and codes that enhance rather than interfere with the application of reasonable alternatives.

The application of basic principles of engineering *per se* is not enough to ensure the best technology in health care. The clinical engineer must be particularly alert to avoid blind or indiscriminate application of recommendations even though the recommendations appear sound as general principles. Ignoring sound alternatives can impose a serious and unnecessary financial burden on health-care facilities.

In the safety field, there has been too much emphasis placed on certain types of hazards that are indeed possible but that do not—because of many factors—exist very high on the scale of probabilities. The administration of technology requires recognizing that factors directly associated with the nature of the health-care setting serve to actually reduce hazard incidence and probabilities that may very well be of serious proportions in other kinds of occupancies. The administration of technology, as well as the development and promulgation of codes, requires that proper credit be given to the fact that hospitals are staffed by competent people, that surveillance is of a high order, that the presence of clinical engineers is a safety system that operates continuously through selection, evaluation, maintenance, and repair, and that given the condition of the patient and the things that have to be done to prolong life, there is no safer place in the real world than in a hospital operating room or critical-care area. Unfortunately, too many code and standard makers have a tendency to ignore some of these realities. Rather than blame them, however, it must be recognized that there is a serious lack of research to provide hard data to take the place of supposition that often results in overkill. During the past several years health-care facilities have suffered financially from *pro forma* application of certain recommendations related to design and construction without commensurate gain in safety or quality of care.

While the technical merits of such recommendations may be legitimate, and in some applications may even be necessary, the ''totality of the means employed'' must be considered in the context of nonengineering requirements such as cost effectiveness and the realization that money spent unnecessarily may be depriving the facility of the means for providing the best in health care for the greatest number of those who need it.

Administration of health-care technology requires a definite program that will maintain integration and cohesiveness of all of the elements involved. These include the mission of the hospital, the state-of-the-art instrumentation needed, the physical capabilities of the facility, the staffing available, and the economic factors that may well dictate the parameters of the final result.

Consistent and intelligent liaison with architects and design engineers, hospital administration, medical, nursing and technical staffs, and the authorities having jurisdiction related to code compliance is essential. The logical person to provide this liaison is the clinical engineer. In hospitals that are able to support a clinical engineering department, the responsibility becomes that of the administrative clinical engineer.

The clinical engineer is always aware that in health care the state-of-the-art is only as of the moment and that he is a participant in a constantly changing situation. He must have a willingness and ability to seek improvement in the tools of his profession, whether it involves circuit design and its application, devices, or the rules laid down to use them. This concept is validated by the acceptance of industry and code-making agencies of clinical engineering input leading to significant improvement in devices, instrumentation, and requirements.

Proper administration of technology requires that the operators and end users of equipment and systems utilize the knowledge and experience of the clinical engineer in acquisition and design. The objectivity of the engineer is needed to balance the enthusiasm of the salesman and sometimes the sales-induced enthusiasm of the staff. The constant pressure of health-care economics is best served by the cooperative and combined advice of the medical and nursing staff and the clinical engineer working with hospital administration.

Safety is really the name of the game, whether it is applied to mitigating the hazards of electricity, medicines, the structure itself, or inadequacies of staff training. The clinical engineer is the safety specialist in the field of instrumentation and system safety and in specialized teaching. To fulfill this role, he must constantly seek facts and exercise sound judgment in evaluating assumptions where hard data is lacking. The administration of technology in a safe environment is enhanced when the clinical engineer is a direct participant in the development and testing of codes and standards and in the education of users. This kind of education should extend beyond the hospital staff and include the architect and design engineers.

The practice of health care is part art, part science, and possibly part luck. It may never be practically possible to measure the value of codes and standards and the part they play in this practice. It is, however, possible to quantify their negative impact when their implementation requires expenditure of health-care dollars without returning commensurate benefits in the quality and quantity of health care or safety.

Implementation of most or all of these concepts will make a very significant contribution to realization of the goals of health care.

While the clinical engineer feels a great deal of satisfaction when he participates as an active member of the total health-care team, this feeling is always strengthened when it is possible to find some measure of proof that ideas and concepts really work.

SELECTED BIBLIOGRAPHY

1. Ackerman, E. "Biophysical Science." Prentice Hall, Englewood Cliffs, New Jersey, 1965.
2. Alt, F. "Biomedical Sciences Instrumentation." Plenum Press, New York, 1963.
3. American Hospital Association, "Hospital Engineering Handbook." Chicago, 1974.
4. Anderson, J., and Begon, F. "Medical Informatics." Taylor and Francis, London, 1976.
5. Armstrong, P. A., Bashshur, R. L., and Youssef, Z. I. "Telemedicine: Explorations in the Use of Telecommunications in Health Care." Thomas, Springfield, Illinois, 1975.
6. Bailey, G. L. "Hemodialysis Principles and Practice." Academic Press, New York, 1972.
7. Bennett, K. C. "Methods Improvement in Hospitals." Lippincott, Philadelphia, 1964.
8. Benton, J. G., and Gubner, R. S. "Education in the Health-Related Professions." New York Academy of Sciences, New York, 1969.
9. Berkely, C. "Automated Multiphasic Health Testing." The Engineering Foundation, New York, 1971.
10. Blesser, W. B. "A System Approach to Biomedicine." McGraw-Hill, New York, 1969.
11. Bronwell, A. "Engineering and National Policy." University of Connecticut, Storrs, Connecticut, 1973.
12. Blumberg, M. S. "Shared Services for Hospitals." American Hospital Association, Chicago, Illinois, 1966.
13. Brown, J. H. U., and Gann, D. S., "Engineering Principles in Physiology." Academic Press, New York, 1973.
14. Brown, J. H. U., Jacobs, J. E., and Stark L. "Biomedical Engineering." Davis, Philadelphia, Pennsylvania, 1971.
15. Brown, P. B., Maxfield, B. W., and Moraff H. "Electronics for Neurobiologists," MIT Press, Cambridge, Massachusetts, 1972.
16. Bugliarello, G. "Bioengineering—An Engineering View." San Francisco Press, San Francisco, 1968.
17. Bugliarello, G., and Simon, H. A. "Technology, The University and the Community." Pergamon Press, New York, 1976.
18. Bukstein, E. J. "Medical Electronics." Frederick Ungar, New York, 1959.
19. Bukstein, E. J. "Electronics for Medical Personnel." Howard W. Sams, New York, 1972.
20. Bukstein, E. J. "Introduction to Biomedical Electronics." Howard W. Sams, New York, 1973.
21. Caceres, C. A. "Biomedical Telemetry." Academic Press, New York, 1965.

22. Caceres, C. A., and Dreifus, L. S. "Clinical Electrocardiography and Computers." Academic Press, New York, 1970.
23. Caceres, C. A., and Perry, L. "The Innocent Murmur." Little, Brown, Boston, Massachusetts, 1967.
24. Caceres, C. A., and Rikli, A. E. "Diagnostic Computers." Thomas, Springfield, Illinois, 1969.
25. Chen, K. "Technology and Social Institutions." IEEE Press, New York, 1974.
26. Chung, E. K. "Now-Invasive Cardiac Diagnosis." Lea and Febiger, Philadelphia, Pennsylvania, 1976.
27. Clynes M., and Milsum, J. H. "Biomedical Engineering Systems." McGraw-Hill, New York, 1970.
28. Collen, M. F. "Hospital Computer Systems." Wiley, New York, 1974.
29. Cobbold, R. S. "Transducers for Biomedical Measurements." Wiley, New York, 1974.
30. Cooney, D. O. "Biomedical Engineering Principles." Marcel Dekker, New York, 1976.
31. Cromwell, L., Weibell, F. J., Pfeiffer, E. A., and Usselman, L. B. "Biomedical Instrumentation and Measurements." Prentice-Hall, Englewood Cliffs, New Jersey, 1973.
32. Cromwell, L. "Medical Instrumentation for Health Care." Prentice Hall, Englewood Cliffs, New Jersey, 1976.
33. Cuadra, C. A. "Annual Review of Information Science and Technology." Encyclopaedia Britannica, Chicago, Illinois, 1971.
34. Damon, A., Stoudt, H. W., and McFarland, R. A. "The Human Body in Equipment Design." Harvard University Press, Cambridge, Massachusetts, 1966.
35. Dallow, R. L. "Television Opthalmoscopy." Thomas, Springfield, Illinois, 1970.
36. Defares, J. G., and Sneddon, I. N. "An Introduction to the Mathematics of Medicine and Biology." Yearbook Publishers, Chicago, Illinois, 1960.
37. DeMellow, W. C. "Electrical Phenomena in the Heart." Academic Press, New York, 1972.
38. Department of Health, Education and Welfare. "Automated Multiphasic Health Testing and Services." Washington, D.C., 1970.
39. Department of Health, Education and Welfare, Center for Disease Control. "Quality Control—Clinical Chemistry." Atlanta, Georgia, 1971.
40. Dewhurst, D. J. "Physical Instrumentation in Medicine and Biology." Pergamon Press, Oxford, 1966.
41. Dewhurst, D. J. "An Introduction to Biomedical Instrumentation," 2nd ed. Pergamon Press, Oxford, 1975.
42. Dickson, J. F., and Brown, J. H. U. "Future Goals of Engineering in Biology and Medicine." Academic Press, New York, 1969.
43. Dixon, W. J., and Massey, J. F. "Introduction to Statistical Analysis." McGraw-Hill, New York, 1957.
44. Dodson, B., and Latimer, B. W. "Strategies for Clinical Engineering through Shared Services." 1976.
45. Drucker, P. F. "Technology, Management and Society," Harper and Row, New York, 1970.
46. Driggs, M. F. "Problem-Directed and Medical Information Systems." Intercontinental Medical Book Corp., New York, 1973.
47. Eden, M., and Padwo, S. "Federal Agency Development in Medical Engineering." National Academy of Engineering, Washington, D.C., 1972.
48. Elder, A. T., and Neill, D. W. "Biomedical Technology in Hospital Diagnosis." Pergamon Press, Oxford, 1972.
49. Enslein, K. "Data Acquisition and Processing in Biology and Medicine." Pergamon Press, New York, 1964.
50. Escher, D., and Furman, S., eds. "Modern Cardiac Pacing—A Clinical Overview." Charles Press, Bowie, 1975.
51. Feinberg, B. N., and Fleming, D. G. "Handbook of Bioengineering in Medicine and Biology." CRC Press, Cleveland, Ohio, 1976.

52. Fields, W. S. "Neural Organization and its Relevance to Prosthetics." Intercontinental Medical Book Corp., New York, 1973.
53. Fogel, L. J., and George, F. W. "Progress in Biomedical Engineering." Macmillian, London, 1967.
54. Flook, E. E., and Sanazaro, P. J. "Health Services Research and R&D in Perspective." Health Administration Press, Ann Arbor, Michigan, 1973.
55. Garrett, R. D. "Hospitals—A Systems Approach." Auerbach, Philadelphia, Pennsylvania, 1973.
56. Geddes, L. A., and Baker, L. E. "Principles of Applied Biomedical Instrumentation." Wiley, New York, 1975.
57. Ghista, D. N., Mirsky, I., and Sandler, H. "Cardiac Mechanics," Wiley, New York, 1974.
58. Glasser, O. "Medical Physics," Vol. 1. Yearbook Publishers, Chicago, Illinois, 1944.
59. Glasser, O. "Medical Physics," Vol. 2. Yearbook Publishers, Chicago, Illinois, 1950.
60. Glasser, O. "Medical Physics," Vol. 3. Yearbook Publishers, Chicago, Illinois, 1960.
61. Gordon, B. L. "Simplified Medical Records System." Publishing Sciences Group, Acton, Massachusetts, 1975.
62. Gross, J. F., Kaufmann, R., and Wetterer, E. "Modern Techniques in Physiological Sciences." Academic Press, New York, 1973.
63. Haga, E. "Computer Techniques in Biomedicine and Medicine." Auerbach, Philadelphia, Pennsylvania, 1973.
64. Harris, S. E. "The Economics of American Medicine." Macmillan, New York, 1964.
65. Harrison, D. C., and Miller, H. A. "Biomedical Electrode Technology: Theory and Practice." Academic Press, New York, 1974.
66. Health Computer Information Bureau. "Health Computer Applications in Canada," Ottawa, Canada, 1975.
67. Hebert, N. C. "Ion-Selective Microelectrodes." Plenum Press, New York, 1974.
68. Hiestand, D. L. "Changing Careers after Thirty-five." Columbia University Press, New York, 1971.
69. Hill, D. W. "Electronic Measurement Techniques in Anesthesia and Surgery." Butterworths, London, 1970.
70. Hill, D. W., and Bushman, J. A. "Biomedical Computer Technology," Peter Peregriums, London, 1976.
71. Hill, D. W., and Dolan, A. M. "Intensive Care Instrumentation." Academic Press, New York, 1976.
72. Inbar, G. F. "Signal Analysis and Pattern Recognition in Biomedical Engineering." Wiley, New York, 1975.
73. Jacobson, B., and Webster, J. G. "Medicine and Clinical Engineering." Prentice-Hall, Englewood Cliffs, New Jersey, 1977.
74. Jacquez, J. A. "Computer Diagnosis and Diagnostic Methods." Thomas, Springfield, Illinois, 1972.
75. J. Lloyd Johnson Associates, "Clinical Laboratory Computer Systems a Comprehensive Evaluation." (College of American Pathologists), Northbrook, Illinois, 1971.
76. Joint Commission on Accreditation of Hospitals. "J.C.A.H. Accreditation Manual." Chicago, Illinois, 1976.
77. Klarman, H. E. "The Economics of Health." Columbia University Press, New York, 1965.
78. Kenedi, R. M. "Perspectives in Biomedical Engineering." University Park Press, Baltimore, Maryland, 1973.
79. Kline, J. "Biological Foundations of Biomedical Engineering." Little, Brown, Boston, Massachusetts, 1976.
80. Krasnoff, S. O. "Computers in Medicine." Thomas, Springfield, Illinois, 1967.
81. Kronenthal, R. L., Oser, A., and Martin E. "Polymers in Medicine and Surgery." Plenum Press, New York, 1975.
82. La Londe, W. S. "Professional Engineer's Examination—Questions and Answers." McGraw-Hill, New York, 1966.

83. Levine, S. N. "Advances in Biomedical Engineering and Medical Physics." Wiley, New York, 1968.
84. Levitt, T. "Innovation in Marketing." McGraw-Hill, New York, 1962.
85. Lindberg, D. A. B. "The Computer and Medical Care." Thomas, Springfield, Illinois, 1968.
86. Lion, K. S. "Instrumentation in Scientific Research." McGraw-Hill, New York, 1959.
87. Longmore D., and Ross-MacDonald M. "Machines in Medicine." Aldus, London, 1969.
88. Ludwig, H. "Computer Applications and Techniques in Clinical Medicine." Wiley, New York, 1974.
89. Mackay, R. S. "Bio-Medical Telemetry." Wiley, New York, 1968.
90. Matarazzo, J. M., and Kyed, J. M. "Scientific, Engineering and Medical Societies Publications in Print, 1976–1977." Jacques Cattel Press, Tempe, Arizona, 1976.
91. Mather, K. "Statistical Analysis in Biology." Methuen, London, 1964.
92. McCutcheon, E. P. "Chronically Implanted Cardiovascular Instrumentation." Academic Press, New York, 1973.
93. McLachlan, G., and Shegog, R. A. "Computers in the Service of Medicine." Oxford, 1968.
94. Miller, H. A., and Harrison, D. C. "Biomedical Electrode Technology—Theory and Practice." Academic Press, New York, 1974.
95. Mitre Corporation. "Symposium on Advanced Systems for Health Care Delivery, Education and Information." McLean, Virginia, 1973.
96. Mendelsohn, E., Swazey, J. P., and Taviss, I. "Human Aspects of Biomedical Innovation." Harvard University Press, Cambridge, Massachusetts, 1971.
97. Morris, A. C. "A Physician's Introduction to Electronics." Pergamon Press, Oxford, 1961.
98. National Academy of Engineering. "A Study of Technology Assessment." Washington, D.C., 1969.
99. National Academy of Engineering. "Engineering and Medicine." Washington, D.C., 1970.
100. National Academy of Engineering. "An Assessment of Industrial Activity in the Field of Biomedical Engineering." Washington, D.C., 1971.
101. National Science Foundation. "A Selected and Technology in State and Local Government." Washington, D.C., 1972.
102. Nose, Y. "Cardiac Engineering." Wiley, (Interscience), New York, 1970.
103. Oakes, J. B. "Proceedings of the Conference on Clinical Engineering Education." Baltimore, Maryland, 1976.
104. Ockenden, J. M., and Bodenham, K. E. "Focus on Medical Computer Development." Oxford University Press, London, 1970.
105. Park, B. "An Introduction to Telemedicine, Interactive Television for Delivery of Health Services." The Alternate Media Center at New York University, 1974.
106. Pickett, R. M., and Triggs, T. J. "Human Factors in Health Care." Heath, Lexington, Massachusetts, 1975.
107. Piller, L. W. "Electronic Instrumentation Theory of Cardiac Technology." Thomas, Springfield, Illinois, 1970.
108. Poyer, J., Herrick, J., and Weber, T. B. "Biomedical Sciences Instrumentation," Vol. 3. Plenum Press, New York, 1967.
109. Ray, C. D. "Medical Engineering." Yearbook Publishers, Chicago, Illinois, 1974.
110. Rosen, R. "Optimality Principles in Biology." Plenum Press, New York, 1967.
111. Roth, H. H., Teltscher, E. J., and Kane, I. M. "Electrical Safety in Health Care Facilities." Academic Press, New York, 1975.
112. Rushmer, R. F. "Medical Engineering—Projections for Health Care Delivery." Academic Press, New York, 1972.
113. Ryan, G. A., and Monroe, K. E. "Computer Assisted Medical Practice: The AMA's Role." American Medical Association, Chicago, Illinois, 1971.
114. Salkovitz, E., Gerende, L., and Wingard, L. "Dimensions of Biomedical Engineering." San Francisco Press, San Francisco, 1968.
115. Sances, A., and Larson, S. J. "Electroanesthesia." Academic Press, New York, 1975.

116. Sayers, B. M., Watson, B. W., and Swanson, S. A. V. "Engineering in Medicine." Oxford University Press, London, 1975.
117. Schmitt, O. H., and Caceres, C. A. "Electronic and Computer-Assisted Studies of Bio-Medical Problems." Thomas, Springfield, Illinois, 1964.
118. Scott, F. D. "Instruments in Clinical Medicine." F. A. Davis, Philadelphia, Pennsylvania. 1967.
119. Seely, S. "An Introduction to Engineering Systems." Pergamon Press, New York, 1972.
120. Segal, B. L., and Kilpatrick, D. G. "Engineering in the Practice of Medicine." Williams and Wilkins, Baltimore, Maryland, 1967.
121. Siler, W., and Lindberg, D. "Computers in Life Science Research." Plenum Press, New York, 1975.
122. Simmons, D. A. "Medical and Hospital Control Systems." Little, Brown, Boston, 1972.
123. Springer, E. W. "Automated Medical Records and the Law." Aspen Systems Corp., Pittsburgh, 1971.
124. Suckling, E. E. "Bioelectricity." McGraw-Hill, New York, 1961.
125. Technical Education Research Center. "Development of Career Opportunities for Biomedical Equipment Technicians." Cambridge, Massachusetts, 1970.
126. Thomas, H. E. "Handbook of Biomedical Instrumentation and Measurement." Prentice-Hall, Englewood Cliffs, New Jersey, 1974.
127. U.S. House of Representatives, 92nd Congress, Second Session. "Public Technology. A Report to the Committee on Science and Astronautics." Washington, D.C., 1973.
128. Van Cott, H. P., and Kinkade, R. G. "Human Engineering Guide to Equipment Design." American Institutes for Research, Washington, D.C., 1972.
129. Ware, C. G. "Basic Electronics for Biologists." Churchill, London, 1967.
130. Weed, L. L. "Medical Records Medical Education, and Patient Care." Case Western Reserve, Cleveland, Ohio, 1970.
131. Wolff, H. S. "Biomedical Engineering." McGraw-Hill, New York, 1970.
132. Yanof, H. M. "Biomedical Electronics." F. A. Davis, Philadelphia, Pennsylvania, 1972.

INDEX